Oral Signs of Systemic Disease

Nasim Fazel
Editor

Oral Signs of Systemic Disease

Springer

Editor
Nasim Fazel
Department of Dermatology
University of California, Davis
Sacramento, CA
USA

ISBN 978-3-030-10861-8 ISBN 978-3-030-10863-2 (eBook)
https://doi.org/10.1007/978-3-030-10863-2

This Springer imprint is published by the registered company Springer Nature Switzerland AG
The registered company address is: Gewerbestrasse 11, 6330 Cham, Switzerland

To my beautiful children, Sina and Monah, who inspire me to persevere through any challenge and bring so much love and joy into my life.

Foreword

Oral Signs of Systemic Disease provides valuable insight into solving diagnostic challenges. Careful oral examination can provide such clues to the learned observer. However, the medical education and training of most physicians and other healthcare providers does not emphasize the oral cavity. This results in a lack of familiarity with normal and abnormal features and the diagnostic clues they can provide. By contrast, dental education provides the necessary skills to distinguish between normal and abnormal findings. However, the dental clinician may not be skilled in placing abnormal features in the context of a mucocutaneous or systemic condition. Thus, this contribution serves to educate both physicians and dentists.

Dr. Nasim Fazel is an eminently well-suited editor for *Oral Signs of Systemic Disease*. She is a DDS graduate of Northwestern University Dental School and an MD graduate of the University of Michigan Medical School. This education was followed by residency training in dermatology at Henry Ford Hospital in Detroit, Michigan. Dr. Fazel has been a faculty member at the University of California, Davis in the Department of Dermatology for more than a decade and a half, where she has developed an oral dermatology practice and has served as Dermatology Residency Program Director. As a dual-trained dentist and dermatologist, as well as a consummate educator, Dr. Fazel brings great knowledge and experience to bear on the topic.

The contributors to this textbook are scholars from broad areas of expertise including dentistry, pediatric dermatology, oral dermatology, oral medicine, oral pathology, microbiology, and medical genetics. Each brings a depth of knowledge and understanding of the relevance of their topics to the problem-solving algorithm for the patient with troublesome oral lesions. Dermatologists know that the skin is often a mirror of systemic diseases. Those skilled in the diagnosis of challenging oral diseases know that the mouth is, similarly, a mirror of systemic diseases.

This book will be a valuable addition to medical libraries as a reference volume and to the personal library of the clinician whose patient has a vexing oral disease.

Roy S. Rogers
Professor of Dermatology
Mayo Clinic College of Medicine
Scottsdale, AZ, USA

Preface

The conception of *Oral Signs of Systemic Disease* came about with the intention to provide a practical reference for the day-to-day practice of clinicians in the fields of dermatology, dentistry, oral medicine, and otolaryngology. In addition, the comprehensive nature of this textbook can serve as an educational tool for students, residents, and fellows in training with the goal of learning the fundamentals of oral mucosal disease.

Oral Signs of Systemic Disease provides descriptive clinical and oral manifestations and differential diagnoses, including principles of therapy of major entities, while maintaining a uniform chapter format. I am greatly appreciative of the authors for their contributions, without whom this textbook would not have been possible. I would also like to thank Portia Wong, Diane Lamsback, and Rebekah Collins at Springer Publishing for their time and support.

Sacramento, CA, USA — Nasim Fazel

Contents

Contributors

Silvio Alencar-Marques, MD, PhD Department of Dermatology and Radiotherapy, Botucatu School of Medicine – São Paulo State University (UNESP), Botucatu, Brazil

Danielle N. Brown, MD Department of Pediatrics, Massachusetts General Hospital for Children, Boston, MA, USA

Alison J. Bruce, MD Department of Dermatology, Mayo Clinic, Jacksonville, FL, USA

Parastoo Davari, MD Department of Dermatology, University of California, Davis, Sacramento, CA, USA

Scott S. De Rossi, DMD Department of Oral Medicine, Augusta University Dental College of Georgia, Augusta, GA, USA

Nasim Fazel, MD, DDS Department of Dermatology, University of California, Davis, Sacramento, CA, USA

Elda Giansante, MD University Hospital Caracas, Central University of Venezuela, Caracas, Venezuela

Antonio Guzmán-Fawcett, MD Pierre Fauchard Faculty of Dentistry, Autonomous University of Paraguay, Asunción, Paraguay

Jennifer L. Hand, MD Department of Dermatology, Mayo Clinic and Foundation, Rochester, MN, USA

Kenisha R. Heath Air Force Institute of Technology, Wright-Patterson AFB, OH, USA

Ramya Kollipara, MD Dermatology, Cosmetic Laser Dermatology, San Diego, CA, USA

Julia S. Lehman, MD Departments of Dermatology and Laboratory Medicine and Pathology, Mayo Clinic, Rochester, MN, USA

Diana V. Messadi, DDS, MMSc, DMSc Section of Oral Medicine and Orofacial Pain, Division of Oral Biology and Medicine, UCLA School of Dentistry, Los Angeles, CA, USA

Ginat W. Mirowski, DMD, MD Department of Oral Pathology Medicine, Radiology, Indiana University School of Dentistry, Indianapolis, IN, USA

Department of Dermatology, Indiana University School of Medicine, Indianapolis, IN, USA

Ricardo Pérez-Alfonzo, MD Dermatologic Program, "Jacinto Convit" Institute of Biomedicine, Central University of Venezuela, Caracas, Venezuela

Roy Steele Rogers III, MD Department of Dermatology, Mayo Clinic Arizona, Scottsdale, AZ, USA

Julio C. Sartori-Valinotti, MD Department of Dermatology, Mayo Clinic and Foundation, Rochester, MN, USA

Emily W. Shelley, DO Cleveland Medical Center, University Hospitals, Cleveland, OH, USA

Thomas P. Sollecito, DMD, FDS, RCS The Robert Schattner Center, University of Pennsylvania School of Dental Medicine, Philadelphia, PA, USA

John C. Steele, MB ChB, BDS, FDS(OM)RCSEd, FHEA The Leeds Teaching Hospitals NHS Trust, Leeds, UK

Faculty of Medicine and Health, University of Leeds, Leeds, UK

Jaisri R. Thoppay, BDS, MBA, MS Department of Oral and Maxillofacial Surgery, VCU School of Dentistry at VCU Medical Center, Virginia Commonwealth University, Richmond, VA, USA

Stanislav N. Tolkachjov, MD Surgical Dermatology Group, Birmingham, AL, USA

Rochelle R. Torgerson, MD, PhD Departments of Dermatology and Obstetrics and Gynecology, Mayo Clinic, Rochester, MN, USA

Stephen Tyring, MD Department of Dermatology, University of Texas Health Sciences Center at Houston, Houston, TX, USA

Michael Z. Wang, MD Department of Dermatology, Mayo Clinic, Rochester, MN, USA

Introduction

1

Parastoo Davari and Nasim Fazel

Introduction

Oral signs and symptoms can be a presenting feature of many systemic diseases, which can aid the clinician in establishing a definitive diagnosis. Immunologic and infectious conditions, hematologic disorders, vitamin deficiencies, and endocrinopathies, in addition to psychological disorders and physiologic conditions such as pregnancy, can present with oral signs and symptoms. Oral signs such as mucosal inflammation or infection, discoloration, decreased salivary flow, dental caries, and bleeding can be indicative of a systemic condition. However, these oral signs can be overlooked without thorough examination of the oral mucosa, thus increasing the likelihood of delayed diagnosis or misdiagnosis.

Competence in the diagnosis of oral diseases and recognition of their signs and symptoms is relevant to all practitioners. However, adequate knowledge and understanding of oral diseases is particularly important for specialists such as dermatologists, dentists, and otolaryngologists. In this introductory chapter, we briefly review the anatomy, histology, physiology, and microbiology of the oral mucosa.

P. Davari · N. Fazel (✉)
Department of Dermatology, University of California, Davis, Sacramento, CA, USA
e-mail: nfazel@ucdavis.edu

Anatomy and Histology

The oral cavity includes four main components: the mucosa, tongue, dentition, and salivary glands.

Oral Mucosa

The oral cavity is lined by stratified squamous epithelium. Merkel cells and melanocytes can also be found throughout the oral mucosa [1]. The turnover time of the epithelial mucosa ranges from 14 to 24 days, for the buccal mucosa and the hard palate, respectively [2]. Various degrees of keratinization are observed in the epithelium of different regions of the oral cavity. The gingiva and hard palate are exposed to friction and mechanical stress during mastication. Hence, these areas are lined by a keratinized epithelium, which is tightly adherent to the underlying tissues. The dorsal tongue has a specialized mucosa composed of a mosaic of keratinized and nonkeratinized epithelium that is firmly attached to the underlying tongue muscles [2, 3]. The epithelium of the floor of the mouth, buccal mucosa, and the ventral tongue is nonkeratinized allowing for movements that are required for functions such as mastication, swallowing, and phonation. In addition, the underlying connective tissue is more flexible than the masticatory regions of the oral cavity. The specialized mucosa of the dorsal tongue represents approximately 15% of the surface area of the oral cavity,

N. Fazel (ed.), *Oral Signs of Systemic Disease*, https://doi.org/10.1007/978-3-030-10863-2_1

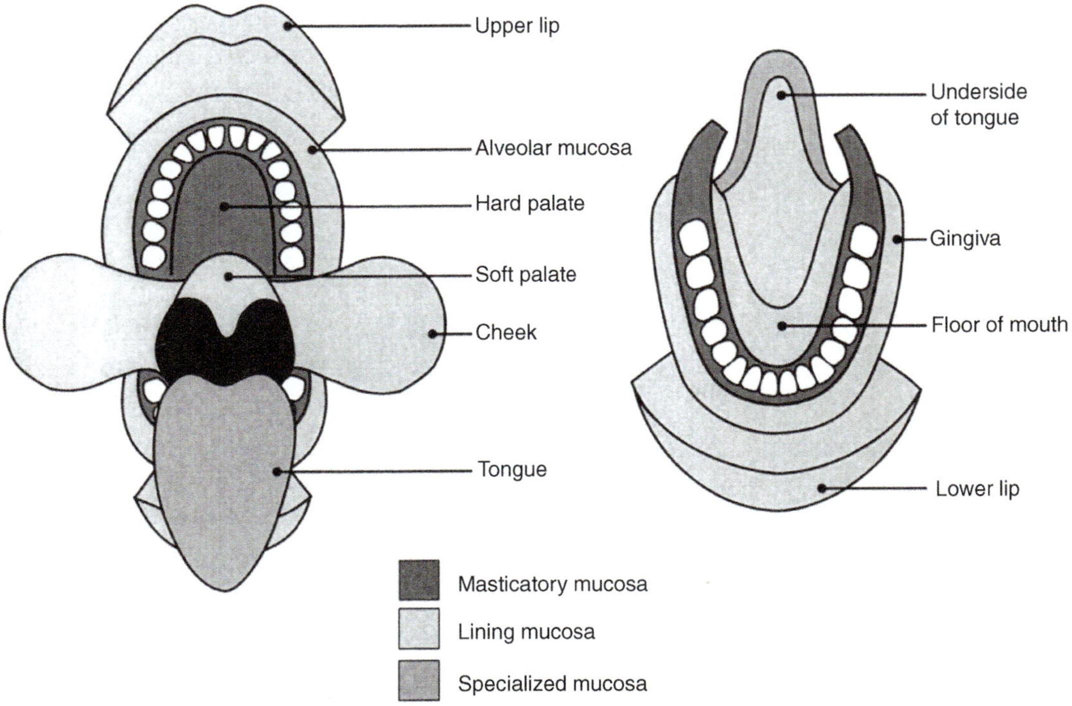

Fig. 1.1 Oral cavity regions. (Reprinted with permission from Squier and Kremer [2])

while the nonkeratinized surfaces (i.e., labial mucosa, buccal mucosa, and floor of the mouth) and masticatory mucosa cover approximately 60% and 25% of the surface area, respectively (Fig. 1.1) [2].

The Tongue

The tongue is a muscular organ that is entirely covered by a specialized mucosa, which is attached to the floor of the mouth via the lingual frenulum. A tuft of mucosa (sublingual caruncles) on either side of the lingual frenulum harbors the opening of the sublingual and submandibular salivary gland ducts. The median sulcus divides the tongue into two parts: right and left halves. Figure 1.2 demonstrates that the sulcus terminalis is a V-shaped groove that divides the tongue into the body (anterior two-thirds) and the root (posterior one-third) [4].

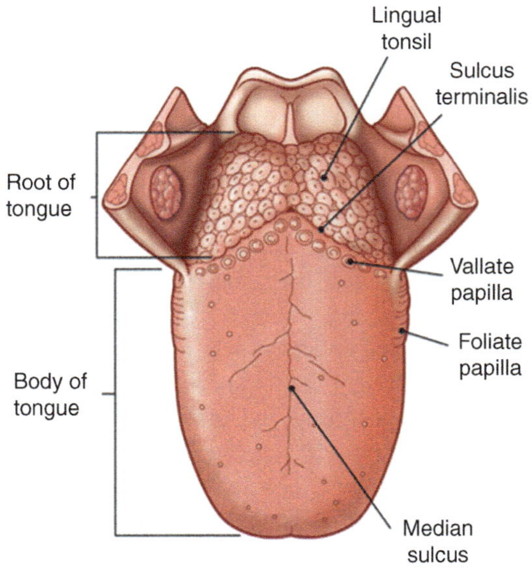

Fig. 1.2 The tongue is divided by the sulcus terminalis into two parts: the body and the root. The circumvallate papillae are located anterior to the sulcus terminalis. (Reprinted with permission from Weaker [4])

The dorsum of the tongue is lined by lingual papillae that are lamina propria projections covered by keratinized epithelium. Foliate papillae are small and found on the lateral surfaces of the tongue. Filiform papillae are the most numerous papillae of the tongue. Fungiform papillae are mushroom-shaped, fewer in number, and dispersed in between the filiform papillae. Circumvallate papillae, the most prominent and largest papillae, are located in a V-shaped configuration anterior to the sulcus terminalis. Taste buds are present in foliate, circumvallate, and fungiform papillae as well as the soft palate and pharynx [4, 5].

Dentition

The permanent dentition consists of 8 incisors, 4 canines, 8 premolars, and 12 molars (Fig. 1.3). Each tooth is divided into a root and a crown. The crown includes enamel and dentin enclosing the pulp, while the root contains only dentin surrounding the pulp and is covered by cementum. Enamel is the hard, highly mineralized outer surface of the tooth that protects the dentin and pulp and serves as the grinding surface during mastication. The interior chamber of the root contains the radicular pulp, whereas the interior chamber of the crown houses the coronal pulp. Nerves, blood vessels, and lymphatics pass through the apical foramen (Fig. 1.4). The periodontal ligament attaches the tooth to the surrounding bony structures of the maxilla and mandibular alveolar processes. The teeth are enclosed by the gingiva including the free, attached, papillary, and marginal gingiva. The interdental papilla is found between two adjacent teeth. The marginal gingiva lines the space between the teeth and the gingiva. The mucogingival line separates the gingiva from the alveolar mucosa [4].

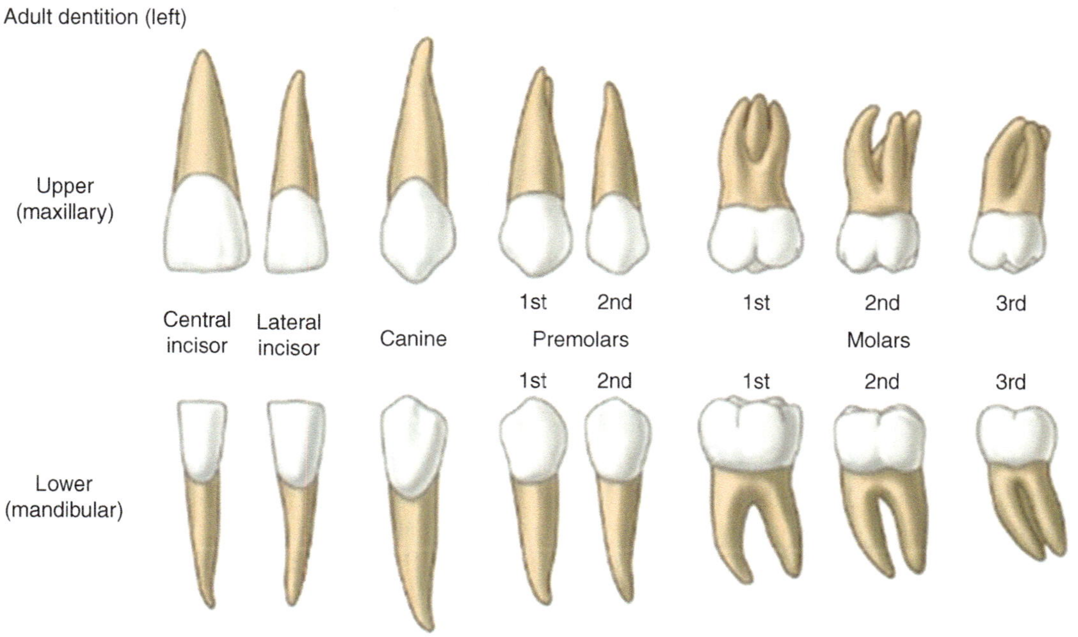

Fig. 1.3 The adult dentition is composed of two incisors, one canine, two premolars, and three molars in each quadrant. (Reprinted with permission from Weaker [4])

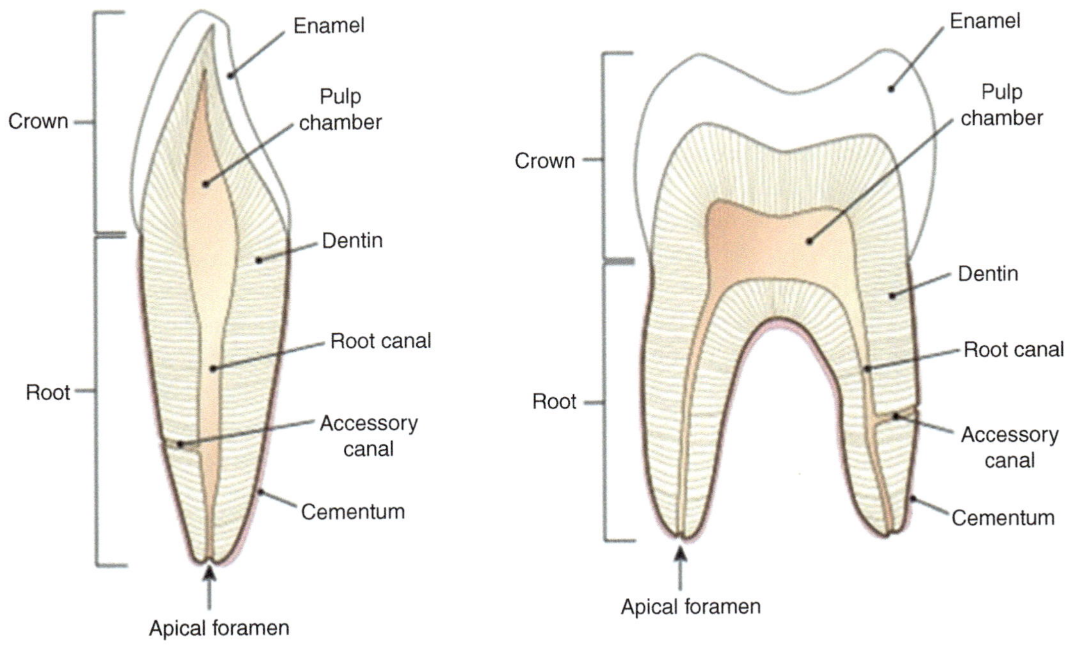

Fig. 1.4 Cross-section of a tooth showing two main parts: the crown and the root. The crown is composed of enamel, dentin, and the pulp chamber, which harbors the blood vessels, nerves, and lymphatics of the pulp. Dentin surrounds the pulp of the root and is covered by cementum. (Reprinted with permission from Weaker [4])

Salivary Glands

The parotid, submandibular, and sublingual salivary glands are the major salivary glands, which are paired and secrete 95% of the saliva. The parotid is the largest salivary gland. It is a serous gland, producing 30% of the saliva, and has a triangular shape with its base facing the zygomatic arch and its apex extending to the angle of mandible. Diseases of the parotid can affect the major anatomical structures passing through the gland: the facial nerve, retromandibular vein, and external carotid artery.

The submandibular gland is found in the submandibular triangle, which produces approximately 60%–65% of the saliva. It contains both mucous and serous fluids; however, serous secretion is more predominant. The sublingual gland, the smallest major salivary gland, is located in the floor of the mouth. It is a mixed gland with predominantly mucinous secretion. Minor salivary glands are concentrated in the submucosa throughout the walls of the oral cavity. The soft and hard palate, the labial and buccal mucosa, and the tongue contain several minor salivary glands [2, 6].

Physiology

The major functions of the oral cavity are mastication, taste, and phonation. The lips prevent the saliva from drooling and the food from spilling from the mouth. The tongue has both motor and sensory functions and plays a central role in swallowing. Molar teeth are necessary for chewing food. The lips, tongue, and palate are essential for phonation and articulation. A major function of the oral mucosa is to protect underlying structures from mechanical and chemical injuries. The epithelium also prevents fluid loss and entry of environmental toxins and microbial agents. The masticatory stratum corneum endures the mechanical forces and shearing stress. The continuous shedding of the oral mucosa also limits colonization of microbial agents [2]. Saliva lubricates the oral mucosa, which facilitates the functions of phonation, mastication, food bolus formation, and swallowing. It also protects the oral mucosa from mechanical injuries such as abrasion and contains enzymes that aid in the digestion of carbohydrates. In addition to its antimicrobial properties, saliva enhances the removal of microorganisms and desquamated cells from the oral mucosa and has a protective role in the prevention of dental caries. As a buffer, it modulates the pH and protects the oral mucosa and teeth from the acidic environment caused by the ingestion of food or gastroesophageal reflux [7].

Oral Microbiome

Despite constant desquamation of the oral mucosa, the oral cavity contains a dense population of microorganisms including bacteria, viruses, protozoa, fungi, and archaea [8]. The oral cavity is a suitable environment for microbial agents to thrive due to its stable temperature, pH and the presence of saliva as a medium [9]. Carbohydrates, lipids, and proteins in dietary food and salivary glycoproteins in addition to exuded serum proteins from the gingival sulci provide nutrients for the oral microbiota [10]. The microbiome composition of the oral cavity varies in different sites. The tongue has the highest density of microorganisms containing different microbial communities such as *Veillonella atypica* and *Porphyromonas gingivalis*, while the tooth surface provides a unique microenvironment for microbial biofilms containing *Streptococcus mutans*, *Actinomyces*, *Eubacterium*, and *Peptostreptococcus*. Figure 1.5 demonstrates the heterogeneity of the oral microbiome within the different anatomical areas of the oral cavity [9]. Bacteria are frequently responsible for the major microbiome-related diseases of the oral cav-

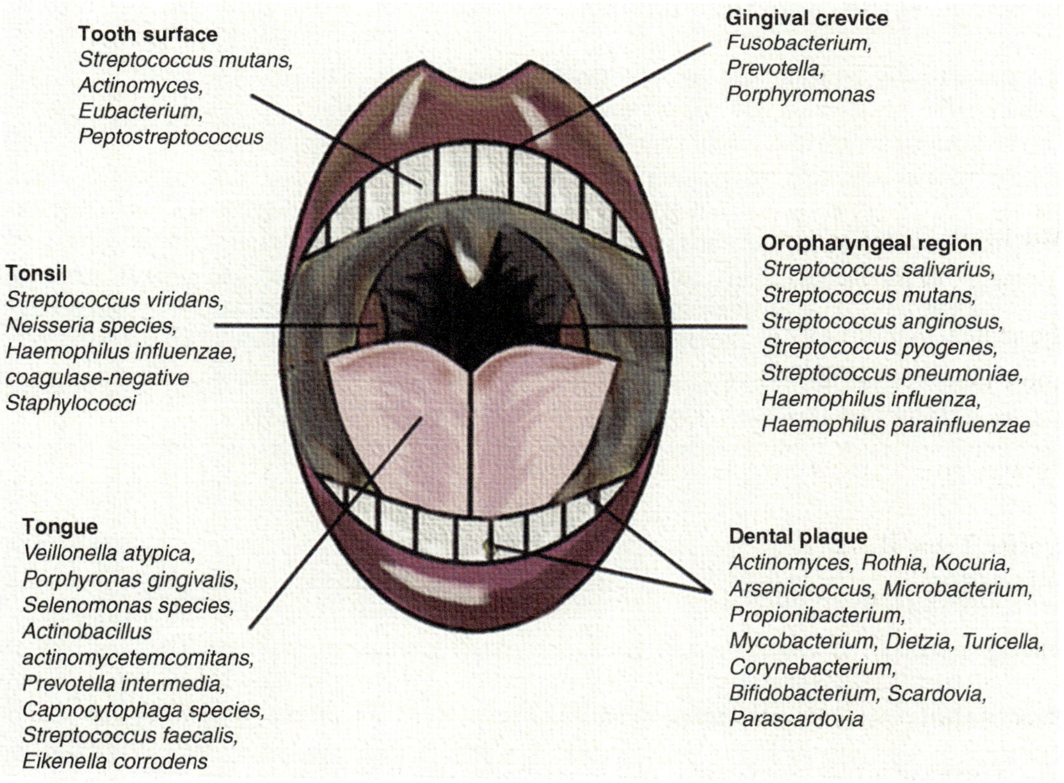

Fig. 1.5 Major microbial agents residing in the oral cavity and oropharyngeal region. (Reprinted with permission from Lim et al. [9])

ity including dental caries, endodontic infections, gingivitis, and periodontitis. The correlation between oral diseases and systemic conditions such as cardiovascular diseases, head and neck cancers, and diabetes mellitus warrants further characterization of the oral microbiome [8, 9]. The commensal microbiome provides a healthy environment in the oral cavity and prevents overgrowth of pathogens such as candida and *Staphylococcus aureus*. Some microbial species such as *Streptococcus salivarius* have shown protective effects against periodontitis and halitosis in in vitro and in vivo studies, respectively [11, 12]. Nitrate-reducing bacteria such as *Actinomyces* and *Veillonella* convert nitrates to nitrites, which may lower the risk of dental caries. Acidified nitrites may restrict the growth of cariogenic bacteria via the antimicrobial effect of oxides of nitrogen such as nitric oxide [13–15].

Principles of the Oral Examination

Comprehensive examination of the oral cavity includes visual inspection and palpation of the various anatomical structures within the oral cavity. Partial and complete removable prostheses should be removed prior to examination of the oral mucosa. Adequate lighting and proper positioning of the patient is of significant importance in conducting an oral examination. The patient's head should be stable and well positioned to allow visualization of all mucosal surfaces. A tongue blade or a cotton gauze is used to retract the tongue and allow adequate exposure to various sites within the oral cavity [16].

Inspection

The lips, dorsal and ventral tongue, hard and soft palates, buccal mucosa, gingiva, and the floor of the mouth are visually inspected for the presence of any abnormal growths, inflammation, ulceration, discoloration, or bleeding. Visual inspection is performed by using a tongue blade or dental mirror to retract the lips and cheeks and evaluate the buccal mucosa, teeth, and alveolar ridges. The patient should be asked to raise the tongue and touch the palate to adequately examine the floor of the mouth and the ventral tongue. The lateral tongue and floor of the mouth are best observed by retracting the tongue using a tongue blade or a gauze wrapped around the tip of the tongue. The posterior oropharynx can be inspected using a dental mirror. The presence of hypoglossal and glossopharyngeal nerve palsy can be assessed, if the patient's condition warrants it. To detect hypoglossal palsy, the examiner should initially look for signs of atrophy, fasciculation, or tongue deviation while the tongue is in a resting position. The tongue deviates toward the affected side when the patient protrudes the tongue. The glossopharyngeal nerve can be assessed by inducing the gag reflex. Movement of the soft palate and uvula should be also assessed; in hypoglossal nerve palsy, the soft palate and uvula deviate to the unaffected side while the patient says "Ah" [16].

Palpation

If an abnormality is noted on visual inspection, the suspected area should be palpated to assess the consistency, texture, and depth of the lesion. The face and neck should also be palpated for any abnormalities to include palpation of the anterior/posterior cervical, submandibular, and supraclavicular lymph nodes [16].

Summary

Clinical competence in detecting abnormalities within the oral cavity, familiarity with common manifestations of systemic disorders, and the pathophysiology of those conditions are important elements of the comprehensive clinical exam. A thorough history and meticulous oral exam can play a crucial role in the early diagnosis and prompt treatment of various systemic diseases.

References

1. Stelow E, Mills S. Normal anatomy and histology. In: Stelow E, Mills S, editors. Biopsy interpretation of the upper aerodigestive tract and ear. Philadelphia: Lippincott Williams & Wilkins; 2013. p. 1–16.
2. Squier CA, Kremer MJ. Biology of oral mucosa and esophagus. J Natl Cancer Inst Monogr. 2001; 29:7–15.
3. Qin R, Steel A, Fazel N. Oral mucosa biology and salivary biomarkers. Clin Dermatol. 2017;35(5):477–83.
4. Weaker F. Oral cavity. In: Weaker F, editor. Structures of the head and neck. Philadelphia: F. A. Davis; 2014. p. 124–43.
5. Pramod J. Structure of the oral mucous membrane. In: Pramod J, editor. Textbook of oral medicine. New Delhi: Jaypee Brothers Medical Publishers (P) Ltd.; 2014. p. 39–50.
6. Weaker F. Salivary glands. In: Weaker F, editor. Structures of the head and neck. Philadelphia: F. A. Davis; 2014. p. 144–53.
7. Dawes C, Pedersen AM, Villa A, Ekström J, Proctor GB, Vissink A, et al. The functions of human saliva: a review sponsored by the World Workshop on Oral Medicine VI. Arch Oral Biol. 2015;60(6): 863–74.
8. Wade WG. The oral microbiome in health and disease. Pharmacol Res. 2013;69(1):137–43.
9. Lim Y, Totsika M, Morrison M, Punyadeera C. Oral microbiome: a new biomarker reservoir for oral and oropharyngeal cancers. Theranostics. 2017;7(17):4313–21.
10. Costalonga M, Herzberg MC. The oral microbiome and the immunobiology of periodontal disease and caries. Immunol Lett. 2014;162(2 Pt A):22–38.
11. Burton JP, Chilcott CN, Moore CJ, Speiser G, Tagg JR. A preliminary study of the effect of probiotic Streptococcus salivarius K12 on oral malodour parameters. J Appl Microbiol. 2006;100(4):754–64.
12. Wescombe PA, Heng NC, Burton JP, Chilcott CN, Tagg JR. Streptococcal bacteriocins and the case for Streptococcus salivarius as model oral probiotics. Future Microbiol. 2009;4(7):819–35.
13. Allaker RP, Stephen AS. Use of probiotics and oral health. Curr Oral Health Rep. 2017;4(4):309–18.
14. Doel JJ, Benjamin N, Hector MP, Rogers M, Allaker RP. Evaluation of bacterial nitrate reduction in the human oral cavity. Eur J Oral Sci. 2005;113(1):14–9.
15. Silva Mendez LS, Allaker RP, Hardie JM, Benjamin N. Antimicrobial effect of acidified nitrite on cariogenic bacteria. Oral Microbiol Immunol. 1999;14(6):391–2.
16. Grevers G, Probst R. Oral cavity and pharynx. In: Probst R, Grevers G, Iro H, editors. Basic otorhinolaryngology: a step-by-step learning guide. New York: Thieme; 2006. p. 68–95.

2 Oral Signs of Gastrointestinal Disease

John C. Steele

Inflammatory Bowel Disease

Crohn's disease and ulcerative colitis are the most commonly recognized inflammatory bowel diseases (IBD), and both can initially present with oral manifestations. It is estimated that up to 1.4 million people in the United States suffer from inflammatory bowel disease [1] with as many as 70,000 new cases being diagnosed annually [2].

Crohn's disease and orofacial granulomatosis

Crohn's disease and orofacial granulomatosis (OFG) have been grouped together in this section since there is much debate in the literature as to whether the latter is a reflection of oral Crohn's disease or indeed is an entity entirely on its own [3–5]. More recently, a systematic review of pediatric cases of OFG identified a high prevalence of Crohn's disease and concluded that OFG may be a subtype of Crohn's disease [6].

OFG was initially described in 1985 and is an uncommon, chronic inflammatory, granulomatous disorder of the orofacial region [7]. Others have used synonyms for OFG including granulomatous cheilitis, cheilitis granulomatosa, cheilitis granulomatosis, and oral granulomatosis. For the purposes of this chapter, OFG is the preferred nomenclature.

There is also speculation whether OFG without gastrointestinal signs/symptoms, Melkersson-Rosenthal syndrome (triad of facial swelling, facial palsy, and fissured tongue), and cheilitis granulomatosa are a spectrum of the same disease [4, 8, 9]. Cheilitis granulomatosa (Meischer's cheilitis) is monosymptomatic and characterized by lip swelling only.

Epidemiology

The worldwide incidence of Crohn's disease varies from 0.1 to 6/100,000 [1] with an increased incidence in smokers. There have been a few studies examining the prevalence of oral manifestations in Crohn's disease patients [8], and the presence varied from 0.5% to 60%.

Etiopathogenesis

The etiopathogenesis of OFG is uncertain with a number of postulated theories: genetic predisposition, hypersensitivity/allergy to dietary components/dental materials, microbiological agents/infection, and inflammatory/immunological factors.

Genetic

Limited small case series have suggested that there is a genetic link with OFG being seen in families and there being a human leucocyte

J. C. Steele (✉)
The Leeds Teaching Hospitals NHS Trust, Leeds, UK

Faculty of Medicine and Health, University of Leeds, Leeds, UK
e-mail: johncraigsteele@nhs.net

N. Fazel (ed.), *Oral Signs of Systemic Disease*, https://doi.org/10.1007/978-3-030-10863-2_2

antigen (HLA) association. However, there has not been enough evidence for a conclusive link to be made [8, 9].

Hypersensitivity/Allergy

A recent study [10] demonstrated that prevalence rates of allergy were significantly greater in patients with OFG (82%) than in the general population (22%). This has been supported by other studies showing OFG patients to have higher rates of atopy [8]. A number of food additives and substances have been implicated in evoking a delayed-type contact hypersensitivity. These include, among others, cinnamaldehyde (also found in toothpaste) and benzoates. Adhering to a specific cinnamon and benzoate exclusion diet has been shown to improve the clinical features of OFG [11]. Allergy to dental materials has been proposed as an etiological factor in OFG; however, there has not been any conclusive evidence to support this [9].

Microbiological/Infection

An infective etiology has been proposed based on the fact that certain microorganisms (bacteria) have been implicated in other chronic granulomatous conditions such as sarcoidosis, Crohn's disease, and tuberculosis [8, 9]. Research has focused on mycobacteria, *Saccharomyces*, spirochetes, and *Borrelia* species. There appears to be conflicting evidence from small studies as to whether there is a relationship with OFG or not, and so a recent review concludes that there is insufficient evidence to support the role of infection as a cause of OFG [9].

Inflammatory/Immunological

An immunological basis for OFG has not been supported in the literature by studies of appropriate power, and although the theory is plausible, further work is required. There is a hypothesis that OFG is not driven by a single antigen but by a random influx of inflammatory cells [9].

Clinical Manifestations

Crohn's disease can affect any part of the gastrointestinal tract from the mouth at the proximal end to the anus at the distal. The small intestine is most often involved with the terminal ileum being the commonest site. "Skip lesions" of normal non-diseased mucosa may be present. Symptoms include abdominal pain, diarrhea +/− bleeding per rectum, stricture formation, and lesions affecting the anus, perianal region, and the mouth. There is an increased risk of fistulae and abscess formation as well as hematinic deficiencies (B12 and iron). Signs of the disease can be seen clinically, radiologically, and by direct endoscopic visualization. Pathological features include transmural inflammation and the presence of noncaseating granulomas.

Oral Signs and Symptoms

The most common oral complaint is of swelling, which predominantly affects the lips, although other orofacial structures such as the buccal mucosa may also be involved. The physical disfigurement can be detrimental to the psychosocial quality of life of the individual (Fig. 2.1a, b).

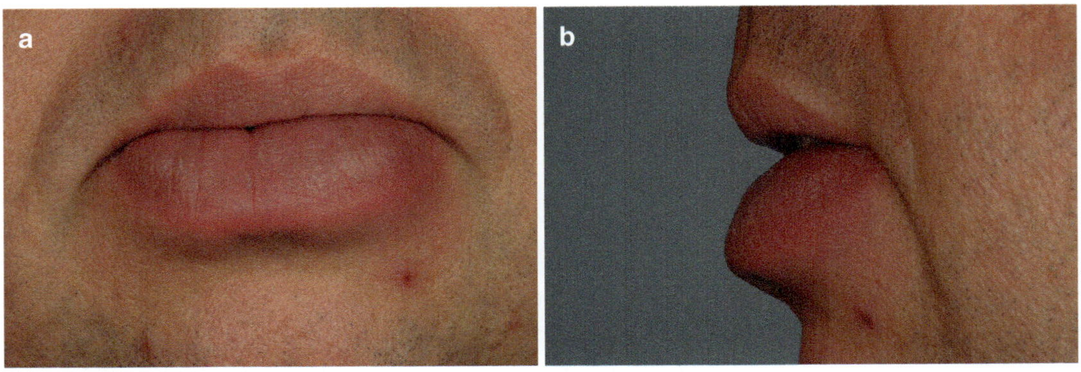

Fig. 2.1 (**a**) OFG – This figure shows swelling of the lower lip (anterior view). (**b**) OFG – This figure shows swelling of the lower lip (lateral view)

Table 2.1 Clinical features of OFG

Extraoral: lip/facial swelling (Fig. 2.1a, b)
Angular cheilitis
Lip fissuring (vertical)
Perioral erythema
Cervical lymphadenopathy
Intraoral: cobblestoning of the buccal mucosa (Fig. 2.2)
Mucosal tags (Figs. 2.3 and 2.4)
Full width gingivitis/hyperplastic gingivitis/ granulomatous gingivitis (Fig. 2.3)
Linear "slit-like" ulceration (Fig. 2.5) or aphthous-like ulcers (round/oval)
"Staghorning" of the submandibular ducts (Fig. 2.6)
Tongue fissuring
Neurological: facial palsy

There have been a few reasonably large case series of OFG patients reported in the literature (Al Johani 2009 – 49 cases [12], McCartan 2011 – 119 cases [13], Campbell 2011 – 207 cases [4]), which aimed to characterize the most common clinical features. Lip swelling was the most common feature (51%, 77%, and 91%, respectively) observed, and this can be either recurrent or persistent. Cobblestoning of the buccal mucosa ranged from 27% to 63% [4, 13]. The mucosal ulcerations associated with OFG can either be aphthous-like (shallow round ulcers with an erythematous border) in appearance or deep and linear. The latter commonly appear in the buccal sulci with hyperplastic mucosal edges and tend to be persistent [14, 15]. Swelling of the area around the submandibular/sublingual gland orifices results in a "staghorn" appearance and was noted in 10% of the largest case series [4]. Neurological manifestations have been reported including recurrent relapsing and remitting facial palsy [9, 12].

Table 2.1 summarizes the most commonly observed extra- and intraoral features associated with OFG, and Figs. 2.1, 2.2, 2.3, 2.4, 2.5, and 2.6 demonstrate some of these presentations.

Pyostomatitis vegetans can present as the sole oral manifestation of Crohn's disease. Please see the section on *Pyostomatitis vegetans* for further information.

Differential Diagnosis

The differential diagnosis for the orofacial swelling associated with OFG includes immunological conditions, infection, and inflammatory disease [9, 12]. Please see Table 2.2.

The following investigations should be considered to help ascertain a definitive diagnosis: CBC, iron studies, inflammatory markers, ACE

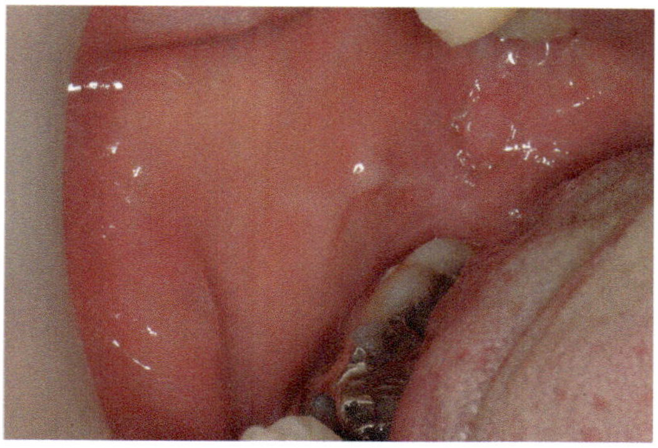

Fig. 2.2 OFG – Cobblestoning of the buccal mucosa can be seen on the anterior right buccal mucosa

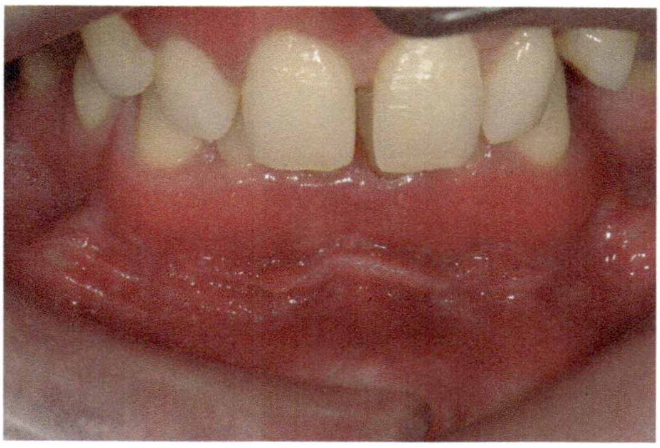

Fig. 2.3 OFG – This figure demonstrates a full-width gingivitis and mucosal tags affecting the anterior mandibular gingivae

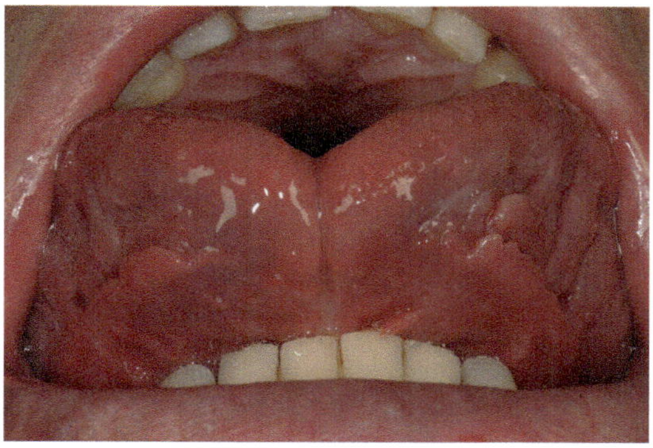

Fig. 2.4 OFG – Mucosal tags can be seen on the ventral surfaces of the tongue

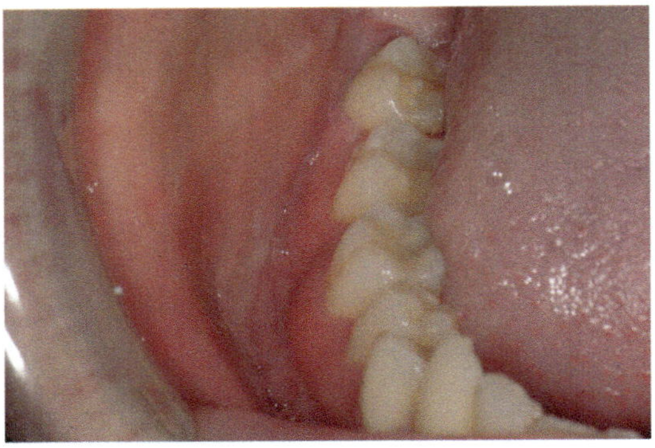

Fig. 2.5 OFG – A healing linear "slit-like" ulcer can be seen in the right buccal sulcus

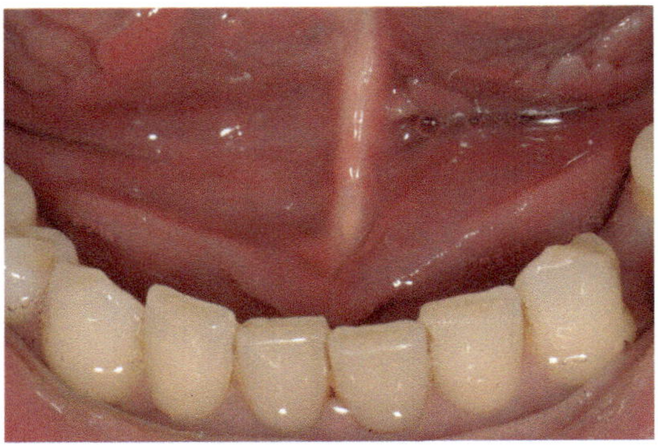

Fig. 2.6 OFG – This figure shows "staghorning" of the submandibular ducts

Table 2.2 Differential diagnosis of orofacial swelling

Immunological	Angioedema – hereditary and acquired/c1-esterase inhibitor deficiency
Infections	Tuberculosis
	Deep fungal infections
	Leprosy
Inflammatory disease	Crohn's disease
	Foreign body and delayed hypersensitivity reactions
	Cheilitis granulomatosa (Meischer's cheilitis)
	Sarcoidosis
	Melkersson-Rosenthal syndrome

levels, chest x-ray, and a deep incisional biopsy of any swollen oral mucosa.

The characteristic histopathological features of OFG [4] are of noncaseating epithelioid granulomas, lymphedema of the corium, and dilated lymphatics, which can be virtually indistinguishable from Crohn's disease or systemic sarcoidosis [9].

Table 2.3 Management/treatment options for OFG

Angular cheilitis	Topical/systemic antimicrobial agents
Diet	Cinnamon- and benzoate-free diet (low phenolic acid diet)
Lip fissure	Emollients
	Antimicrobial/combined antimicrobial and corticosteroid
Lip swelling	Local
	Intralesional corticosteroid injection
	Topical corticosteroid
	Systemic
	Dietary modification
	Immunosuppression (off-label)
Generalized inflammation	Immunosuppression (off-label)
	Azathioprine
	Anti-TNFα therapy
Oral ulceration	Topical
	Corticosteroids (various preparations)
	Analgesics
	Antiseptic mouthwash
	Systemic
	Corticosteroids (rescue therapy)
	Immunosuppression (off-label)

Treatment Recommendations

The aim of treatment for OFG depends on the presenting symptom. In the majority of cases, the patient is concerned about the cosmetic appearance of any facial swelling. Patients are also concerned about pain and impact on their quality of life from oral ulcers. Management/treatment options are listed in Table 2.3. The undertaking of much larger randomized controlled trials is needed since much of the evidence is based on small case series.

Intralesional corticosteroid injection has been shown to be effective in treating persistent lip swelling; however, multiple injections are often required [9]. The injection itself can be painful, and consideration should be given to injecting local anesthetic prior to injecting the corticosteroid.

Many different types of immunosuppressants have been used off-label to manage the clinical manifestations of OFG. These include colchicine, dapsone, hydroxychloroquine, infliximab, methotrexate, tacrolimus, and thalidomide among others

[6]. Two small case series using anti-TNFα treatment have been reported showing a good short-term response in the management of recalcitrant OFG with infliximab [16] and thalidomide [17]. Unfortunately, a significant number of those taking infliximab lost efficacy over time.

Dietary modification can be of significant benefit. An initial study published in 2006 involving 32 patients showed a statistically significant improvement in global lip and oral inflammatory scores after 8 weeks adhering to a cinnamon- and benzoate-free diet [11]. A review of the literature by the same research group in 2011 demonstrated that this diet can be beneficial in 54–78% of patients with 23% requiring no adjunctive therapies [18]. They also noted that the results of patch testing for cinnamaldehyde and benzoates did not predict success or failure in adhering to this diet. More recently, the same group has tested a low phenolic acid diet with micronutrient supplementation [19] since phenolic acids are among the constituents restricted in a cinnamon- and benzoate-free diet. The conclusion was that this new diet holds potential promise but larger-scale studies are required.

The clinician should consider referral to gastroenterology, especially in children, for a thorough work-up to rule out inflammatory bowel disease.

Ulcerative Colitis

Ulcerative colitis (UC) is a chronic inflammatory bowel disease that mainly affects the large intestine (colon) and rectum (proctitis).

Epidemiology

The worldwide incidence of UC varies from 0.5 to 24.5/100,000 [1]. There is a decreased incidence of UC in smokers. In the USA, UC affects between 250,000 and 500,000 people with an annual incidence of two to seven per 100,000 [20].

Etiopathogenesis

An inflammatory cell infiltrate affects only the mucosa and submucosa. The current theory is that the mucosal immune system becomes dysregulated, which results in normal microflora inducing an excessive immunological response [20].

Clinical Manifestations

The main symptom is of diarrhea with associated blood and mucous. Other symptoms include abdominal pain, nausea, fever, rectal urgency, and tenesmus [1, 20]. UC is associated with an increased incidence of chronic active hepatitis, primary biliary cirrhosis, sclerosing cholangitis, and colon cancer. Toxic megacolon may develop possibly necessitating an urgent colectomy.

Oral Signs and Symptoms

There are no oral signs and symptoms specific to UC. However, there can be oral signs of iron deficiency anemia if there is significant blood loss such as aphthous ulcers, angular cheilitis, and glossitis. Pyostomatitis vegetans can present as the sole oral manifestation of UC. Please see the section on *Pyostomatitis vegetans* for further information. A recent small case-control study [21] examining the oral manifestations of UC patients versus a control group without gastrointestinal disease reported that the presence of a tongue coating and the symptoms of dry mouth, halitosis, and taste changes were more common in the former group.

Differential Diagnosis

Please see the next section on *Pyostomatitis vegetans*.

Treatment Recommendations

The main medication classes used to treat UC include aminosalicylates, corticosteroids, immunosuppressants, and antibiotics. Surgery, as mentioned above, has a role and can "cure" UC following total colectomy [1].

Correction of any underlying iron deficiency can help control the symptoms of oral ulcers, angular cheilitis, or glossitis. Topical corticosteroids and analgesics can be prescribed to manage the pain and discomfort associated with ulcers. Antimicrobials can be prescribed to manage angular cheilitis depending on the implicated organism, which are usually either a *Candida* species or *Staphylococcus aureus*.

Pyostomatitis vegetans

Pyostomatitis vegetans (PV) is a rare, benign, chronic condition that is strongly associated with and considered a highly specific marker of IBD [22–24]. It is more commonly seen in UC than in Crohn's disease. It is considered the mucosal equivalent of pyodermatitis vegetans and is also associated with pyodermatitis gangrenosum. IBD commonly presents before the onset of oral lesions by a period of months to years [22].

Epidemiology

There is a male predilection [14, 22] for PV with a ratio of 2–3:1. PV can be seen in patients of any age but is most commonly seen in young-middle-aged patients between 20 and 59 years of age with a mean of 34 years [14].

Etiopathogenesis

The etiopathogenesis of PV is unknown and poorly understood. Immune dysregulation, microbial factors, or a nutritional deficiency have been implicated in the etiology [22].

Components of a complete blood count (CBC) and features seen on histopathological examination may support the immunological reaction theory. Raised lymphocyte and eosinophil counts are often seen as well as atypical immunofluorescence being observed at the basement membrane although this may be due to tissue damage [22]. A further theory concerns cross-reacting antigens of the bowel and skin [24].

Microbial factors have been considered since the cutaneous equivalent of PV, pyodermatitis vegetans, occurs in areas where microbial growth is encouraged (e.g., skin folds) and PV is a disorder included in the chronic pyodermas group. However, bacterial, fungal, and viral cultures of PV lesions are consistently negative [22, 24]. An additional hypothesis is that infections and their effect on the immune system may be implicated in the pathogenesis of IBD [22]. Interestingly, it has been noted that peripheral eosinophilia is present in 90% of reported cases [22].

Clinical Manifestations

PV usually runs in parallel with underlying IBD and has been considered a reliable marker of intestinal activity by some research groups [25]. Please see the preceding sections on Crohn's disease and ulcerative colitis for information on the clinical manifestations.

Oral Signs and Symptoms

Oral lesions present as multiple friable, gray-yellow pustules on an erythematous and thickened mucosal base. The pustules tend to rupture easily, producing erosions and fissures, and may coalesce, resulting in the appearance of "snail-track" ulceration and vegetations. All areas of the oral cavity can be affected with the most commonly affected sites being the labial and buccal mucosa, hard and soft palate, gingivae, and sulci. The tongue and floor of the mouth are least likely to be affected [23, 24].

Differential Diagnosis

The differential diagnosis [14, 22, 23] is summarized in Table 2.4. Histopathological examination including immunofluorescence studies can help differentiate immunobullous disease from PV.

Treatment Recommendations

In the absence of any underlying IBD, topical corticosteroids can successfully treat PV [22]. There are various preparations available including mouthwashes prepared by dissolving corticosteroid tablets, sprays, and ointments although many of these preparations are used off-label as they may not be indicated for oral use.

Table 2.4 Differential diagnosis of pyostomatitis vegetans

Behçet's disease
Bullous drug eruption
Bullous pemphigoid
Dermatitis herpetiformis
Erythema multiforme
Epidermolysis bullosa acquisita
Herpes simplex infection
Pemphigus vegetans/vulgaris

It would be sensible to refer a patient with PV who does not have any IBD symptoms for a gastroenterology consultation to exclude any silent disease [15, 24].

In the presence of IBD, medical or surgical interventions (total colectomy for UC) are the main management considerations.

There have been a number of case reports/small case series [22, 23] reporting that the following systemic treatments may be helpful in the management of PV: corticosteroids, dapsone, sulfasalazine, sulfamethoxypyridazine, azathioprine, cyclosporine, and isotretinoin. A single case report found success with topical tacrolimus [26].

Celiac Disease (Sprue)

Celiac disease (also known as sprue) is an autoimmune, T-cell-mediated, gluten-sensitive enteropathy seen in genetically susceptible individuals. It is the most common genetically based food intolerance worldwide [27, 28].

Gluten is a substance rich in glutamine and proline residues that is unable to be fully digested in celiac disease [27]. It is found in wheat (gliadin), barley (hordein), and rye (secalin) and seen in foods such as pasta, cereals, and grains [29]. Celiac disease often develops when solid food is introduced into the diet and therefore usually presents after the sixth month of life during transition to solid foods such as cereals [29].

There are different presentations of celiac disease: typical (with gastrointestinal symptoms), atypical (having extraintestinal manifestations), and the silent form (asymptomatic) [30].

Antibody testing is used as a screening tool with the current recommendation being to use the serum immunoglobulin A tissue transglutaminase (tTG) antibody test, which has a sensitivity and specificity >90% [28, 31]. This would identify those who would then need a diagnostic endoscopic small bowel biopsy [28].

Epidemiology

The estimated incidence of celiac disease is 3–13 cases per 1000 with an overall prevalence of 1% [28]. Only 10–15% of this population have been diagnosed and treated; therefore a large number of cases remain undiagnosed [27, 31]. There is a higher prevalence among relatives of patients with celiac disease, and this has been calculated at 1:22 for first-degree relatives and 1:39 for second-degree relatives [28, 32]. In a recently published large study, the prevalence of celiac disease in the United States was calculated at 0.71% (1 in 141), but the authors acknowledged that most cases were in fact undiagnosed [33].

Etiopathogenesis

There is a genetic and environmental basis to the development of celiac disease.

Genetic

It is acknowledged that under the influence of environmental factors, genetically susceptible individuals develop celiac disease with two HLA class II genes (HLA-DQ2 and HLA-DQ8) having been identified [27, 28].

Environmental

Celiac disease does not develop without dietary exposure to gluten. Some studies have reported that children introduced to gluten in the first 3 months of life were at greater risk of celiac disease. Interestingly, prolonged breastfeeding is associated with a smaller risk of developing the disease [27].

Clinical Manifestations

In typical celiac disease, the most common symptom is abdominal pain. Other gastrointestinal symptoms include diarrhea (chronic or intermittent), vomiting, abdominal distension, and constipation [27, 28]. Failure to thrive or weight loss can be a sign of celiac disease. Cachexia and severe malnutrition can be observed in a delayed or late diagnosis [28].

In atypical celiac disease, the most common extraintestinal sign is iron deficiency anemia [27]. Dermatitis herpetiformis, which is a symmetrical chronic, pruritic blistering rash affecting the extensor surfaces of the elbows and knees and the buttocks, is the cutaneous manifestation of celiac disease [27]. Other signs and symptoms include deficiencies in vitamin D leading to osteoporosis, short stature, malabsorption resulting in hematinic deficiencies, extreme weakness, fatigue, myalgias, headaches, liver function abnormalities, menstrual irregularities, infertility, and adverse pregnancy outcomes [28, 29, 31].

Celiac disease is often associated with other conditions, most notably Type 1 diabetes mellitus and autoimmune thyroiditis as they have a common genetic background [30]. Other associations include selective IgA deficiency and various chromosomal disorders including Down syndrome, Turner syndrome, and Williams syndrome [27].

Oral Signs and Symptoms

Celiac disease can be suspected in individuals with both oral mucosal and dental signs and symptoms.

Aphthous ulcers (Fig. 2.7) are associated with celiac disease although the cause is unknown. The ulcers may be due to malabsorption leading to a hematinic deficiency [31]. The highest prevalence that has been observed in celiac patient subgroups has been in children, adolescents, and women and measures approximately 20% [29].

Dermatitis herpetiformis, the cutaneous manifestation of celiac disease, can present in the oral cavity in the form of erosions and desquamative gingivitis.

Another oral soft tissue sign that has been noted is papillary atrophy of the tongue, which can appear red and be painful. It is postulated that this is due to malabsorption of hematinics [29].

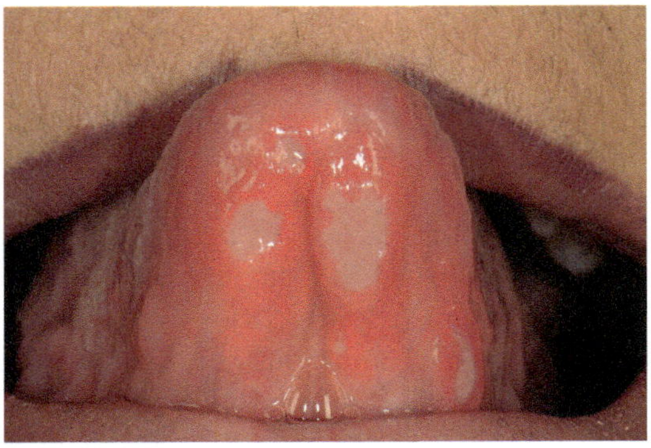

Fig. 2.7 Aphthous ulcers on the ventral surface of the tongue

Enamel defects (enamel hypoplasia, pitting, grooving, and partial/complete loss of enamel) have been observed in celiac disease patient cohorts [27, 31]. The prevalence of dental enamel hypoplasia among celiac patients is reported to be in the range 10–97% according to various studies [27, 28], although there is debate in the literature as to whether there is a true association [34]. There are two theories as to how enamel defects arise. The first concerns malabsorption of calcium and phosphorus during enamel formation, which leads to nutritional deficiencies such as hypocalcemia resulting in hypomineralization [35]. The second relates to immune disturbances against the enamel organ itself during enamel formation [28, 31, 34]. An association between delayed eruption of teeth [27] has been identified in up to 27%.

A case-control study involving 300 celiac patients reported that 33% were affected by enamel hypoplasia and 8.3% by recurrent aphthous ulcers and 20% had experienced a delay in dental eruption. The results for the control group were 11%, 3%, and 8%, respectively [34].

Differential Diagnosis

The differential diagnoses for the cause of enamel defects [29, 31] and other factors predisposing to the formation of aphthous-like ulcers [36, 37] are seen in Tables 2.5 and 2.6, respectively.

Treatment Recommendations

Adhering to a strict gluten-free diet for life is the mainstay of treatment in the management of both typical and atypical celiac disease. Compliance can be difficult especially in teenagers [28]. Aphthous ulcers often regress when patients are on a gluten-free diet [28], but topical agents (steroids, analgesics, and antiseptics) may have to be considered in the interim while a patient is adapting to a new diet.

Table 2.5 Differential diagnosis for enamel defects

Amelogenesis imperfecta
Enamel fluorosis
Localized infection
Nutritional disorders during enamel formation
Hypocalcaemia
Malnutrition
Vitamin D deficiency
Trauma

Table 2.6 Factors predisposing to the formation of aphthous-like ulcers

Behçet's disease
Cyclic neutropenia
Hematinic deficiencies
HIV disease
MAGIC syndrome (mouth and genital ulcers with inflamed cartilage)
PFAPA (periodic fever, aphthous stomatitis, pharyngitis, and cervical adenitis)
Sweet's syndrome
Trauma

Consideration should be given to referring a patient to a dentist for restorative treatment if there is a concern regarding enamel defects or missing teeth.

Gardner's syndrome

Gardner's syndrome (GS) is a rare autosomal dominant inherited disorder that is considered a subtype of familial adenomatous polyposis (FAP). GS comprises the triad of potentially malignant (high risk) intestinal adenomatous polyps, cutaneous lesions, and osteomas [38, 39].

Epidemiology

The incidence of GS ranges from 1 in 4000 to 1 in 12000 [40]. In comparison, the incidence of FAP ranges between 1 in 8300 and 1 in 14,025 live births with equal sex distribution and uniform worldwide distribution [39]. Intestinal polyps usually occur prior to puberty and become more generalized in early adulthood [39, 40]. If these polyps are not treated, all (100%) patients will develop cancer of the large intestine before the age of 40 [39].

Etiopathogenesis

GS is an autosomal dominant disorder with almost complete penetrance of 80% [41]. It is caused by a mutation in the *APC* gene located on the long arm of chromosome 5 (5q21) [39–41].

Clinical Manifestations

Polyps can develop at any site in the gastrointestinal tract but are particularly located in the distal colon [40].

Table 2.7 Orofacial signs of Gardner's syndrome

Dental	Congenitally missing teeth
	Dentigerous cysts
	Hypodontia
	Hypercementosis
	Impacted/unerupted teeth
	Odontomas
	Supernumerary teeth
Osteomas	Can affect the maxilla or mandible
Soft tissue	Epidermoid cysts
	Fibromas

Soft tissue manifestations include epidermoid, dermoid, and sebaceous cysts with the latter being present in 60% of patients with GS [38]. In 15–30% of patients, fibromas are noted.

Oral Signs and Symptoms

There are a number of dental anomalies that are associated with GS, and these can be present in 17–75% of GS patients [38, 40]. Supernumerary teeth, unerupted teeth, and odontomas (compound) usually affect the anterior parts of the jaws with the molar regions being rarely affected [15]. Osteomas affecting the mandible are more common than those affecting the maxilla and tend to be larger in size [39]. They are generally asymptomatic but can lead to facial asymmetry and therefore aesthetic concerns for the patient [40]. Soft tissue lesions, as mentioned above, can also affect the oral and maxillofacial region. The majority of soft tissue lesions are of multiple benign epidermoid cysts affecting the face, scalp, and extremities [40, 42]. Fibromas have been noted to infiltrate the masticatory and suprahyoid musculature [38]. Orofacial signs are summarized in Table 2.7.

Differential Diagnosis

Conditions that can have multiple radiopaque masses/odontomas on plain film radiographs as well as supernumerary and impacted teeth include the following rare conditions: cleidocranial dysplasia, osteo-cemental dysplasia, and periapical osteo-cemental dysplasia [38].

The differential diagnosis for intestinal polyposis includes a number of different syndromes of varying incidence, and these are listed below in Table 2.8.

Table 2.8 Differential diagnosis of intestinal polyposis syndromes

Basal cell nevus syndrome
Bannayan-Ruvalcaba-Riley syndrome
Cowden's syndrome
Cronkhite-Canada syndrome
Familial adenomatous polyposis (FAP) syndrome
Familial juvenile polyposis
Hereditary mixed polyposis
Hyperplastic polyposis syndrome
MYH-associated polyposis (MAP)
Peutz-Jeghers syndrome
Turcot's syndrome

Treatment Recommendations

The high risk of colorectal cancer developing from an intestinal polyp necessitates screening and endoscopic surveillance, but often prophylactic colectomy is required to ensure that the risk is minimized [38, 39]. Osteomas are surgically excised if they result in functional or cosmetic problems. Sebaceous cysts may be removed at the request of the patient, if they have a detrimental effect on their appearance. Fibromas/fibromatous tumors are sometimes excised, if they locally infiltrate the musculature [38].

Peutz-Jeghers syndrome

Peutz-Jeghers syndrome (PJS) is a rare condition of autosomal dominant inheritance that is associated with the development of hamartomatous polyposis mainly of the small intestine and mucocutaneous oral/perioral pigmentation. There is an associated increased cancer risk related to the polyps but also in relation to other malignancies.

The diagnosis of PJS is made clinically and is based on the presence of benign hamartomatous polyps, mucocutaneous pigmentation, and family history. The diagnostic criteria for PJS is based on any one of the following findings [43]:

- Three or more histologically confirmed benign hamartomatous polyps
- Family history of PJS and any number of hamartomatous polyps
- Family history of PJS and mucocutaneous pigmentation
- Any number of hamartomatous polyps and mucocutaneous pigmentation

Epidemiology

There are various estimates for the prevalence of PJS, which range from 1 in 8500 live births to 1 in 200,000 live births depending on the population sampled. There is no discrepancy based on sex or ethnicity [43, 44].

Etiopathogenesis

Half of all PJS cases are attributed to a mutation of a serine-threonine kinase (STK11/LKB1) gene, which is located on the short arm of chromosome 19p13.3 [43–45].

Clinical Manifestations

Seventy to 90% of patients have polyps present in the small intestine [45] with the jejunum being the most common location [43]. Colorectal polyps are present in 50% of patients and 25% have gastric polyps [45].

A significant increase in the size of a polyp can result in intussusception (especially in younger patients) as well as bowel obstruction. This can present clinically as severe abdominal pain and bleeding both from within the gastrointestinal tract and rectally, which can result in anemia [43].

There is a 2–3% incidence of gastrointestinal adenocarcinoma in PJS. There is also an increased risk of malignancies of the breast, pancreas, thyroid gland, genitourinary tract, lung, and testis. An estimated 48% of patients with PJS will succumb to malignancy by the average age of 57 [42].

Oral Signs and Symptoms

Melanotic macules classically present on or around the lips and appear in up to 95% of all PJS patients [46]. The vermillion border is also affected in 95% of patients [42]. They can vary in size from 1 to 5 mm and also in color incorporating different

Table 2.9 Differential diagnosis of mucocutaneous oral pigmentation

Becker's nevi
Carney complex
Cowden syndrome
Laugier-Hunziker syndrome
Leopard syndrome
Melanotic macules/ephelides/nevi/lentigines
Nevi of Ota

shades of brown and black [44]. They first appear in infancy and can also affect other oral sites including the buccal mucosa, labial mucosa, palate, and tongue [43, 44]. Lentigines can present periorally on the skin as well as other sites including perianally and on the fingers and toes [46].

Anemia as a result of gastrointestinal/rectal bleeding can be indicated by the presence of oral ulcers, glossitis, or angular cheilitis.

Differential Diagnosis

The differential diagnosis of intestinal polyposis [38, 43, 45] and mucocutaneous oral pigmentation [43] are summarized in Tables 2.8 (see section on Gardner's Syndrome) and 2.9, respectively.

Treatment Recommendations

There is no medically indicated requirement to remove any mucocutaneous pigmentation although the appearance may be cosmetically unappealing and, thus, has a psychosocial impact on the patient [15]. Camouflage makeup can be used to conservatively cover up any hyperpigmentation. Various modalities have been used to remove such pigmentation; however, there is no definitive treatment recommendation to be made.

Approaches utilized include filtered intense pulse light, Q-switch ruby laser, and CO_2-based lasers [46].

Surveillance is the key to managing the intestinal polyps. A recent review paper [46] acknowledges that there is no consensus as to how and when this is undertaken. The role of surveillance is to detect large polyps that may predispose to obstruction/intussusception or bleeding and also to detect any cancerous changes as early as possible [46]. The authors conclude that a baseline colonoscopy and upper gastrointestinal endoscopy are indicated at age 8 years and video capsule endoscopy should be performed every 3 years, if polyps are found at the initial examination. Polypectomy of enlarging polyps is the surgical intervention of choice.

Malabsorption Conditions

Malabsorption is a term that encompasses various processes with many causes whereby nutrients are not fully absorbed from the gastrointestinal tract. Malabsorption can arise from maldigestion, mucosal or mural problems, or microbial causes [47]. A consequence of malabsorption is malnutrition. Hematinic (ferritin, folate, and vitamin B_{12}) deficiencies caused by malabsorption can lead to oral signs and symptoms.

The most common causes of hematinic malabsorption that can present with oral manifestations include Crohn's disease, celiac disease, and pernicious anemia.

The different causes of malabsorption that can contribute to each of the aforementioned hematinic deficiencies are outlined in Table 2.10 [47–49].

The epidemiology and etiopathogenesis of Crohn's disease and celiac disease have been elaborated on earlier in this chapter. To discuss all of the other less common causes mentioned in Table 2.10 in detail would be beyond the scope of this chapter. However, a brief description of pernicious anemia follows.

Pernicious anemia is an autoimmune macrocytic anemia that is caused by vitamin B_{12} (cobalamin) deficiency. Intrinsic factor, which is produced by gastric parietal cells, is required to absorb vitamin B_{12}. Autoantibodies act against both gastric parietal cells and intrinsic factor resulting in a deficiency of B_{12} [48, 50]. Pernicious anemia is associated with the development of gastric adenocarcinoma and atrophic body gastritis [50].

Clinical Manifestations

General signs of malabsorption include unintentional weight loss or failure to thrive in

Table 2.10 Malabsorptive causes of hematinic deficiencies

B_{12}	Atrophic gastritis
	Blind loop syndrome
	Celiac disease
	Crohn's disease
	Gastrectomy – partial/total
	Ileal resection/disease
	Long-term use of acid-reducing drugs
	Parasitic/bacterial infections of the small intestine
	Bacterial overgrowth
	Fish tapeworm (diphyllobothriasis)
	Giardiasis
	Pernicious anemia
	Tropical sprue
	Zollinger-Ellison syndrome
Ferritin	Celiac disease
	Crohn's disease
Folate	Celiac disease
	Tropical sprue

children. The main clinical manifestations of malabsorption with respect to hematinics are those of anemia such as fatigue, lethargy, pallor, and breathlessness.

Oral Signs and Symptoms

Hematinic deficiencies (ferritin, folate, and vitamin B_{12}) are implicated in the development of recurrent oral ulceration (aphthous ulcers), a susceptibility to developing infection (angular cheilitis), a burning sensation of the oral mucosal tissues (stomatodynia), and the development of atrophic glossitis (beefy red tongue), which can be painful [15].

Differential Diagnosis

Please see Table 2.6 for factors predisposing to the formation of aphthous-like ulcers. Please see Table 2.11 for the differential diagnosis of an oral burning sensation.

Treatment Recommendations

Management/treatment depends primarily on addressing the underlying cause. It may also be necessary to replace deficient nutrients. Treatment for oral ulcers and angular cheilitis is outlined in the section entitled Crohn's disease and orofacial granulomatosis.

Table 2.11 Differential diagnosis for an oral burning sensation

Local causes	Allergy/contact sensitivity
	Dry mouth
	Infection (fungal/viral)
	Mucosal lesions (e.g., geographic tongue, oral lichen planus)
	Pain conditions (e.g., postherpetic neuralgia)
	Trauma (friction from grinding/clenching teeth/loose dentures)
Systemic causes	Endocrine (diabetes/hypothyroidism)
	Hematinic deficiency
	HIV disease
	Medication side effects
	Sjögren's syndrome (dry mouth)

Gastroesophageal Reflux Disease

Gastroesophageal reflux disease (GERD) is a chronic disease and occurs when there is involuntary projection of gastric acid from the stomach upwards through the esophagus. The acid can be regurgitated into the oral cavity. There are many reasons as to why this occurs, but it is more commonly seen in obesity, pregnancy, patients with a hiatal hernia, smokers, and a high-fat diet.

Epidemiology

It is estimated that seven million people in the United States have some symptoms of GERD and that 50% of those diagnosed are between the ages of 45 and 64 [51].

Etiopathogenesis

Problems with the lower esophageal sphincter such as transient relaxation or hypotonia can result in GERD. Other etiological factors include changes to the gastroesophageal anti-reflux barrier, which may occur with a slipping hiatal hernia and inadequate esophageal peristalsis [52].

Clinical Manifestations

The main clinical manifestations of GERD include dyspepsia (indigestion), heartburn, odynophagia, regurgitation of acid/foodstuffs into the pharynx/oral cavity, and a dry cough particularly at nighttime when lying flat. Complications of long-standing acid reflux into the esophagus include metaplastic changes as seen in Barrett's esophagus, which is a potentially malignant condition and the formation of strictures.

Oral Signs and Symptoms

Acid reflux into the oral cavity can lead to erosion of the dentition [53], halitosis, and a burning sensation of the oral soft tissues through direct contact [54]. Dental erosion, which is one of the types of non-carious loss of tooth structure along with attrition and abrasion, can affect posterior teeth and the palatal surface of anterior teeth [53]. This can lead to an irreversible loss of tooth substance and increased sensitivity especially pain with consuming cold substances. The enamel can become smooth and shiny, and with significant erosion, the yellow appearance of the underlying dentin can be visualized [15].

Differential Diagnosis

The differential diagnosis for an oral burning sensation and the causes of dental erosion are outlined in Tables 2.11 and 2.12, respectively.

Treatment Recommendations

Avoiding precipitants such as alcohol or specific foodstuffs (e.g., spicy foods) should be advised.

Medical management entails the use of drugs that inhibit gastric acid secretion. Proton pump inhibitors are the most potent and effective. Histamine 2 receptor antagonists and antacids are alternatives but much less effective [55, 56]. A formal gastroenterology consultation may also need to be sought.

The surgical procedure of choice, if medical intervention fails, would be a fundoplication.

Referral for a dental consultation should be considered if there is evidence of significant dental erosion in order to facilitate restorative treatment.

Table 2.12 Differential diagnosis for causes of dental erosion

Alcoholism	Chronic vomiting
	Consuming low pH alcoholic drinks
Eating disorders	Anorexia nervosa
	Bulimia
Dietary erosion	Acidic foods (e.g., vinegars)
	Low pH carbonated drinks
	Fruit juices

References

1. Inflammatory Bowel Disease. Centers for Disease Control and Prevention. (CDC); 2014. http://www.cdc.gov/ibd/ Accessed 02 Oct 2014.
2. The Facts about Inflammatory Bowel Diseases. Crohn's and Colitis Foundation of America; 2011. http://www.ccfa.org/assets/pdfs/ibdfactbook.pdf. Accessed 02 Oct 2014.
3. Sanderson J, Nunes C, Escudier M, Barnard K, Shirlaw P, Odell E, et al. Oro-facial granulomatosis: Crohn's disease or a new inflammatory bowel disease? Inflamm Bowel Dis. 2005;11(9):84–846.
4. Campbell H, Escudier M, Patel P, Nunes C, Elliott TR, Barnard K, et al. Distinguishing orofacial granulomatosis from Crohn's disease: two separate disease entities? Inflamm Bowel Dis. 2011;17(10):2109–15.
5. Zbar AP, Ben-Horin S, Beer-Gabel M, Eliakim R. Oral Crohn's disease: is it a separable disease from orofacial granulomatosis? A review. J Crohns Colitis. 2012;6:135–42.
6. Lazzerini M, Bramuzzo M, Ventura A. Association between orofacial granulomatosis and Crohn's disease in children: systematic review. World J Gastroenterol. 2014;20(23):7497–504.
7. Wiesenfeld D, Ferguson MM, Mitchell DN, MacDonald DG, Scully C, Cochran K, et al. Oro-facial granulomatosis – a clinical and pathological analysis. Q J Med. 1985;54(213):101–13.
8. Tilakaratne WM, Freysdottir FF. Orofacial granulomatosis: review on aetiology and pathogenesis. J Oral Pathol Med. 2008;37:191–5.
9. Grave B, McCullough M, Wiesenfeld D. Orofacial granulomatosis – a 20-year review. Oral Dis. 2009;15:46–51.
10. Patel P, Brostoff J, Campbell H, Goel RM, Taylor K, Ray S, et al. Clinical evidence for allergy in orofacial granulomatosis and inflammatory bowel disease. Clin Transl Allergy. 2013;3(1):26.
11. White A, Nunes C, Escudier M, Lomer MCE, Barnard K, Shirlaw P, et al. Improvement in orofacial granulomatosis on a cinnamon- and benzoate-free diet. Inflamm Bowel Dis. 2006;12(6):508–14.
12. Al Johani K, Moles DR, Hodgson T, Porter SR, Fedele S. Onset and progression of clinical manifestations of orofacial granulomatosis. Oral Dis. 2009;15:214–9.
13. McCartan BE, Healy CM, McCreary CE, Flint SR, Rogers S, Toner ME. Characteristics of patients with orofacial granulomatosis. Oral Dis. 2011;17(7):696–704.
14. Lankarani KB, Sivandzadeh GR, Hassanpour S. Oral manifestation in inflammatory bowel disease: a review. World J Gastroenterol. 2013;19(46):8571–9.
15. Daley TD, Armstrong JE. Oral manifestations of gastrointestinal diseases. Can J Gastroenterol. 2007;21(4):241–4.
16. Elliott T, Campbell H, Escudier M, Poate T, Nunes C, Lomer M, Mentzer A, et al. Experience with

anti-TNF-α therapy for orofacial granulomatosis. J Oral Pathol Med. 2011;40:14–9.
17. Hegarty A, Hodgson T, Porter S. Thalidomide for the treatment of recalcitrant oral Crohn's disease and orofacial granulomatosis. Oral Surg Oral Med Oral Pathol Oral Radiol Endod. 2003;95(5):576–85.
18. Campbell HE, Escudier MP, Patel P, Challacombe SJ, Sanderson JD, Lomer MCE. Review article: cinnamon- and benzoate-free diet as a primary treatment for orofacial granulomatosis. Aliment Pharmacol Ther. 2011;34:687–701.
19. Campbell HE, Escudier MP, Milligan P, Challacombe SJ, Sanderson JD, Lomer MC. Development pf a low phenolic acid diet for the management of orofacial granulomatosis. J Hum Nutr Diet. 2013;26(6):527–37.
20. Langan RC, Gotsch PB, Krafczyk MA, Skillinge DD. Ulcerative colitis: diagnosis and treatment. Am Fam Physician. 2007;76(9):1323–30.
21. Elahi M, Telkabadi M, Samadi V, Vakili H. Association of oral manifestations with ulcerative colitis. Gastroenterol Hepatol Bed Bench. 2012;5(3):155–60.
22. Hegarty AM, Barrett AW, Scully C. Pyostomatitis vegetans. Clin Exp Dermatol. 2004;29(1):1–7.
23. Konstantopoulou M, O'Dwyer EM, Steele JC, Field EA, Lewis MAO, Macfarlane AW. Pyodermatitis-pyostomatitis vegetans complicated by methicillin-resistant *Staphylococcus aureus* infection. Clin Exp Dermatol. 2005;30(6):666–8.
24. Femiano F, Lanza A, Buonaiuto C, Perillo L, Dell'Ermo A, Cirillo N. Pyostomatitis vegetans: a review of the literature. Med Oral Patol Oral Cir Bucal. 2009;14(3):E114–7.
25. Nico MM, Hussein TP, Aoki V, Lourenco SV. Pyostomatitis vegetans and its relation to inflammatory bowel disease, pyoderma gangrenosum, pyodermatitis vegetans, and pemphigus. J Oral Pathol Med. 2012;41(8):584–8.
26. Werchniak AE, Storm CA, Plunkett RW, Beutner EH, Dinulos JG. Treatment of pyostomatitis vegetans with topical tacrolimus. J Am Acad Dermatol. 2005;52(4):722–3.
27. Rivera E, Assiri A, Guandalini S. Celiac disease. Oral Dis. 2013;19(7):635–41.
28. Guandalini S, Assiri A. Celiac disease. JAMA Pediatr. 2014;168(3):272–8.
29. Ferraz EG, Campos Ede J, Sarmento VA, Silva LR. Pediatr Dent. 2012;34(7):485–8.
30. Nenna R, Guandalini S, Popp A, Kurppa. Coeliac disease. Autoimmune Dis. 2014;2014:623784.
31. Rashid M, Zarkadas M, Anca A, Limeback H. Oral manifestations of celiac disease: a clinical guide for dentists. J Can Dent Assoc. 2011;77:b39.
32. Fasano A, Berti I, Gerarduzzi T, et al. Prevalence of celiac disease in at-risk and not-at-risk groups in the United States. Arch Intern Med. 2003;163(3):268–92.
33. Rubio-Tapia A, Ludvigsson JF, Brantner TL, Murray JA, Everhart JE. The prevalence of celiac disease in the United States. Am J Gastroenterol. 2012;107(10):1538–44.
34. Costacurta M, Maturo P, Bartolino M, Docimo R. Oral manifestations of coeliac disease. A clinical-statistic study. Oral Implantol (Rome). 2010;3(1):12–9.
35. Elli L, Pigatto PD, Guzzi G, Bardella MT. New dental enamel defects in coeliac disease. Clin Exp Dermatol. 2011;36(3):309–10.
36. Jurge S, Kuffer R, Scully C, Porter SR. Mucosal disease series. Number VI. Recurrent aphthous stomatitis. Oral Dis. 2006;12(1):1–21.
37. Chavan M, Jain H, Diwan N, Khedkar S, Shete A, Durkar S. Recurrent aphthous stomatitis: a review. J Oral Pathol Med. 2012;41(8):577–83.
38. Chimenos-Küstner E, Pascual M, Blanco I, Finestres F. Hereditary familial polyposis and Gardner's syndrome: contribution of the odonto-stomatology examination in its diagnosis and a case description. Med Oral Patol Oral Cir Bucal. 2005;10(5):402–9.
39. Smud D, Augustin G, Kekez T, Kinda E, Majerovic M, Jelincic Z. Gardner's syndrome: genetic testing and colonoscopy are indicated in adolescents and young adults with cranial osteomas: a case report. World J Gastroenterol. 2007;13(28):3900–3.
40. Cankaya AB, Erdem MA, Isler SC, Cifter M, Olgac V, Kasapoglu C, et al. Oral and maxillofacial considerations in Gardner's syndrome. Int J Med Sci. 2012;9(2):137–41.
41. Cristofaro MG, Giudice A, Amantea M, Riccelli U, Giudice M. Gardner's syndrome: a clinical and genetic study of a family. Oral Surg Oral Med Oral Pathol Oral Radiol. 2013;115(3):e1–6.
42. Woo VL, Abdelsayed R. Oral manifestations of internal malignancy and paraneoplastic syndromes. Dent Clin N Am. 2008;52(1):203–30.
43. Higham P, Alawi F, Stoopler ET. Medical management update: Peutz Jeghers syndrome. Oral Surg Oral Med Oral Pathol Oral Radiol Endod. 2010;109(1):5–11.
44. Riegert-Johnson D, Gleeson FC, Westra W, Hefferon T, Wong Kee Song LM, Spurck L, et al. In: Riegert-Johnson DL, Boardman LA, Hefferon T, Roberts M, editors. Cancer syndromes [internet]. Bethesda: National Center for Biotechnology Information (US); 2009.. 2008 Jul 18 [updated 2008 Aug 09]. http://www.ncbi.nlm.nih.gov/books/NBK1826/ Accessed 19 Sept 2014.
45. Omundsen M, Lam FF. The other colonic polyposis syndromes. ANZ J Surg. 2012;82:675–81.
46. Beggs AD, Latchford AR, Vasen HFA, Moslein G, Alonso A, Aretz S, et al. Peutz-Jeghers syndrome: a systematic review and recommendations for management. Gut. 2010;59:975–86.
47. Owens SR, Greenson JK. The pathology of malabsorption: current concepts. Histopathology. 2007;50(1):64–82.
48. Bizzaro N, Antico A. Diagnosis and classification of pernicious anemia. Autoimmun Rev. 2014;13(4–5):565–8.

49. Hunt A, Harrington D, Robinson S. Vitamin B12 deficiency. BMJ. 2014;349:g5226. https://doi.org/10.1136/bmj.g5226.
50. Lahner E, Annibale B. Pernicious anemia: new insights from a gastroenterological point of view. World J Gastroenterol. 2009;15(41):5121–8.
51. Acid Reflux (GERD) Statistics and Facts. Healthline Networks Inc; 2012. http://www.healthline.com/health/gerd/statistics. Accessed 11 Nov 2014.
52. Henry MA. Diagnosis and management of gastroesophageal reflux disease. Arq Bras Cir Dig. 2014;27(3):210–5.
53. Pace F, Pallotta S, Tonini M, Vakil N, Bianchi Porro G. Systematic review: gastro-oesophageal reflux disease and dental lesions. Aliment Pharmacol Ther. 2008;27:1179–86.
54. Liberali SAC. Oral impact of gastro-oesophageal reflux disease: a case report. Aust Dent J. 2008;53:176–9.
55. NICE guidelines (CG184). Dyspepsia and gastro-oesophageal reflux disease. Investigation and management of dyspepsia, symptoms suggestive of gastro-oesophageal disease, or both. www.nice.org.uk/guidance/cg184. Accessed 26 Oct 2014.
56. Roman S, Kahrilas PJ. The diagnosis and management of hiatus hernia. BMJ. 2014;349:g6154.

Oral Signs of Hematologic Disease

3

Diana V. Messadi and Ginat W. Mirowski

Introduction

Oral manifestations of blood dyscrasias are variable and sometimes resemble other local or systemic conditions. The mucous membranes, periodontal tissues, salivary glands, and perioral skin may be impacted. The oral manifestations include hemorrhage, infections, ulcerations, and cellular infiltration of tissues. This chapter will cover the common oral manifestations of hematologic conditions starting with disorders of the white blood cells including leukemias, lymphomas, cyclic hematopoiesis (cyclic neutropenia), plasma cell dyscrasias, and Langerhans cell disorders. A discussion of the impact of red blood cell disorders including anemias and less common red cell dyscrasias (sickle cell disease and hemochromatosis as well as thrombocytopenia will follow [1]).

Leukemia

Etiopathogenesis

Leukemia is a malignancy affecting the white blood cells of the bone marrow. This neoplastic process results in a marked increase in circulating immature or abnormal white blood cells, leading to suppression of normal hematopoiesis, causing secondary anemias, thrombocytopenia, and a deficiency of normal functioning leukocytes [2].

The etiology of leukemia, in most cases, is unknown, but exposure to large doses of ionizing radiation, certain chemicals (benzene), infections (Epstein-Barr virus and human lymphotropic virus), and genetic disorders (Down, Klinefelter's, and Fanconi' s syndromes) have an increased risk of developing leukemia [3].

Leukemia is classified either by its clinical course (acute or chronic) or according to the progenitor cell lineage (lymphoid or myeloid). Acute leukemias are divided into two major groups: acute lymphocytic leukemia (ALL) and acute myelogenous leukemia (AML). ALL commonly affects children, while AML is present more frequently in adults. The two major types of chronic leukemias are chronic myelocytic leukemia (CML) and chronic lymphocytic leukemia (CLL), which predominantly affects adults [4].

D. V. Messadi (✉)
Section of Oral Medicine and Orofacial Pain, Division of Oral Biology and Medicine, UCLA School of Dentistry, Los Angeles, CA, USA
e-mail: dmessadi@dentistry.ucla.edu

G. W. Mirowski
Department of Oral Pathology Medicine, Radiology, Indiana University School of Dentistry, Indianapolis, IN, USA

Department of Dermatology, Indiana University School of Medicine, Indianapolis, IN, USA

N. Fazel (ed.), *Oral Signs of Systemic Disease*, https://doi.org/10.1007/978-3-030-10863-2_3

Clinical Manifestations

Fatigue, pallor, bleeding, and easy bruising are common. Impaired leucocyte function may result in lymphadenopathy, recurrent infection, and bone and abdominal pain. Infiltration of leukemic cells into the skin, leukemia cutis, presents as firm and rubbery, papules, plaques, and nodules and may precede systemic leukemia. Ulcers and blisters occur less commonly. Myelogenous leukemias, chloromas or granulocytic sarcomas may present as dermal nodules with a green hue [5].

Oral Signs and Symptoms

Oral manifestations are more prevalent in acute (versus chronic) and myeloid (versus lymphoid) leukemias. Findings include gingival hypertrophy, petechiae, ecchymosis, ulcers, and hemorrhage especially spontaneous gingival bleeding. Viral, fungal, and bacterial oral infections are a common consequence of immunosuppression [6]. The direct effect of chemotherapeutic drugs on the oral mucosa may result in ulcers that must be differentiated from herpes simplex virus (HSV) or cytomegalovirus (CMV) [7]. Mental nerve neuropathy, "numb chin syndrome," is a rare presenting complaint [8].

Gingival hyperplasia is most commonly associated with AML and acute promyelocytic leukemia. The gingiva appears markedly edematous, erythematous, and friable (Fig. 3.1). Gingival hyperplasia improves with chemotherapy [9].

Complications of hematopoietic stem cell transplantation (HSCT) include lichenoid or keratotic papules and plaques, desquamative gingivitis, atrophy, and ulcerations [10].

Differential Diagnosis

A biopsy of the hypertrophic gingival tissues will confirm the diagnosis of leukemic infiltrates. The clinical differential of acquired medication-induced gingival hyperplasia (anticonvulsants, calcium channel blockers, and immunosuppressants) must be ruled out by a thorough medication history. Furthermore, cultures and cytologic smears with fluorescent antibody smears should be obtained in order to differentiate oral ulcers of viral etiology in patients receiving immunosuppressive chemotherapy [10].

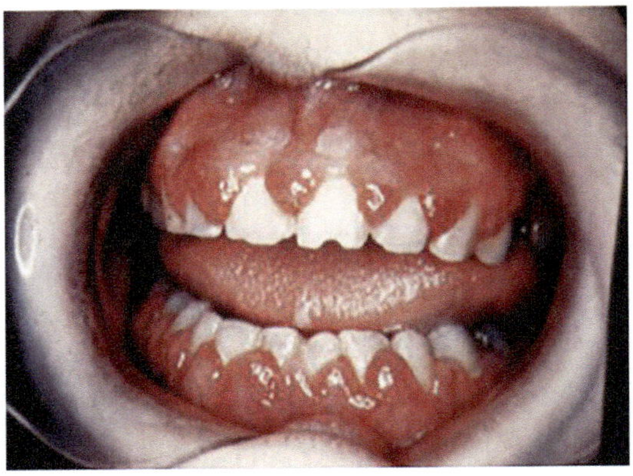

Fig. 3.1 Diffuse gingival hyperplasia in a 53-year-old male with acute myelogenous leukemia (AML). (Courtesy of Indiana University School of Dentistry Teaching Collection)

Treatment Recommendations

In general, treatment of the underlying disease with chemotherapy and/or HSCT will improve the oral manifestations of leukemia. Secondary infections must be treated appropriately. Supportive care with kaolin and pectin plus diphenhydramine oral rinses can be used to reduce mucosal pain.

Lymphomas

Etiopathogenesis

Lymphomas are solid tumor malignancies involving B and T lymphocytes and monocytes. These tumors develop most commonly in the lymph nodes and less frequently in extra-nodal sites. The etiology is unknown, but identified risk factors include immunodeficiency states, viral infections, and chemical exposures [11].

One classification scheme differentiates Hodgkin lymphoma (HL) from non-Hodgkin lymphoma (NHL) [12]. HL predominantly affects adolescents and young adults with an additional prevalence peak in middle age. HL used to be a uniformly fatal disease, but modern modes of diagnosis and treatment have given a newly diagnosed patient a more than 90% chance of cure. NHL typically presents in middle-aged to older individuals. Both HL and NHL occur more commonly in men [13].

Clinical Manifestations

Clinical manifestations of lymphomas are diverse but frequently include painless lymphadenopathy, hepatosplenomegaly, and secondary infections. The symptoms of fever, night sweats, and weight loss (B-cell lymphoma symptoms) as well as pruritus suggest advanced disease and portend a poor prognosis. The diagnosis is based on histologic (Fig. 3.2) and immohistochemical findings in diseased tissues [11].

Oral Signs and Symptoms

Oral signs and symptoms are far more likely to occur in NHL, particularly Burkitt's lymphoma and AIDS-associated lymphoma [14, 15]. In NHL, oral involvement preferentially affects the lymphoid tissues of Waldeyer's ring as well as the vestibule and gingivae. Painless, soft masses, with or without traumatic ulceration, may also involve the palate and buccal mucosa. These lesions have been described as slow-growing, painless, bluish soft masses; palatal lesions have been confused with minor salivary gland tumors (Fig. 3.3). Intraosseous lesions maybe associated with loose teeth and paresthesia of the face. Major salivary gland enlargement may also be a presenting sign of NHL [16].

AIDS-associated lymphoma is typically a non-Hodgkin B-cell lymphoma that presents as a

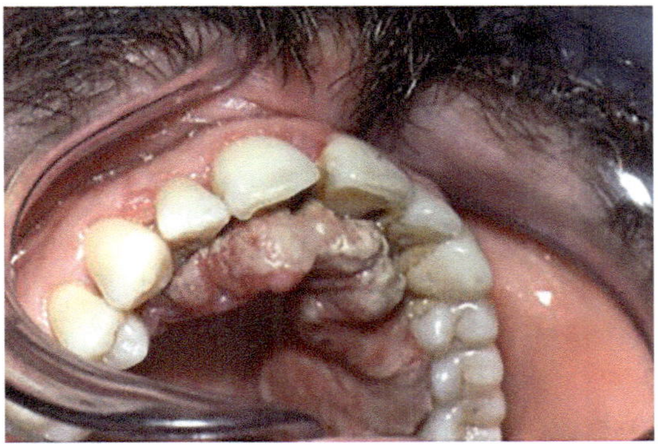

Fig. 3.3 HIV positive man presenting with a bleeding palatal mass. Histology confirmed a B-cell lymphoma (Courtesy of Dr. Mirowski's private collection)

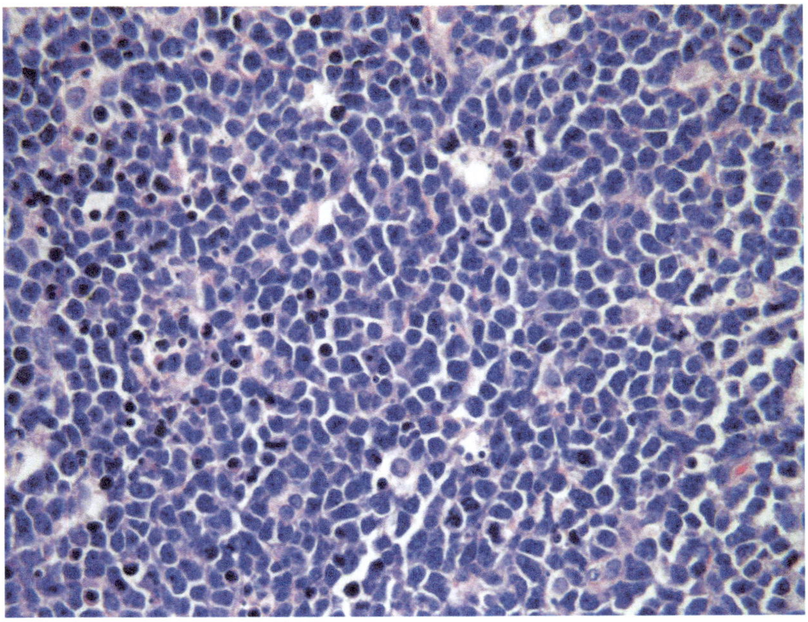

Fig. 3.2 High-power micrograph (400x) of uniform neoplastic cells of lymphocytic series with minimal cytoplasm in B cell lymphoma. (Courtesy of Dr. YiLing Lin UCLA School of Dentistry)

papule, nodule, or tumor that may be ulcerated; this entity typically affects Waldeyer's ring or the gingivae. AIDS-associated lymphoma typically manifests with CD4 count <50/IJI and portends a poor prognosis [15].

Burkitt's lymphoma is an aggressive pediatric lymphoma that is commonly associated with oral manifestations. The Epstein-Barr virus has been implicated in its pathogenesis. Burkitt's lymphoma presents as a rapidly expanding mass causing bone and adjacent soft tissue destruction resulting in painful loosening of the teeth; it more commonly affects the maxilla than the mandible [14].

Oral lesions have also been described in patients with cutaneous T-cell lymphoma (mycosis fungoides). These lesions are described as indurated plaques with a red or white surface or ulcerated tumors. The most common site of involvement is the tongue and usually follows skin lesions.

Differential Diagnosis

When lymphoma is included in the differential diagnosis of an oral lesion, a biopsy specimen should be taken from the center of the lesion and special stains and markers should be applied to classify the NHL type [17].

Biopsy and immunohistopathology markers are the hallmark for lymphoma classification and diagnosis. The most recent WHO classification, published in 2008, stresses the importance of integrating the morphological, immunophenotypic, molecular, cytogenetic, and clinical findings in order to accurately diagnose lymphomas [12].

Treatment Recommendations

Radiation and chemotherapy are the most successful modes of treatment for all lymphomas. Localized NHL is highly radiosensitive. Intensive combinations of chemotherapeutic drugs are the treatment of choice for intermediate and high-grade NHL. The specific regimen used depends on the result of clinical staging and classification [11, 18].

Cyclic Neutropenia (Cyclic Hematopoiesis)

Etiopathogenesis

Neutrophils, also known as polymorphonuclear leukocytes (PMNs), are part of the innate immune system against bacterial pathogens, accounting for 50–70% of the circulating white blood cell population. Neutrophil activation releases myeloperoxidase, a heme protein that produces cytotoxic oxidants and impacts nitric oxide-dependent signaling within the vascular endothelium. Cyclic neutropenia, a rare disorder with variable expression, is characterized by periodic failure of hematopoietic progenitor cells resulting in dramatic oscillations in neutrophil, monocyte, eosinophil, platelet, and reticulocyte counts [19].

Both the autosomal dominant (AD) form of the disease and sporadic cases are caused by a mutation in the gene for neutrophil elastase (*ELA2*, now called ELANE, on chromosome 19p13.3) [20, 21]. These mutations disrupt granulopoiesis and induce apoptosis. Similar mutations maybe found in severe congenital neutropenia (SCN). Unlike SCN, cyclic neutropenia is not associated with malignant transformation to AML [22].

Clinical Manifestation

Cyclic neutropenia commonly affects infants and children, although adult onset may also occur. Generally, disease manifestations recede with age. Clinical presentation can vary in severity and tends to occur when the neutrophil count drops below 500 cells/μL. Patients with this disease typically experience transient fever, oral ulcerations, and recurrent skin infections and pharyngitis in conjunction with the neutropenia that occurs at intervals of 15–35 days (most commonly 21 days) [23]. The hallmark of the clinical presentation is the very predictable recurrence of symptoms.

Oral Signs and Symptoms

Oral lesions are common in cyclic neutropenia and may be the major clinical manifestation of the

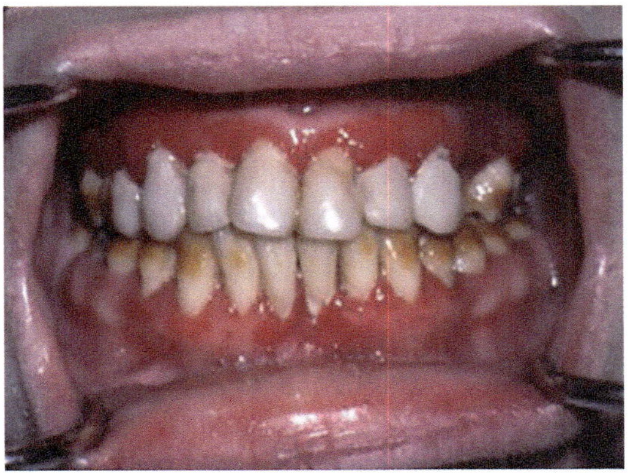

Fig. 3.4 Cyclic neutropenia presenting with recurrent gingival erosions. (Courtesy of Dr. Jack Schaaf, Indiana University School of Dentistry)

disease. The oral manifestations include recurrent aphthous stomatitis (RAS), recurrent gingivitis, and periodontitis (Fig. 3.4). RAS arises during the nadir and resolves spontaneously as the neutrophil count improves. The periodontal manifestations range from marginal gingivitis to rapidly advancing periodontal bone loss caused by bacterial infection of the supporting dental structures. The finding of RAS with or without periodontal disease, particularly in a child, should raise the suspicion of cyclic neutropenia [24].

Differential Diagnosis

Diagnostic evaluation entails serial measurement of circulating neutrophils. The diagnosis may be established by demonstrating at least 2 cycles of neutropenia [23]. Cyclic episodes of fever due to cyclic neutropenia must be differentiated from the periodic fever syndromes (Familial Mediterranean Fever, TNF receptor-1-associated periodic syndrome, hyper-IgD syndrome) disorders that are not associated with neutropenia.

Treatment Recommendations

The regular administration of recombinant granulocyte colony-stimulating factor (G-CSF) diminishes the frequency and severity of symptoms, reduces gingival and dental complications, and reduces the risk of sepsis during periods of severe neutropenia. Bone density should be monitored for development of osteoporosis, a well-known side effect during prolonged treatment with G-CSF [25].

Plasma Cell Dyscrasias

Plasma cell dyscrasias are a diverse group of diseases characterized by the proliferation of a single clone of cells producing a monoclonal immunoglobulin or immunoglobulin fragment. This group includes multiple myeloma, amyloidosis, Waldenström macroglobulinemia, heavy chain disease, and benign monoclonal gammopathy [1]. Histologically, the malignant cells usually display a plasma cell morphology, but rarely lymphocytic or lymphoplasmacytic features are noted.

Multiple Myeloma

Etiopathogenesis

Multiple myeloma (MM) is a malignant plasma cell dyscrasia that results in the overproduction of immunoglobulin light chains. It is a relatively uncommon malignancy of plasma cells that appears to have a multicentric origin in bone. MM makes up 1% of all malignancies, 10–15% of hematologic malignancies, and nearly 50% of all malignancies (excluding metastatic disease) involving bone. The abnormal plasma cells are monoclonal and probably arise from a single malignant precursor cell. These monoclonal cells produce the same immunoglobulin that is nonfunctional and tends to accumulate as amyloid. MM typically presents in middle-aged and older adults with a gender predilection in men and a higher prevalence in African-Americans [26]. Amyloidosis confers a poorer prognosis in patients with MM [27].

Clinical Manifestations

The most common presenting symptom in MM is bone pain caused by osteolytic lesions or pathologic fractures due to bone destruction. Anemia and petechial hemorrhages may also be seen [28]. Hemorrhage and infection are major concerns in patients with MM. Bleeding may result from several causes, including thrombocytopenia, abnormal platelet function, or abnormal coagulation [29].

Patients may also present with hypercalcemia, proteinuria, renal failure, or thrombocytopenia. The radiographic finding of multiple "punched-out" well-defined or ragged radiolucencies is highly suggestive of advanced MM (Fig. 3.5). These may be especially evident on skull films. Renal failure may be the presenting sign as a result of tumor produced immunoglobulin accumulation in the kidneys. Light chains (Bence Jones protein) may be found in the urine in 30–50% of patients [30].

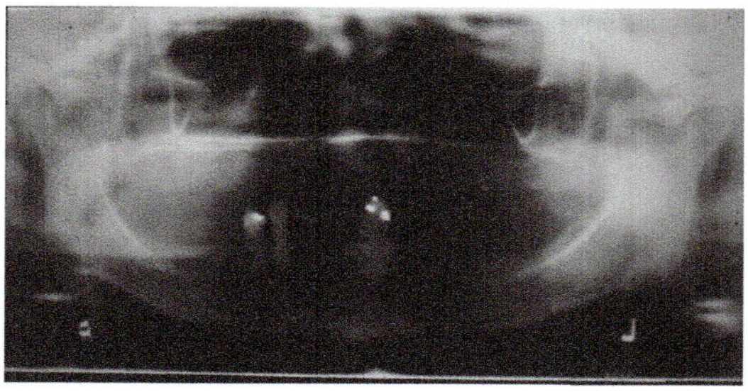

Fig. 3.5 Panoramic radiograph in a patient with multiple myeloma, illustrating typical punch out ragged radiolucencies. (Courtesy of Dr. Fariba Younai UCLA, School of Dentistry)

Oral Signs and Symptoms

A variety of oral manifestations in MM have been described. Up to 30% of patients will have involvement of the mandible with associated swelling, pain, paresthesias, and tooth loss. Additionally, gingival bleeding or oral petechiae may be seen, if bone marrow infiltration by malignant plasma cells causes thrombocytopenia. In rare instances, MM can produce extramedullary plasmacytomas. When located in the oral cavity, these lesions are most commonly found on the gingivae or hard palate and appear as dome-shaped masses that have a tendency to ulcerate.

Differential Diagnosis

The diagnosis of MM requires evidence of end-organ damage (lytic bone lesions, anemia, hypercalcemia, or renal insufficiency), bone marrow aspiration or biopsy to demonstrate plasma cell proliferation in the marrow, and the detection of monoclonal protein in the serum or urine. The presence of an "M spike" indicates massive overproduction of one abnormal immunoglobulin by the neoplastic plasma cells [31]. Monotonous sheets of crowded atypical plasma cells may be seen histologically (Fig. 3.6).

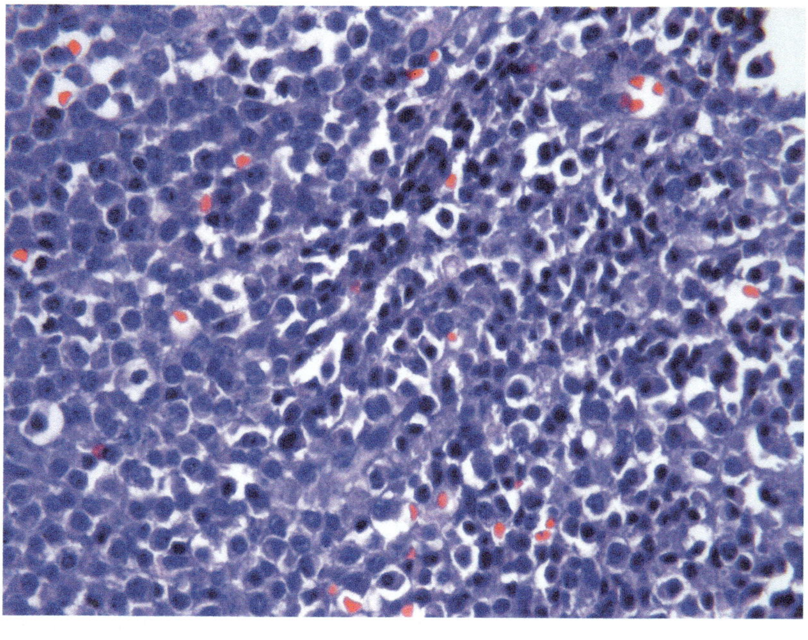

Fig. 3.6 High-power micrograph (400x) showing sheets of malignant plasma cells in a patient with multiple myeloma. (Courtesy of Dr. Yi-Ling Lin UCLA, School of Dentistry)

Treatment Recommendations

Treatment of MM consists of chemotherapy with prednisone and approximately 60% of patients will initially respond. Radiation therapy is useful for palliation only. Prognosis is poor but younger patients do better than older individuals. Median survival of 30–36 months after onset of symptoms can be expected. The survival rate remains at 10% after 5 years. The survival rate is only marginally improved with aggressive chemotherapy and bone marrow transplantation [26].

Amyloidosis

Etiopathogenesis

Amyloidosis is a heterogeneous group of conditions characterized by the deposition of an extracellular proteinaceous substance. Amyloidosis is classified according to the type of protein produced and whether the protein deposition is local or systemic [32].

Localized amyloidosis, affects a single tissue of the body impairing its function, while systemic amyloidosis can cause serious changes in virtually any organ of the body. Systemic amyloidosis are categorized as primary (AL), secondary (AA), or hereditary (ATTR). Amyloidosis may be a primary disorder, or it can be a secondary manifestation of neoplastic (multiple myeloma) or chronic inflammatory disorders (rheumatoid arthritis, tuberculosis) [33].

Clinical Manifestations

AL is the most common systemic amyloidosis. Due to AL's extensive range of organ and tissue involvement, the clinical manifestations are numerous. Some signs and symptoms include fatigue, weight loss, edema, renal failure, autonomic and peripheral neuropathy, and rapidly evolving congestive heart failure due to a restrictive cardiomyopathy [34].

Oral Signs and Symptoms

The oral cavity is most commonly involved in AL amyloidosis; however, localized amyloidosis may also produce oral lesions. Localized amyloidosis of the oral cavity is relatively rare. Patients may present with one or more soft, red, yellow, purple, or blue nodules involving the buccal mucosa, tongue, gingivae, or, less commonly, the hard palate [35].

The oral manifestations of AL amyloidosis include macroglossia, edema, submucosal hemorrhage, glossodynia, taste disturbance, and xerostomia (due to destruction of salivary glands by amyloid deposits). Macroglossia is found in 20% of patients making it the most widely documented oral finding. Macroglossia is not typically found in other systemic amyloidosis [35]. Macroglossia presents with enlargement (localized, nodular, or diffuse) and/or stiffening of the tongue (Fig. 3.7). Scalloping of the lateral tongue borders results from counter pressure exerted by the teeth as the tongue enlarges. On occasion, macroglossia can be severe enough to compromise the airway [36]. In some patients with AL amyloidosis, firm, yellowish nodules composed of amyloid may also occur on the gingivae, buccal mucosa, or hard palate.

Differential Diagnosis

The diagnosis of amyloidosis requires histologic examination of involved tissues. Amyloid

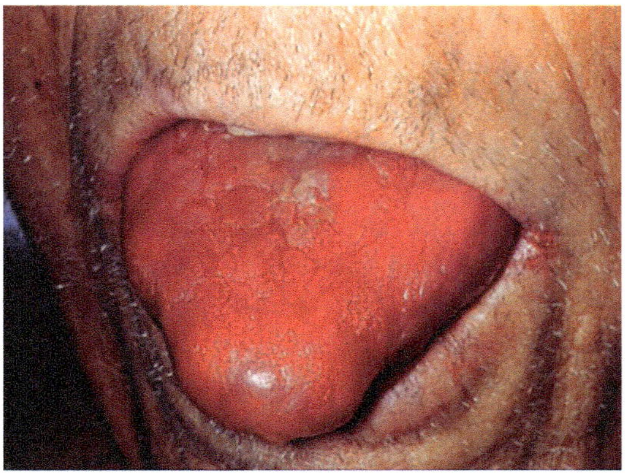

Fig. 3.7 A firm enlarged woody tongue in a patient with amyloidosis (Courtesy of Dr. Mirowski's Private collection)

deposits may be seen on H and E and are confirmed by Congo red, Thioflavin T, or crystal violet stains. Once histologic specimens are stained with Congo red, they are examined with polarized microscopy to demonstrate the characteristic apple green birefringence. Immunohistochemical stains may include kappa and lambda light chain, beta-amyloid A4 protein, transthyretin, and beta 2-microglobulin to demonstrate extracellular amyloid deposits. Immunofixation electrophoresis of serum or urine may also be used to detect and characterize circulating proteins [37].

Treatment Recommendations

No effective therapy is available for most forms of amyloidosis. Surgical debulking of the tongue is done with limited success [38]. Treatment with antibiotics and anti-inflammatory agents will aid in the control of secondary amyloidosis. Renal transplantation may stop the progress of hemodialysis-associated amyloidosis, but it will not reverse deposits in bones and joints.

Treatment of primary and multiple myeloma-associated amyloidosis with colchicine, prednisone, and melphalan may improve the prognosis in patients without renal or cardiac involvement.

Langerhans Cell Histiocytosis

Etiopathogenesis

Langerhans cell histiocytosis (LCH) formerly known as histiocytosis X is a rare condition of unknown etiology and pathogenesis characterized by destructive tissue infiltration by abnormal histiocytes mixed with lymphocytes and eosinophils. LCH was thought to be derived from the morphologically similar Langerhans cells, which are specialized dendritic cells found in the skin and mucosa. However, gene expression array data have shown that the skin Langerhans cell is not the cell of origin for LCH. Rather, it is a myeloid dendritic cell that expresses the same antigens (CD1a, CD207) as the skin Langerhans cell. Peripheral monocytes found in normal blood can differentiate into macrophages and interstitial dendritic cells that may travel through lymphatics to draining lymph nodes. There are probably two populations of circulating myeloid dendritic cells that can differentiate into committed dendritic cells. Expression array results support the notion that one of these could become the pathologic dendritic cell in LCH [39].

Clinical Manifestations

LCH has a broad spectrum of clinical manifestations depending on the site and extent of organ involvement. There are three forms of LCH, the diffuse form previously referred to as *Letterer-Siwe disease* and the localized variant previously referred to as *Hand-Schüller-Christian disease*, while the third form, *eosinophilic granuloma*, is the most common form. LCH is a rare disease that predominantly affects infants and children and rarely adults [40]. Diffuse LCH most commonly affects infants and is characterized by widespread involvement of the viscera, potentially leading to death. Skin lesions are common and include papules, plaques, vesicles, and hemorrhagic nodules, all of which may manifest in a pattern similar to that of seborrheic dermatitis [41]. The localized variant is a childhood disease that consists of the triad of diabetes insipidus, lytic bone lesions, and proptosis [42]. Eosinophilic granuloma presents in young adults. Radiolucent bone lesions can occur anywhere but are most common in flat bones [43]. Some patients have mild, localized pain due to isolated bone lesions, whereas others develop rapidly progressive systemic disease involving nearly every organ system. Definitive diagnosis of LCH requires histologic confirmation [44].

Oral Signs and Symptoms

LCH commonly affects bone, with 10–20% of patients having involvement of the maxilla or mandible, the symptoms of which can mimic an odontogenic infection or periodontal disease [45].

Oral manifestations include irregular ulcerations of the hard palate, which may be the primary manifestation of the disease [46]. Osteolytic lesions may cause edema and ulceration of the overlying mucosa. Lesions in alveolar bone can produce gingival inflammation, necrosis, and recession as well as increased tooth mobility and premature tooth loss. Within the radiographic lucency that results from osteolytic destruction, the teeth have a characteristic floating appearance [41, 46].

In rare cases, LCH may cause ulceration of the oral mucosa in the absence of underlying bone lesions. Oral ulcers tend to be painful with inflamed borders and are most commonly localized to the buccal mucosa, gingiva, hard palate, and floor of the mouth, along with a necrotizing gingivitis [42, 47]. Solitary oral lesions may be part of a multisystem disease, and oral/periodontal disease may also be an early sign of disease reactivation [48].

Differential Diagnosis

Biopsy is necessary to establish a diagnosis because the inflammation and ulcerations are clinically nonspecific. Histology reveals pale Langerhans cells with bi-lobed nuclei, which resemble coffee beans. Clusters of eosinophils also may be present. The diagnosis of LCH is confirmed by the characteristic morphology and the presence of CD1a or CD207 (Langerin) positive histiocytic cells [39, 44].

Evaluation of the patient with LCH should include whole-body radiographic skeletal survey or bone scintigraphy and serum studies to assess for diabetes insipidus and hypercalcemia [47].

Treatment Recommendations

The choice of therapy is generally made based upon the site of involvement and number of lesions aiming at minimizing toxicity. Treatment options include single-agent prednisone, or the combination of vinblastine and prednisone, curettage of bone lesions, and topical therapy for skin lesions [49, 50].

Red Blood Cell Disorders

Red blood cell disorders include anemias and red blood cell (RBC) dyscrasias (sickle cell disease and hemochromatosis as well as thrombocytopenia). Anemias are categorized by the size of RBC. In microcytic anemias, the RBCs are smaller than normal, while macrocytic anemia is associated with an increased size of RBC. Microcytic anemia can result from a lack of iron (due to deficiency, chronic diseases, or defects in heme synthesis (sideroblastic anemias) or defects in the production of hemoglobin protein (thalassemia).

Clinically, pallor, fatigue, dyspnea, tachycardia, glossitis, glossodynia, and stomatitis characterize all anemias regardless of the etiology. These findings may precede a fall in hemoglobin or change in mean corpuscular volume particularly when the anemia is due to deficiency of iron, folate, or vitamin B_{12}.

Platelet Disorders

Platelets are small, non-nucleated cells in the blood that play a critical role in hemostasis [51]. Fragmentation of megakaryocytes results in platelet formation. Thrombocytopenia is characterized by a reduction in platelet count (±2 standard deviations from normal, where normal is typically 150,000–450,000 platelets per microliter). Thrombocytopenia may occur due to autoimmune destruction (including connective tissue disease), splenic sequestration, bone marrow infiltration by tumor cells, and infection (infectious mononucleosis) or as an adverse drug reaction. Pseudothrombocytopenia is the result of in vitro platelet clumping and should be differentiated from true thrombocytopenia.

Epidemiology

Data regarding the incidence and prevalence of thrombocytopenia is variable depending upon whether the study is of acutely ill patients in the intensive care unit or in asymptomatic patients without evidence of systemic disease [52].

Etiopathogenesis

Impaired platelet production may result from bone marrow failure due to aplastic anemia, alcoholism, bone marrow infiltration by tumor cells, infections, myelodysplastic syndrome, and drug- or chemotherapy-induced thrombocytopenia. Increased destruction is seen in disseminated intravascular coagulation (DIC) and thrombotic angiopathy. Splenic sequestration can be seen in congestive splenomegaly due to portal hypertension, heparin-induced thrombocytopenia, or autoimmune destruction (including connective tissue disease). Other conditions associated with thrombocytopenia include burns, cardiopulmonary bypass, extracorporeal membrane oxygenation, HIV, hyperthyroidism, hypothermia, intra-aortic balloon pump, nutritional deficiencies, pregnancy, renal replacement therapy, sepsis/infection, systemic lupus erythematosus, or vasculitis [51, 53, 54].

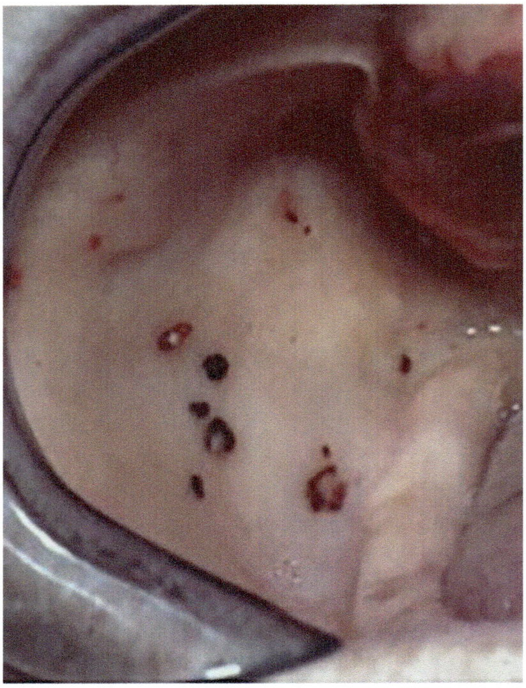

Fig. 3.8 Multiple petechiae on the buccal mucosa in a patient with thrombocytopenia, (Courtesy of Dr. Mirowski's Private collection)

Clinical Manifestations

Presentations consist of petechiae, purpura, and bleeding including epistaxis, hematuria, menorrhagia, gastrointestinal bleeding, and intracranial hemorrhage. Other findings include organomegaly or skeletal abnormalities. Neurologic defects and joint or extensive soft tissue bleeding suggest a coagulation defect as in DIC. Ischemic limbs or skin necrosis raises the specter of heparin-induced thrombocytopenia.

In addition to spontaneous bleeding that occurs when the platelets fall below 10,000–20,000 platelets per microliter, thrombocytopenia can complicate or prevent the effective treatment of a variety of condition such as chemotherapy or antiviral therapy for hepatitis C or surgery.

Oral Signs and Symptoms

Gingival bleeding, as a result of minor trauma such as brushing or flossing, may be the first sign of thrombocytopenia. Other early signs include petechiae and ecchymoses on the soft palate or buccal mucosa (Fig. 3.8). Purpura and mucocutaneous bleeding resulting in hemorrhagic bullae that appear deep red to black are associated with very low platelet counts [1].

Differential Diagnosis

The associated clinical findings may help to focus the differential: fever suggests infection, sepsis, or DIC; lymphadenopathy may be associated with infection, lymphoma, or other malignancy; thrombosis may be due to heparin, antiphospholipid antibodies, or paroxysmal nocturnal hemoglobinuria; neurologic findings may be associated with vitamin B_{12} or copper deficiency [51].

Treatment Recommendations

Effort should be made to maintain platelet levels greater than 50,000 platelets per microliter so as to limit bleeding. Specific treatment recommendations depend on the degree of thrombocytopenia and the procedure indicated. For dermatologic procedures and/or dental extractions, platelet transfusion and application of local measures (such as fibrinolytic mouth rinses or absorbable hemostat) during extraction are safe and effective to limit postoperative bleeding [55].

Thalassemias

Thalassemias are a group of inherited diseases that are characterized by genetic defects in hemoglobin production resulting in ineffective erythropoiesis and subsequent hemolysis.

Epidemiology

The thalassemias affect 4.83% of the world's population with a worldwide prevalence of alpha and beta thalassemia trait of 1.7% [56]. Males and females are equally affected. The epidemiology of specific diseases depends on the geographic area and the diseased population being studied. Most affected individuals are from Africa, the Mediterranean area, and Southeast Asia.

Etiopathogenesis

Hemoglobin is composed of two alpha globin and two beta globin protein molecules. The predominant hemoglobin in adults is hemoglobin A. Four types of alpha thalassemia and three forms of beta thalassemia have been described.

Clinical Manifestations

Clinical findings in the thalassemias are related to reduction in oxygen carrying capacity and resultant anemia. This may vary from asymptomatic or silent carriers in individuals with alpha thalassemia, fatigue in patients with mild anemia, and progressive symptoms such as reduced growth and delayed puberty, bone pain, brittleness, and increased fractures in patients who require bone marrow expansion in patients with beta thalassemia major. Children with severe anemia appear pale and listless, have a poor appetite, and exhibit slowed growth and delayed puberty, and their urine may be dark due to hemoglobinuria. Children may also be jaundiced. Bone problems in the face are common [57]. Hydrops fetalis results when there is loss of all four alpha globin genes. Severe anemia resulting in intrauterine demise is typical. Impaired growth and delayed development is common as is extramedullary hematopoiesis and bone deformities [58, 59]. Endocrinologic insufficiencies are due to both chronic anemia and from iron overload secondary to transfusion dependence. In secondary craniosynostosis, the premature sutural fusion is of unknown etiology.

Oral Signs and Symptoms

In addition to the pallor of the mucosa due to anemia and yellowing of the mucosa due to jaundice, the bones of the face and skull may show "hair on end" striations due to vertical trabeculation secondary to expansion of hematopoiesis. The diploic space is enlarged, while the outer plate is thinned [60]. Much less common is involvement of the facial bones resulting in frontal enlargement of the head, expansion of the maxillary bones, and malalignment of the dentition (hemolytic facies) [58].

Treatment Recommendations

Iron overload, in patients who are transfusion dependent (such as in thalassemia), must be avoided by the use of chelating agents.

Megaloblastic Anemia

Megaloblastic anemia is a consequence of defective DNA synthesis during erythropoiesis and most commonly results from vitamin B_{12} (cobalamin, cyanocobalamin) or folate deficiency.

Etiopathogenesis

Vitamin B_{12} is an essential water-soluble nutrient that is a naturally occurring cobalamin (contains cobalt). Fifty percent of vitamin B_{12} is present in food. Both gastric acid and pepsin help to free the tightly bound vitamin B_{12} from ingested proteins. Intrinsic factor (IF) helps bind vitamin B_{12} soon after leaving the acidic environment of the stomach, and the two are then absorbed in the small intestine. Medications that block acid secretions also hinder the release of protein-bound vitamin B_{12} and thus contribute to decreased absorption. Supplemental vitamin B_{12} is not protein-bound and thus not impacted by proton pump inhibitors that block the secretion of gastric acid [61]. Vitamin B_{12} deficiency is less common than folate deficiency but may be seen in the elderly, vegetarians, and patients with pernicious anemia (see below), HIV, or gastrointestinal disease. Folate is also a water-soluble B vitamin that is present in food but can be supplemented. Folic acid is composed of a p-aminobenzoic molecule linked to a pteridine ring and one molecule of glutamic acid. As a coenzyme, folate helps to transfer single carbons, which is essential in the metabolism of amino acids as well as DNA and RNA synthesis. Potential etiologies of folate deficiency include inadequate dietary intake, malabsorption, or increased folate consumption, which may occur during pregnancy and periods of rapid growth or as a result of chronic inflammation.

Clinical Manifestations

The clinical findings in both megaloblastic anemia and pernicious anemia are very similar. Fatigue, weakness, and difficulty breathing are typical. Patients may notice tingling or a burning sensation of the skin and numbness or weakness of the legs. Mood alteration, disorientation, memory loss, and decrease in cognition may be noted as well. Myelopathy results in uncontrolled spasms and lack of equilibrium. Urinary incontinence is common as well. In the developing fetus, vitamin B_{12} deficiency may result in neural tube defects.

Oral Signs and Symptoms

Megaloblastic anemia presents with symptoms of burning tongue and or lips associated with atrophic glossitis and cheilitis. Occasionally, RAS may be noted. Folate and vitamin B_{12} deficiencies have been implicated as contributing factors to RAS, and in some patients, aphthae will improve following folate and vitamin B_{12} repletion [1, 62–65].

Differential Diagnosis

The diagnosis of vitamin B_{12} deficiency can be distinguished from folate deficiency by direct measurement of serum vitamin B_{12} levels or the detection of elevated serum methylmalonic acid.

Treatment Recommendations

Most patients are treated with exogenous cobalamin or folate. Transfusion therapy is rarely required unless the patient has severe uncompensated or life threatening anemia.

Pernicious Anemia

Pernicious anemia (PA) is a complex clinical condition. Alterations in the IF-mediated vitamin B_{12} absorption due to loss of parietal cells, small intestine disorders, genetic mutations, and/or gastric surgery account for many cases of PA [61]. Autoantibodies targeting gastric parietal cells are found in 90% of cases, but this is of low specificity as anti-parietal cells may be seen in patients without megaloblastic anemia and in other autoimmune disorders. Antibodies that target IF are seen in 60% of patients with PA and are highly specific [66]. It is the IF that is necessary for absorption of the water-soluble essential nutrient vitamin B12.

Epidemiology

PA is seen in 2% of adults [61].

Etiopathogenesis

PA is a complex disorder that involves the blood, immune system, and the gastrointestinal tract. PA occurs in individuals who are unable to absorb vitamin B12 due to lack of IF [67].

Clinical Manifestations

In addition to the usual clinical manifestations of anemia such as fatigue, weakness, and difficulty breathing, neurologic complications may be seen in 90% of vitamin B12-deficient patients. The neuropsychiatric findings include ataxia, loss of vibratory sensation, dementia, or psychosis. Patients may notice tingling or burning feelings on the skin and numbness or weakness of the legs. Mood alteration, disorientation, memory loss, and decrease in cognition may be noted as well. Myelopathy results in uncontrolled spasms, lack of equilibrium, and urinary incontinence. In the developing fetus, vitamin B12 deficiency may result in neural tube defects.

Oral Signs and Symptoms

The classic oral finding in PA is the presence of a painful or burning, atrophic tongue or "bald" tongue [68, 69]. Loss of both the filiform and fungiform papillae results in atrophy of the oral mucosa exhibited by erythema and glossitis. Angular cheilitis may also occur in addition to alterations in taste sensation (dysgeusia) [69].

Differential Diagnosis

PA must be differentiated from other vitamin deficiencies associated with glossitis and an atrophic tongue. The diagnosis requires confirmation of an atrophic gastritis, megaloblastic anemia with hypersegmented neutrophils and reduced absolute IF.

Treatment Recommendations

Treatment options include parenteral administration of vitamin B_{12} and dietary supplementation.

Iron Deficiency Anemia

A diagnosis of iron deficiency anemia is suggested by the finding of microcytic, hypochromic anemia in conjunction with decreased serum iron (<60 μg/dl), decreased serum ferritin (<15 μg/dl), and elevated total iron-binding capacity (>400 μg/dl). Plummer-Vinson syndrome primarily affects middle-aged women and is characterized by iron deficiency anemia, glossitis, glossodynia, and esophageal strictures or webs. These patients have an increased risk of oral and pharyngeal carcinoma.

Epidemiology

Iron deficiency anemia is the most common cause of anemia worldwide. More than a quarter of the world's population is anemic and half of those are iron deficient. Women of reproductive age are most commonly affected as both menstruation and pregnancy increase the propensity to develop iron deficiency [70]. Other populations at risk include athletes, obese patients who have undergone bariatric surgery, and young children [71]. Epidemiological studies show variable association between iron deficiency and RAS, but replacement therapy may not impact the clinical course of RAS [63, 64].

Etiopathogenesis

Iron deficiency anemia may result from insufficient dietary intake or malabsorption of iron, chronic blood loss, hemolysis, and/or pregnancy.

Clinical Manifestations

Iron deficiency anemia presents with weakness, pallor, fatigue, dyspnea, tachycardia, headache, irritability, and telogen effluvium. Pagophagia (ice craving), a form of pica, may be present as well. Iron deficiency anemia tends to produce nail findings such as splitting or spooning (koilonychia). In men and non-menstruating women, the diagnosis of iron deficiency anemia should prompt further investigation for possible gastrointestinal bleeding.

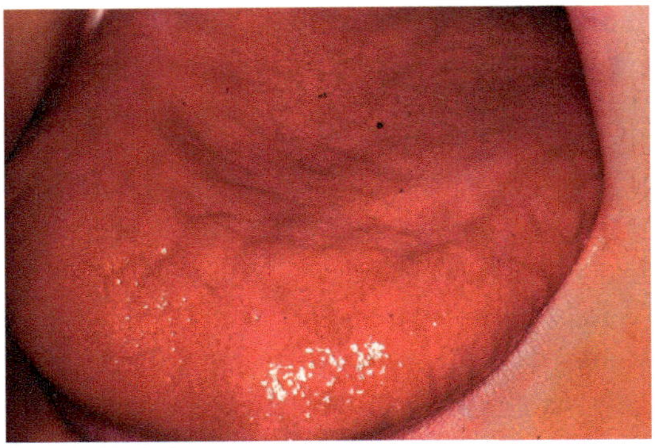

Fig. 3.9 Atrophic "bald" tongue in a 55-year-old female with iron deficiency anemia (Courtesy of Dr. Messadi, UCLA, School of Detistry)

Oral Signs and Symptoms

Oral findings in iron deficiency anemia include mucosal pallor, especially pallor of the gingivae and vermilion border of the lips, angular cheilitis, and atrophic glossitis due to loss of filiform and fungiform papillae of the tongue, causing the tongue to appear smooth and red (Fig. 3.9). The atrophic glossitis may be preceded by pain, burning sensation or dysphagia [62, 72]. Iron deficiency anemia is a predisposing factor for oral candidiasis [62, 73].

Differential Diagnosis

Many vitamin deficiencies, erythematous candidiasis, and viral illnesses may also present with an atrophic erythematous tongue.

Treatment Recommendations

Once the etiology of iron deficiency has been identified, it must be corrected. When iron is to be repleted, increased dietary iron sources are recommended, and iron supplements are prescribed. Iron-rich foods including pork, chicken, fish, liver, and beans are very effective for the treatment of mild iron deficiency anemia. Although iron supplementation is safe, inexpensive, and very effective when ingested, it is poorly tolerated. GI side effects such as constipation or diarrhea, abdominal upset and pain, and nausea and vomiting may contribute to poor compliance. Metallic taste has also been described as a side effect of iron supplementation. Underlying malabsorptive disease may both limit absorption and may be exacerbated by ingestion of iron. Ideally iron should be taken on an empty stomach or with vitamin C to increase absorption; because calcium and fiber block the absorption of iron, dairy products, tea, coffee, or cereals should be avoided [74]. Parenteral iron formulations are now available with decreased toxicity and should be considered in patients who are unable to tolerate oral supplementation or those with poor absorption due to underlying GI disease.

Polycythemia Vera (PV)

PV is a chronic myeloproliferative disorder characterized by clinical, serologic, and bone marrow histological findings. These include an elevation in number of RBCs and hemoglobin or leukocytosis, thrombocytosis, and panmyeloid hyperplasia of the bone marrow [75]. Myelofibrosis and acute leukemia are a natural progression of PV. Chronic myeloproliferative disorders specifically exclude CML because of its relation with the Philadelphia chromosome translocation and its response to both interferon alpha and imatinib mesylate [75].

Epidemiology

The incidence of PV is approximately 2.3/100,000 individuals; the incidence may be higher in some ethnic groups, particularly those of Jewish ancestry [75, 76]. Although PV has been reported in all age groups, most patients are over 60 years of age, and men only slightly outnumber women [75].

Etiopathogenesis

PV appears to be a clonal stem cell disease that affects all three lineages of the bone marrow. No specific genetic abnormality has been elucidated, but nonspecific abnormalities including trisomies of chromosome 9 and 8 and deletions of the long arms of chromosomes 13 and 20 have been noted [75]. In some cases, the cells appear to be erythropoietin independent or erythropoietin hypersensitive.

Clinical Manifestations

Elevated hematocrit and associated hyperviscosity are associated with reduced cerebral blood flow rate and reduced oxygenation. Clinically, patients suffer from constitutional symptoms such as headaches and fatigue as well as microvascular abnormalities. Aquagenic pruritus and erythromelalgia and splenomegaly are common.

Oral Signs and Symptoms

The tongue, gingiva, and other mucosal surfaces are often deep red to violaceous. The gingiva may be edematous and bleed with minimal trauma. Petechial hemorrhages are common [77]. Poor oral hygiene, poor periodontal health, gingival hyperplasia, and easy bruising have been reported [78].

Differential Diagnosis

True PV may be a clonal myeloproliferative disorder or a non-clonal increase in red cell mass that is often mediated by erythropoietin, while apparent polycythemia is due to reduction in plasma volume [75]. Laboratory abnormalities include leukocytosis, thrombocytosis, and microcytosis. The bone marrow is hypercellular with megakaryocytic hyperplasia and clustering.

Treatment Recommendations

Phlebotomy remains the mainstay of treatment of PV, but myelosuppressive therapy may play a role in the very ill patient.

Sickle Cell Disease

Sickle cell disease (SCD) is a group of autosomal recessively inherited disorders of erythrocytes associated with anemia, chronic infections, and episodes of pain. These hemoglobin mutations predispose RBCs to deformation and loss of elasticity in the setting of low oxygen tension. Sickle cell trait (SCT) is not a disease but a condition in which only one of the beta hemoglobin chains is affected by a carrier state. A diagnosis of SCD requires demonstration of hemoglobin S by hemoglobin electrophoresis.

Epidemiology

SCD predominantly affects 70,000–100,000 Africans and African-Americans in the United States, while two million individuals carry the SCT [79]. Numbers in Africa range dramatically from country to country.

Etiopathogenesis

In contrast to normal hemoglobin, which contains two alpha and two beta chains, the beta chains in SCD are altered. Glutamic acid substitution of valine in the beta chain results in susceptibility of the normally biconcave RBCs to morphologic alterations (sickle shape), increased fragility, and increased susceptibility to distortion in the setting of hypoxemia. These altered erythrocytes are unable to pass through normal microvasculature resulting in painful episodes of vaso-occlusion and subsequent damage.

Clinical Manifestations

The clinical manifestations of SCD are diverse. Patients suffer from microthrombi, pain (both acute and chronic), fatigue, and anemia. Generally, patients are at increased risk of osteomyelitis. Acute pain in the long bones, chest, or abdomen, fever, malaise, numbness, weakness, and altered cognition may signify an acute sickle crisis. Patients may suffer from strokes, splenic infarcts, splenic sequestration, and increased susceptibility to infection. Leg ulcers, pulmonary hypertension, and renal end-organ damage are predominantly seen in adults with SCD.

Oral Signs and Symptoms

The most common oral manifestations of SCD are pallor or jaundice particularly involving the soft palate or floor of the mouth. Increased prevalence of dental caries and poor oral hygiene in these patients is associated with low socioeconomic status. No significant role was found in the patients' dietary habits or frequency of tooth brushing [80, 81]. In addition, patients may develop sudden onset of pain or necrosis in previously healthy teeth due to sickle crisis [82]. Overgrowth of the midface, anesthesia of the mandibular nerve, asymptomatic necrosis of the neurovascular canal, and gingival overgrowth are well described [82]. Overgrowth of the midface, frontal bossing, exposure of the maxillary teeth, and maxillary bone overgrowth may result in a depressed nasal bridge with resultant malocclusion in conjunction with a characteristic facial profile. Osteomyelitis of the mandible is a rare complication [83, 84]. Infarction of branches of the mandibular nerve, due to vaso-occlusion, rarely causes persistent anesthesia of the teeth, gingivae, or oral mucosa [85, 86].

Differential Diagnosis

Patients with SCD must be evaluated to rule out other causes of anemia, pain, osteomyelitis, dental abscesses, or facial trauma.

Treatment Recommendations

Correction of anemia prior to any surgery for treatment of fractures or osteomyelitis is recommended. Postoperative antibiotic coverage is also indicated.

Acknowledgment We would like to acknowledge Mr. Michael Gordon for his editorial support.

References

1. Schlosser BJ, Pirigyi M, Mirowski GW. Oral manifestations of hematologic and nutritional diseases. Otolaryngol Clin N Am. 2011;44(1):183–203., vii. https://doi.org/10.1016/j.otc.2010.09.007.
2. Burket LW, Greenberg MS, Glick M, Ship JA. Burket's oral medicine. 11th ed. Hamilton: BC Decker; 2008.
3. Vogel VG, Fisher RE. Epidemiology and etiology of leukemia. Curr Opin Oncol. 1993;5(1):26–34.
4. Swerdlow SH, International Agency for Research on Cancer, World Health Organization. WHO classification of tumours of haematopoietic and lymphoid tissues, World Health Organization classification of tumours. 4th ed. Lyon: International Agency for Research on Cancer; 2008.
5. Cho-Vega JH, Medeiros LJ, Prieto VG, Vega F. Leukemia cutis. Am J Clin Pathol. 2008;129(1):130–42. https://doi.org/10.1309/WYACYWF6NGM3WBRT.
6. Hou GL, Huang JS, Tsai CC. Analysis of oral manifestations of leukemia: a retrospective study. Oral Dis. 1997;3(1):31–8.
7. Weckx LL, Hidal LB, Marcucci G. Oral manifestations of leukemia. Ear Nose Throat J. 1990;69(5):341–2.. 5–6
8. Hiraki A, Nakamura S, Abe K, Takenoshita Y, Horinouchi Y, Shinohara M, et al. Numb chin syndrome as an initial symptom of acute lymphocytic leukemia: report of three cases. Oral Surg Oral Med Oral Pathol Oral Radiol Endod. 1997;83(5):555–61.
9. Cooper CL, Loewen R, Shore T. Gingival hyperplasia complicating acute myelomonocytic leukemia. J Can Dent Assoc. 2000;66(2):78–9.
10. Neville BW, Damm DD, White DK. Color atlas of clinical oral pathology. 2nd ed. Baltimore: Williams & Wilkins; 1999.
11. Word ZH, Matasar MJ. Advances in the diagnosis and management of lymphoma. Blood Lymphat Cancer: Targets Ther. 2012;2012(2):29–55. https://doi.org/10.2147/BLCTT.S15554.
12. Campo E, Swerdlow SH, Harris NL, Pileri S, Stein H, Jaffe ES. The 2008 WHO classification of lymphoid neoplasms and beyond: evolving concepts and practical applications. Blood. 2011;117(19):5019–32. https://doi.org/10.1182/blood-2011-01-293050.
13. Townsend W, Linch D. Hodgkin's lymphoma in adults. Lancet. 2012;380(9844):836–47. https://doi.org/10.1016/S0140-6736(12)60035-X.
14. Molyneux EM, Rochford R, Griffin B, Newton R, Jackson G, Menon G, et al. Burkitt's lymphoma. Lancet. 2012;379(9822):1234–44. https://doi.org/10.1016/S0140-6736(11)61177-X.

15. Bower M. Acquired immunodeficiency syndrome-related systemic non-Hodgkin's lymphoma. Br J Haematol. 2001;112(4):863–73.
16. Kolokotronis A, Konstantinou N, Christakis I, Papadimitriou P, Matiakis A, Zaraboukas T, et al. Localized B-cell non-Hodgkin's lymphoma of oral cavity and maxillofacial region: a clinical study. Oral Surg Oral Med Oral Pathol Oral Radiol Endod. 2005;99(3):303–10. https://doi.org/10.1016/j.tripleo.2004.03.028.
17. Gabarre J, Raphael M, Lepage E, Martin A, Oksenhendler E, Xerri L, et al. Human immunodeficiency virus-related lymphoma: relation between clinical features and histologic subtypes. Am J Med. 2001;111(9):704–11.
18. Canellos GP, Rosenberg SA, Friedberg JW, Lister TA, Devita VT. Treatment of Hodgkin lymphoma: a 50-year perspective. J Clin Oncol. 2014;32(3):163–8. https://doi.org/10.1200/JCO.2013.53.1194.
19. Berliner N, Horwitz M, Loughran TP Jr. Congenital and acquired neutropenia. Hematol/Educ Program Am Soc Hematol Am Soc Hematol Educ Program. 2004:63–79. https://doi.org/10.1182/asheducation-2004.1.63.
20. Dale DC, Bolyard AA, Aprikyan A. Cyclic neutropenia. Semin Hematol. 2002;39(2):89–94.
21. Bellanne-Chantelot C, Clauin S, Leblanc T, Cassinat B, Rodrigues-Lima F, Beaufils S, et al. Mutations in the ELA2 gene correlate with more severe expression of neutropenia: a study of 81 patients from the French Neutropenia Register. Blood. 2004;103(11):4119–25. https://doi.org/10.1182/blood-2003-10-3518.
22. Dale DC. ELANE-related neutropenia. In: Pagon RA, Adam MP, Ardinger HH, Bird TD, Dolan CR, Fong CT et al., editors. GeneReviews (R). Seattle (WA): University of Washington; 1993.
23. Horwitz MS, Duan Z, Korkmaz B, Lee HH, Mealiffe ME, Salipante SJ. Neutrophil elastase in cyclic and severe congenital neutropenia. Blood. 2007;109(5):1817–24. https://doi.org/10.1182/blood-2006-08-019166.
24. Cohen DW, Morris AL. Periodontal manifestations of cyclic neutropenia. J Periodontol. 1961;32(2):159–68.
25. Hammond WP 4th, Price TH, Souza LM, Dale DC. Treatment of cyclic neutropenia with granulocyte colony-stimulating factor. N Engl J Med. 1989;320(20):1306–11. https://doi.org/10.1056/NEJM198905183202003.
26. Falk RH, Comenzo RL, Skinner M. The systemic amyloidoses. N Engl J Med. 1997;337(13):898–909. https://doi.org/10.1056/NEJM199709253371306.
27. Merlini G, Bellotti V. Molecular mechanisms of amyloidosis. N Engl J Med. 2003;349(6):583–96. https://doi.org/10.1056/NEJMra023144.
28. Biewend ML, Menke DM, Calamia KT. The spectrum of localized amyloidosis: a case series of 20 patients and review of the literature. Amyloid. 2006;13(3):135–42. https://doi.org/10.1080/13506120600876773.
29. Stoopler ET, Sollecito TP, Chen SY. Amyloid deposition in the oral cavity: a retrospective study and review of the literature. Oral Surg Oral Med Oral Pathol Oral Radiol Endod. 2003;95(6):674–80. https://doi.org/10.1067/moe.2003.136.
30. Mardinger O, Rotenberg L, Chaushu G, Taicher S. Surgical management of macroglossia due to primary amyloidosis. Int J Oral Maxillofac Surg. 1999;28(2):129–31.
31. Aono J, Yamagata K, Yoshida H. Local amyloidosis in the hard palate: a case report. Oral Maxillofac Surg. 2009;13(2):119–22. https://doi.org/10.1007/s10006-009-0158-4.
32. Hachulla E, Janin A, Flipo RM, Saile R, Facon T, Bataille D, et al. Labial salivary gland biopsy is a reliable test for the diagnosis of primary and secondary amyloidosis. A prospective clinical and immunohistologic study in 59 patients. Arthritis Rheum. 1993;36(5):691–7.
33. Palumbo A, Anderson K. Multiple myeloma. N Engl J Med. 2011;364(11):1046–60. https://doi.org/10.1056/NEJMra1011442.
34. Vela-Ojeda J, Garcia-Ruiz Esparza MA, Padilla-Gonzalez Y, Sanchez- Cortes E, Garcia-Chavez J, Montiel-Cervantes L, et al. Multiple myeloma-associated amyloidosis is an independent high-risk prognostic factor. Ann Hematol. 2009;88(1):59–66. https://doi.org/10.1007/s00277-008-0554-0.
35. Rajkumar SV, Merlini G, San Miguel JF. Haematological cancer: redefining myeloma. Nat Rev Clin Oncol. 2012;9(9):494–6. https://doi.org/10.1038/nrclinonc.2012.128.
36. Rajkumar SV, Dimopoulos MA, Palumbo A, Blade J, Merlini G, Mateos MV, et al. International myeloma working group updated criteria for the diagnosis of multiple myeloma. Lancet Oncol. 2014;15(12):e538–e48. https://doi.org/10.1016/S1470-2045(14)70442-5.
37. Cardoso RC, Gerngross PJ, Hofstede TM, Weber DM, Chambers MS. The multiple oral presentations of multiple myeloma. Support Care Cancer. 2014;22(1):259–67. https://doi.org/10.1007/s00520-013-1960-y.
38. Chou T. Multiple myeloma: recent progress in diagnosis and treatment. J Clin Exp Hematopathol. 2012;52(3):149–59.
39. Allen CE, Li L, Peters TL, Leung HC, Yu A, Man TK, et al. Cell-specific gene expression in Langerhans cell histiocytosis lesions reveals a distinct profile compared with epidermal Langerhans cells. J Immunol. 2010;184(8):4557–67. https://doi.org/10.4049/jimmunol.0902336.
40. Caldemeyer KS, Parks ET, Mirowski GW. Langerhans cell histiocytosis. J Am Acad Dermatol. 2001;44(3):509–11. https://doi.org/10.1067/mjd.2001.109304.
41. Kilborn TN, Teh J, Goodman TR. Paediatric manifestations of Langerhans cell histiocytosis: a review of the clinical and radiological findings. Clin Radiol. 2003;58(4):269–78.

42. Hoover K, Rosenthal D, Mankin H. Langerhans cell histiocytosis. Skelet Radiol. 2007;36(2):95–104. https://doi.org/10.1007/s00256-006-0193-2.
43. Stull MA, Kransdorf MJ, Devaney KO. Langerhans cell histiocytosis of bone. Radiographics. 1992;12(4):801–23.
44. Windebank K, Nanduri V. Langerhans cell histiocytosis. Arch Dis Child. 2009;94(11):904–8. https://doi.org/10.1136/adc.2007.125872.
45. Milian MA, Bagan JV, Jimenez Y, Perez A, Scully C, Antoniades D. Langerhans' cell histiocytosis restricted to the oral mucosa. Oral Surg Oral Med Oral Pathol Oral Radiol Endod. 2001;91(1):76–9. https://doi.org/10.1067/moe.2001.110031.
46. Hicks J, Flaitz CM. Langerhans cell histiocytosis: current insights in a molecular age with emphasis on clinical oral and maxillofacial pathology practice. Oral Surg Oral Med Oral Pathol Oral Radiol Endod. 2005;100(2 Suppl):S42–66. https://doi.org/10.1016/j.tripleo.2005.06.016.
47. Götz G, Fichter J. Langerhans'-cell histiocytosis in 58 adults. Eur J Med Res. 2004;9(11):510–4.
48. Annibali S, Cristalli MP, Solidani M, Ciavarella D, La Monaca G, Suriano MM, et al. Langerhans cell histiocytosis: oral/periodontal involvement in adult patients. Oral Dis. 2009;15(8):596–601. https://doi.org/10.1111/j.1601-0825.2009.01601.x.
49. Abla O, Egeler RM, Weitzman S. Langerhans cell histiocytosis: current concepts and treatments. Cancer Treat Rev. 2010;36(4):354–9. https://doi.org/10.1016/j.ctrv.2010.02.012.
50. Gadner H, Grois N, Potschger U, Minkov M, Arico M, Braier J, et al. Improved outcome in multisystem Langerhans cell histiocytosis is associated with therapy intensification. Blood. 2008;111(5):2556–62. https://doi.org/10.1182/blood-2007-08-106211.
51. Sekhon SS, Roy V. Thrombocytopenia in adults: a practical approach to evaluation and management. South Med J. 2006;99(5):491–8.
52. Priziola JL, Smythe MA, Dager WE. Drug-induced thrombocytopenia in critically ill patients. Crit Care Med. 2010;38(Suppl):S145–54.
53. Aster RH, Boughie DW. Drug-induced immune thrombocytopenia. N Engl J Med. 2007;357:580–7.
54. Israels S, Schwetz N, Boyar R, McNicol A. Bleeding disorders: characterization, dental considerations and management. J Can Dent Assoc. 2006;72(9):827.
55. Fillmore WJ, Leavitt BD, Arce K. Dental extractions in the thrombocytopenic patient. Oral Surg Oral Med Oral Pathol Oral Radiol. 117(4):e300.
56. Rund D, Rachmilewitz E. β-Thalassemia. N Engl J Med. 2005;353:1135–46.
57. Perisano C, Marzetti E, Spinelli MS, Calla C, Graci C, Maccauro G. Physiopathology of bone modifications in β -thalassemia. Hindawi Publishing Corporation Anemia Volume 2012, Article ID 320737, 5 p.
58. Vogiatzi MG, Macklin EA, Fung EB, Cheung AM, Vichinsky E, Olivieri N, et al. Bone disease in thalassemia: a frequent and still unresolved problem. J Bone Miner Res. 2009;24(3):543–57.
59. Javid B, Said-Al-Naief N. Craniofacial manifestations of β-thalassemia major. Oral Surg Oral Med Oral Pathol Oral Radiol. 2015;119(1):e33–40.
60. Azam M, Bhatti N. Hair on end appearance. Arch Dis Child. 2006;91(9):735.
61. Stover PJ. Vitamin B12 and older adults. Curr Opin Clin Nutr Metab Care. 2010;13:24–7.
62. Koybasi S, Parlak AH, Serin E, Yilmaz F, Serin D. Recurrent aphthous stomatitis: investigation of possible etiologic factors. Am J Otolaryngol. 2006;27(4):229–32.
63. Piskin S, Sayan C, Durukan N, Senol M. Serum iron, ferritin, folic acid, and vitamin B12 levels in recurrent aphthous stomatitis. J Eur Acad Dermatol Venereol. 2002;16(1):66–7.
64. Scully C, Gorsky M, Lozada-Nur F. The diagnosis and management of recurrent aphthous stomatitis: a consensus approach. J Am Dent Assoc. 2003;134(2):200–7.
65. Patton LL, Brahim JS, Travis WD. Mandibular osteomyelitis in a patient with sickle cell anemia: report of case. J Am Dent Assoc. 1990;121(5):602–4.
66. Bizarro N. Diagnosis and classification of pernicious anemia. Autoimmun Rev. 2014;13:565–8.
67. Stabler SP. Vitamin B12 Deficiency. New Engl J Med. 2013;368:149–60.
68. Macleod RI, Hamilton PJ, Soames JV. Quantitative exfoliative oral cytology in iron-deficiency and megaloblastic anemia. Anal Quant Cytol Histol. 1988;10(3):176–80.
69. Lee HJ, Jo DY. Images in clinical medicine. A smooth, shiny tongue. N Engl J Med. 2009;360(6):e8.
70. Kassebaum NJ, Jasrasaria R, Naghavi M, Wulf SK, Johns N, Lozano R, et al. A systematic analysis of global anemia burden from 1990 to 2010. Blood. 2014;123(5):615.
71. Love AL, Billett HH. Obesity, bariatric surgery and iron deficiency: true, true true and related. Am J Hematol. 2008;83:403–9.
72. Eisen D, Lynch DP. Oral manifestations of systemic diseases. The mouth: diagnosis and treatment. St. Louis: Mosby; 1998. p. 212–36.
73. Cawson RA, Odell EW. Cawson's essentials of oral pathology and oral medicine. 8th ed. Edinburgh: Churchill Livingstone/Elsevier; 2008.
74. Deloughery TG. Microcytic anemia. N Engl J Med. 2014;371(14):1324–31.. 2010
75. Tefferi AB, Suman VJ, Sobell JL, Codd MB, Silverstein MN, Melton LJ 3rd. Trends in the incidence of polycythemia vera among Olmsted Coutny, Minnesota resident, 1935–1989. Am J Hematol. 1994:4789–93.
76. Najean Y, Rain JD, Billotey C. Epidemiological data in polycythaemia vera: a study of 842 cases. Hematol Cell Ther. 1998;40:159–65.
77. Lele MV. Oral manifestations of polycythaemia rubra vera. J All India Dent Assoc. 1965;37(11):345–8.
78. Ruparella PB, Ruparella KP, Shirolkar R, Tipathy A. Chronic myeloproliferative disorders: a rarest case

with oral manifestations and dental management. J Indian Aca Oral Med Radio. 2012;24(2):155–7.
79. Creary M, Williamson W, Kulkarni R. Sickle cell disease: current activities, health implications, and future directions. J Women's Health (Larchmt). 2007;16:575–82.
80. Laurence B, George D, Woods D, Shosanya A, Katz RV, Lanzkron S, et al. The association between sickle cell disease and dental caries in African Americans. Spec Care Dentist. 2006;26:95–100.
81. Luna AC, Rodrigues MJ, Menezes VA, Marques KM, Santos FA. Caries prevalence and socioeconomic factors in children with sickle cell anemia. Braz Oral Res. 2012;26:43–9.
82. Javed F, Correa FO, Nooh N, Almas K, Romanos GE, Al-Hezaimi K. Orofacial manifestations in patients with sickle cell disease. Am J Med Sci. 2013;345(3):234–7.
83. Shroyer JV 3rd, Lew D, Abreo F, Unhold GP. Osteomyelitis of the mandible as a result of sickle cell disease. Report and literature review. Oral Surg Oral Med Oral Pathol. 1991;72(1):25–8.
84. Friedlander AH, Genser L, Swerdloff M. Mental nerve neuropathy: a complication of sickle-cell crisis. Oral Surg Oral Med Oral Pathol. 1980;49(1):15–7.
85. Gregory G, Olujohungbe A. Mandibular nerve neuropathy in sickle cell disease. Local factors. Oral Surg Oral Med Oral Pathol. 1994;77(1):66–9.
86. Kelleher M, Bishop K, Briggs P. Oral complications associated with sickle cell anemia: a review and case report. Oral Surg Oral Med Oral Pathol Oral Radiol Endod. 1996;82(2):225–8.

Oral Signs of Endocrine and Metabolic Diseases

4

Jaisri R. Thoppay, Thomas P. Sollecito, and Scott S. De Rossi

Addison's Disease

Adrenal insufficiency is caused by either primary adrenal failure (usually related to destruction of the adrenal cortex, predominantly due to autoimmune etiology) or secondary as a result of hypothalamic-pituitary impairment of the corticotropic axis (predominantly due to pituitary disease). Addison's disease is primary hypoadrenocorticism caused by destruction of the adrenal cortex resulting in reduction or insufficient production of adrenal corticosteroid hormone resulting in adrenal insufficiency.

Epidemiology

Addison's disease is an uncommon condition that is more prevalent in women. Diagnosis is predominantly in the fourth to sixth decades of life. The incidence of Addison's disease is 4.7–6.2 per million people in white populations. The prevalence of Addison's disease varies from 39 to 144 per million, which includes 40–60 cases in the United States, 39 cases in Great Britain, 60 cases in Denmark, and 144 cases in Norway per million in population, as per available data. Roughly 80% of cases are caused by autoimmune adrenalitis [1, 2].

Etiopathogenesis

Addison's disease is caused by destruction of the adrenal cortex precipitated by multiple factors as shown in Table 4.1.

These autoimmune disorders can occur as an isolated process or as part of an autoimmune polyendocrine syndrome known as the polyglandular autoimmune syndrome (PGAS) types I and II. PGAS type I is associated with candidiasis, hypoparathyroidism, and adrenal failure. PGAS type II consists of Addison's disease plus either an autoimmune thyroid disease or type 1 diabetes mellitus associated with hypogonadism, pernicious anemia, celiac disease, or primary biliary cirrhosis.

The main characteristic of the autoimmune process in Addison's disease is the presence of serum antibodies (IgG1 or IgG2a subclass) against the steroidogenic enzymes, with antibodies against 21-hydroxylase being the most prevalent. In cases of PGAS, genetic susceptibility

J. R. Thoppay (✉)
Department of Oral and Maxillofacial Surgery, VCU School of Dentistry at VCU Medical Center, Virginia Commonwealth University, Richmond, VA, USA
e-mail: jthoppay@vcu.edu

T. P. Sollecito
The Robert Schattner Center, University of Pennsylvania School of Dental Medicine, Philadelphia, PA, USA

S. S. De Rossi
Department of Oral Medicine, Augusta University Dental College of Georgia, Augusta, GA, USA

N. Fazel (ed.), *Oral Signs of Systemic Disease*, https://doi.org/10.1007/978-3-030-10863-2_4

Table 4.1 Etiopathogenesis of adrenal insufficiency

		Pathologic mechanism
Autoimmune (80%)	Autoimmune adrenalitis	Associations with HLA DR3-DQ2, HLA DR4-DQ8, MICA, CTLA-4, PTPN22, CIITA, CLEC16A, vitamin D receptor
	Polyglandular autoimmune syndrome type I	AIRE gene mutations
	Polyglandular autoimmune syndrome type II	Associations with HLA-DR3, HLA-DR4, CTLA-4
Drug-induced adrenal insufficiency	Phenytoin, rifampicin, troglitazone, ketoconazole, fluconazole, etomidate, aminoglutethimide, trilostane, and phenobarbital	Based on mechanism of action of the medication, which increases cortisol metabolism
	Anticoagulants (heparin, warfarin), and tyrosine-kinase inhibitors (sunitinib)	Destruction of the adrenal cortex secondary to hemorrhage
Infections	Disseminated tuberculosis, cytomegalovirus histoplasmosis, *Cryptococcus*, toxoplasmosis, HIV, and candidiasis	Destruction of the adrenal cortex secondary to infection caused by pathogens
Infiltrative disorders	Amyloidosis, sarcoidosis, and hemochromatosis	Primary adrenal lymphoma, amyloidogenesis, hemochromatosis
Metastatic disease	Mainly cancers of the lung, stomach, breast, and colon	Destruction of glandular cells due to malignant transformation and metastasis

associations with HLA-B8, HLA-DR3, and HLA-DR4 alleles have been observed. However, specific HLA associations have not been identified [1–3].

Clinical Manifestations

Addison's disease patients present with chronic nonspecific signs and symptoms that can often lead to a delay in diagnosis. The disease progression may develop over a period of months. The clinical manifestations of Addison's disease do not begin to appear until at least 90% of the adrenal gland is destroyed. The clinical presentation is secondary to the deficiency of cortisol and aldosterone. Cortisol deficiency leads to altered glucose, fat, and protein metabolism, resulting in weakness, fatigue, weight loss, inability to tolerate stress, and hypotension [4, 5]. General clinical signs and symptoms and related laboratory abnormalities are listed in Table 4.2.

Oral Signs and Symptoms

Darkening of the orofacial skin, vermillion border of the lips along with other areas of sun exposure leading to a bronzing effect is the hallmark of primary adrenal insufficiency. Oral mucosal hyperpigmentation is seen in 80–94% of patients characteristically presenting as diffuse patchy brown macular pigmentation of the buccal mucosa, gingiva, palate, and dorsal and ventral tongue (Fig. 4.1). This appearance is directly related to increased levels of b-lipotropin or ACTH, which stimulates melanocytes, in turn leading to the bronzing effect and hyperpigmentation. This hyperpigmentation may be homogeneous or blotchy and therefore, may be more difficult to discern from physiologic or racial pigmentation [7]. Oral manifestations, particularly oral pigmentation may be the first sign of the disease preceding the cutaneous manifestations.

The oral hyperpigmentation is histologically characterized by an increase in melanin in the basal layer, without an obvious increased number of melanocytes [8]. Cases of oral squamous cell carcinoma have been reported in type I PGAS, which presents in association with candidiasis, hypoparathyroidism, and adrenal failure. The critical pathogenic pathway implicated in squamous cell carcinoma development is unclear; however, speculation regarding the presence of chronic mucocutaneous candidiasis

Table 4.2 Clinical features of Addison's disease

System	Symptoms	Signs	Related diagnostic abnormalities
General	Anorexia	Hypotension	Hyponatremia
	Weight loss	Dehydration	Hyperkalemia
	Fatigue	± Goiter	Azotemia
	Sweating	Pyrexia of unknown origin (occasionally)	Eosinophilia
	Salt craving		Low 9 a.m. cortisol and response to ACTH stimulation
Oral manifestation		Mucosal hyperpigmentation	Elevated 9 a.m. ACTH
			Elevated renin
Cardiovascular/ respiratory		Shock	Low/normal aldosterone
			Elevated urea
Dermatological		Cutaneous hyperpigmentation	Vitamin B12 deficiency
			Elevated thyroid-stimulating hormone
		Vitiligo	Eosinophilia
Neuromuscular	Headache		Lymphocytosis
	Muscle weakness and myalgia		Hypercalcemia
			Normochromic anemia
	Postural dizziness		Adrenal autoantibodies
	Syncope		Chest X-ray for evidence of tuberculosis [TB] or fungal infection
Gastrointestinal	Nausea		Abdominal radiography, CT scan for evidence of adrenal calcification, enlargement or atrophy, TB, or fungal infection
	Vomiting		
	Constipation		Anemia
	Abdominal pain		
	Diarrhea		
Psychological	Depression and behavioral changes		Hypoglycemia
			Hypochoremia and acidosis
Reproductive	Reduced libido, reduced axillary hair	Infertility and premature ovarian insufficiency	Elevated ESR
	Amenorrhea		

Created with data from Refs. [2, 4–6]
ACTH adrenocorticotropic hormone, *ESR* erythrocyte sedimentation rate

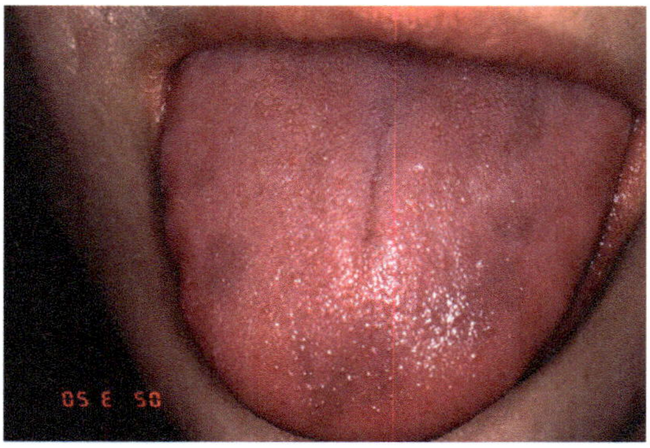

Fig. 4.1 Oral pigmentation in Addison's disease

possibly inducing carcinogenesis has been postulated [9].

Differential Diagnosis

Generally, the coloration of the oral mucosa can vary depending on the presence or absence of keratinization, melanogenic activity of melanocytes, vascularization, and type of submucosal tissue (i.e., muscle, bone, and cartilage) resulting in chromatic variation. Oral hyperpigmentation can present as physiologic pigmentation, or melanin-associated lesions such as the melanotic macule, melanocytic nevi, or malignant melanoma. Various stimuli, such as smoking (i.e., smoker's melanosis), trauma, hormonal changes, medications (such as chloroquine, doxorubicin, and phenothiazines), and radiation therapy, may result in increased production of melanin. Systemic disorders associated with the presence of oral pigmented melanocytic lesions may include Peutz-Jeghers and other familial hamartoma syndromes.

A thorough history will aid the clinician in prompting a diagnostic workup for oral hyperpigmentation to differentiate between various conditions associated with hyperpigmentation. When hyperpigmented areas are diffuse, further examination for underlying diseases or syndromes is warranted. Biopsy can be performed as a gold standard to rule out malignancy in case of an isolated lesion or a lesion that is atypical from the other areas of hyperpigmentation [8].

Treatment Recommendations

Oral hyperpigmentation from Addison's disease is often asymptomatic, and therefore no specific treatment is recommended. However, facial pigmentation may be reduced by minimizing sun exposure and using sunscreen. Periodic monitoring of these lesions is important as malignant lesions have been reported in PGAS type I syndrome [9]. Treatment of the underlying adrenal insufficiency may reverse the mucosal hyperpigmentation.

Hypothyroidism

Hypothyroidism is a condition characterized by a decrease in thyroid hormone (TH) production or by inadequate action of thyroid hormone on its target tissues. A common cause of hypothyroidism is an autoimmune reaction resulting in swelling and inflammation of the thyroid gland cells causing chronic thyroiditis (Hashimoto's disease). Occasionally hypothyroidism may be due to peripheral resistance to TH. A hypothyroid state can present as hypothyroidism or subclinical hypothyroidism (SCH).

Epidemiology

Hypothyroidism is more prevalent in women and increases with advancing age. The prevalence of hypothyroidism is 0.6–12 per 1000 in women and 1.3–4 per 1000 in men. The prevalence of hypothyroidism and SCH in the US population is 0.3% and 4.3%, respectively, as estimated by the National Health and Nutrition Examination Survey III data (http://www.cdc.gov/nchs/nhanes/nh3data.htm Accessed December 2014). Furthermore, head and neck cancer radiation therapy may result in hypothyroidism, which accounts for 10–45% of the cases [10, 11].

Etiopathogenesis

Hypothyroidism can be caused by primary thyroid failure, or it may be secondary to pituitary dysfunction. Common causes of primary thyroid failure are autoimmune thyroiditis, idiopathic atrophy, treatment with radioactive iodide, thyroidectomy, and drug use such as prolonged use of antithyroid drugs, lithium, and amiodarone. Less common causes include congenital dyshormonogenesis, cretinism, and occasionally infiltrative disease. The most common cause of secondary hypothyroidism is centrally mediated deficiency of thyrotropin-releasing hormone or thyroid-stimulating hormone. This can occur as a result of pituitary tumors, infection, and infiltrative disorders such as sarcoidosis, lymphoma, hemochromatosis, and histiocytosis [10, 12].

Clinical Manifestations

Insufficient TH levels cause symptoms such as weight gain, lethargy, cold intolerance, dry cool skin, and puffiness of the face and eyelids. Usually blood pressure is normal, but the heart rate may be bradycardic. The associated clinical signs and symptoms may be vague. Detailed clinical features are listed in the Table 4.3 [12–15].

Oral Signs and Symptoms

Deficiency of TH secretion leads to common oral findings such as macroglossia (Fig. 4.2), dysgeusia, poor periodontal health, salivary gland

Table 4.3 Clinical features of hypothyroidism

System	Symptoms	Signs	Related diagnostic abnormalities
General	Fatigue[a]	Goiter[a]	Thyroid hormone levels:
	Weight gain[a]		TSH:
	Cold intolerance[a]		Primary hypothyroidism –elevated
Oral manifestation	Mouth breathing	Salivary gland enlargement, compromised periodontal health delayed bone resorption, macroglossia (Fig. 4.2)	Secondary hypothyroidism- decreased
	Dysgeusia	Delayed tooth eruption	
		Enamel hypoplasia	T3/T4:
		Anterior open bite	Decreased in primary and secondary
		Micrognathia	
		Thick lips	
Hematological	Fatigue[a]	Megaloblastic anemia -due to gastric atrophy with vitamin B12 malabsorption	Hashimoto's thyroiditis: TSH elevated, T3/T4 may be normal in early disease but decreased in late disease
Cardiovascular/ respiratory		Bradycardia[a]	Associated abnormalities
		Bradypnea and hypoxia	Hyperlipidemia
		Respiratory muscle weakness	Iron-deficiency anemia
		Decreased chest wall and lung compliance	Macrocytic anemia
		Angina	Pernicious anemia
		Cardiac failure	Normochromic, normocytic anemia
		Pericardial effusions	Vitamin B12 deficiency
		Pleural effusions	Hyperprolactinemia
		Coronary artery disease	
		Respiratory failure with Myxedematous coma	
Dermatological	Dry skin[a]	Vitiligo	
		Alopecia	
		Coarse hair	
		Myxedema (local infiltration with hyaluronic acid and mucopolysaccharides)	
Neuromuscular	Aches and pains[a]	Delayed relaxation of reflexes[a]	
	Hoarseness	Myalgia and muscle stiffness	
	Deafness	Carpal tunnel syndrome	
		Cerebellar ataxia	
		Depression	
		Psychosis ("myxedema madness")	
Gastrointestinal	Constipation	Ileus	
		Ascites	
Reproductive	Infertility		
	Menorrhagia		
Developmental/ congenital If untreated can result in cretinism		Growth retardation	
		Mental retardation	
		Delayed puberty	
		Intellectual disability	
		Poor memory	

[a]More common signs and symptoms

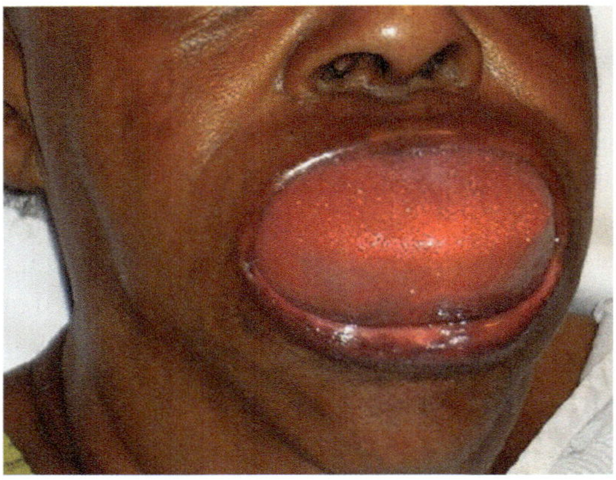

Fig. 4.2 Macroglossia

enlargement, and delayed wound healing. Macroglossia may be seen in 82% of hypothyroid patients.

Untreated childhood hypothyroidism can lead to cretinism, which is characterized by thick lips, delayed tooth eruption, enamel hypoplasia, macroglossia, anterior open bite, and malocclusion. Severe hypothyroidism can result in developmental delay, maxillary and mandibular hypoplasia with a marked reduction in the dimensions of the maxillofacial complex, and dissociation between mandibular growth and dental development. This can lead to prolonged retention of the primary dentition. The long-term effects of severe hypothyroidism on craniofacial growth and dental development may include impacted mandibular second molars. The cause is unclear but may be related to dissociation of mandibular ramus growth with failure of normal resorption of the internal aspect of the ramus, resulting in insufficient space for proper eruption of these teeth. Radiographs (e.g., panoramic) of these patients may display impaired growth of the mandible and maxilla. In addition, retained primary teeth, delayed eruption of permanent teeth and distortion of the roots of the lateral incisors and permanent first molars are notable radiologic findings [15–18]. Lingual thyroid is a rare embryological anomaly and originates from failure of the thyroid gland to descend from the foramen caecum. The ectopic gland located at the base of the tongue is often asymptomatic but may cause local symptoms such as dysphagia, dysphonia, upper airway obstruction, and hemorrhage, often with hypothyroidism [19, 20]. Severe untreated hypothyroidism can result in hypothyroidism or myxedematous coma.

Differential Diagnosis

Hypothyroidism may often present with multiple symptoms and can be nonspecific, but the clinical manifestations may prompt the clinician to pursue further investigations such as thyroid hormone levels and imaging studies. The diagnosis is often based on laboratory values since the clinical manifestations lack specificity.

Treatment Recommendations

Early diagnosis of hypothyroidism in adults and treatment of the underlying etiology may help to prevent oral complications. Symptoms of burning mouth and dysgeusia have been reported in hypothyroid patients [21]. Further, surgical interventions in hypothyroid patients are associated with an increased risk of minor perioperative complications, which should be anticipated and preemptively managed. For example, hemostasis may be impaired due to the presence of excess subcutaneous mucopolysaccharides that may decrease the ability of small blood vessels to constrict when cut or injured. This may result in complications of bleeding. As a result, local pressure for an extended time may be required to control the bleeding from the small vessels. Patients with hypothyroidism may have delayed wound healing, which can in turn increase susceptibility to infection. While, no specific treatment protocols have been reported in the literature, treatment may be provided as per current clinical management standards for the oral manifestations. Also the oral health care provider can play an important role in screening patients by performing a comprehensive oral and head and neck examination. Palpable abnormalities in the thyroid should be referred for endocrinology consultation [22, 23].

Hyperthyroidism

Hyperthyroidism is a pathological metabolic syndrome in which tissue is exposed to excessive amounts of circulating TH resulting in an accelerated metabolic state.

Epidemiology

Hyperthyroidism may be seen in all ages but usually presents with symptoms in the second to fifth decades of life. The prevalence of hyperthyroidism is more common in women with a ratio of 5:1. The reported prevalence is 0.5–2% in women. The most common form of hyperthyroid disease is Grave's disease (aka autoimmune diffuse toxic goiter), which comprises 60–80% of cases. About 1–2% of hyperthyroid patients may experience thyrotoxic emergency characterized by hyperpyrexia, dehydration, organ failure, atrial fibrillation, congestive heart failure, confusion, agitation, delirium, psychosis, seizures, or coma [24, 25].

Etiopathogenesis

The most common causes of hyperthyroidism are Grave's disease, toxic multinodular goiter (Plummer disease), and toxic solitary hyperfunctioning nodules. Occasionally inflammation of the thyroid gland (thyroiditis) results in the release of stored hormone resulting in thyrotoxicosis. Rarely, hyperthyroidism can be secondary to a pituitary adenoma, levothyroxine overdose, inadequate iodine supplementation, drug-induced hyperthyroidism, differentiated thyroid carcinomas and/or their metastases, ectopic thyroid, and familial non-autoimmune hyperthyroidism. During pregnancy a temporary hyperthyroid state may occur due to human chorionic gonadotropin excess with elevation in T3, T4, and suppression of TSH [24, 25].

Clinical Manifestations

The clinical presentation of hyperthyroidism varies from asymptomatic (subclinical) to life threatening (thyroid storm). Pathophysiologic clinical manifestations are a result of increased metabolic activity and enhanced beta adrenergic activity. Patients with hyperthyroidism may be subclinical with mild presentations of subtle neck swelling, eye changes, and other vague generalized signs and symptoms. A detailed list of clinical signs and symptoms is illustrated in Table 4.4.

Oral Signs and Symptoms

Hyperthyroidism during the development and eruption of primary teeth can lead to early exfoliation of primary teeth and premature eruption of permanent teeth. Though limited evidence is available in humans (due to the complexity of metabolic diseases), animal studies support the correlation [26]. Also there is limited data available on hyperthyroidism and its association with periodontal disease [27]. Although rare, hyperthyroidism can be caused by an ectopic thyroid gland presenting as a mass at the base of the tongue. This may be diagnosed as an incidental finding on routine oral examination or by the patient who may complain of pain or dysphagia. Osteoporosis secondary to hyperthyroidism may affect the maxilla and mandible. Oral burning and salivary gland enlargement have also been reported [22, 28].

Differential Diagnosis

Patients may present with unequivocal clinical manifestations of the disease such as a thyroid mass or ophthalmic changes that may prompt workup for hyperthyroidism. Some patients may have fewer and less obvious clinical signs, as in subclinical cases. Other manifestations may include osteoporosis and cardiovascular disease such as atrial fibrillation and tachycardia.

Treatment Recommendations

In order to provide optimal oral health care to these patients, clinicians should understand the disease, its treatment, and the disease impact on

Table 4.4 Clinical features of hyperthyroidism

System	Symptoms	Signs	Related diagnostic abnormalities
General	Weight loss	Cachexia	Nonspecific changes in routine laboratory tests
	Heat intolerance	Diaphoresis	
	Sweating	Hyperthermia	Hypokalemia
	Fatigue	Tremor	Hypercalcemia
		Insomnia	
Head and neck	Double vision	Goiter	Hyperthyroidism – TSH is decreased
		Eyelid swelling	T3 and T4 will be increased
		Exophthalmia neck swelling	
		Periorbital edema	
		Conjunctival injection	
		Lid lag	
		Proptosis	
		Chemosis	
Oral manifestation		Dental caries	
		Maxillary or mandibular osteoporosis	
		Accelerated dental eruption	
Cardiovascular/ respiratory	Palpitations	Tachycardia	
	Dyspnea	Atrial fibrillation	
		Tachypnea	
		Exacerbation of angina pectoris	
Dermatological	Discoloration	Dermal thickening	
		Non pitting edema	
		Elephantiasis	
		Hyperpigmentation	
		Fine hair, soft nails	
		Palmar erythema	
		Rosy complexion	
Musculoskeletal	Difficulty rising from chair	Proximal muscle weakness	
	Difficulty combing hair	Myalgia	
		Osteoporosis	
Gastrointestinal	Diarrhea, nausea vomiting	Abdominal tenderness	
Reproductive	Irregular menstrual cycle	Oligomenorrhea	
		Amenorrhea	
		Breast enlargement	
		Gynecomastia	
		Erectile dysfunction	
Psychiatric	Nervousness restlessness	Anxiety	

Created with data from Refs. [15, 24, 25]

oral structures. Cardiac complications are an important consideration with surgical procedures as hyperthyroidism may be associated with atrial fibrillation, congestive heart failure, angina, and pulmonary hypertension. Preventive measures should be considered while treating elderly patients with thyroid dysfunction. A thorough history (including current management for hyperthyroidism), physical examination, and thyroid hormone levels should be obtained while treating these patients. Patient should be assessed for any limitations or contraindications to local anesthetic with epinephrine for dental procedures [22, 29].

Hyperpituitarism

Hyperpituitarism is defined as the hypersecretion of pituitary hormones. This can be secondary to pituitary adenomas, which are classified based on size as microadenomas (<1 cm), or macroadenomas (>1 cm). Pituitary adenomas can be functional, associated with excess hormone with clinical manifestations or nonfunctional, which do not produce excess hormone [30]. Macroadenomas can result in an overactive pituitary gland that can result in target organ hormonal dysfunctions. The most common cause of hyperpituitarism is an adenoma arising in the anterior lobe.

Epidemiology

Pituitary adenomas comprise 10% of all intracranial neoplasms with a prevalence of less than 1% of the US population. The overall age-adjusted incidence of pituitary tumors in the USA is 0.9 per 100,000 person-years. About one-third of pituitary adenomas are associated with multiple endocrine neoplasia (MEN-1), a familial disorder of the endocrine system affecting the pituitary gland [11]. Commonly involved hormones are prolactin, ACTH, growth hormone, and thyroid-stimulating hormone. Prolactinoma comprise of 40–45%, and somatotroph adenomas are about 20%, which involve growth hormone +/− prolactin. Corticotroph adenomas are about 10–12% involving ACTH +/− other hormones. Thyrotroph adenomas comprise of 1–2% involving TSH +/− growth hormone [31]. Given the high frequency of pituitary adenomas and their potential for causing clinical sequelae, early diagnosis and treatment of pituitary adenomas can have far-reaching benefits.

Etiopathogenesis

Pituitary adenomas can result from hypothalamic dysfunction. Evidence indicates that intrinsic pituicyte alterations may lead to tumor formation. Mutation of the GNAS1 gene, which results in constitutive activation of a stimulatory guanine nucleotide-binding protein (G protein), is one of the more common genetic alterations [32].

Clinical Manifestations

Pituitary adenomas produce complex signs and symptoms as they control other endocrine glands and relative functions. The signs and symptoms of hyperpituitarism are illustrated in Table 4.5.

Oral Signs and Symptoms

Growth hormone-secreting adenomas cause acromegaly, which in turn leads to various orofacial and dental manifestations. The most common craniofacial skeletal changes are protruded glabella, increased anterior facial height, mandibular prognathism, and jaw thickening. The facial changes occur as a result of deposition of periosteal bone in response to excess growth hormone. Dental malocclusion may occur as a result of changes in craniofacial structures. Buccal tipping of the dentition can occur as a consequence of macroglossia and pressure exerted on the dentition. Patients tend to demonstrate downward mandibular advancement that may result in a cross bite, extension of the ascending ramus causing downward displacement of the mandible, and bimaxillary alveolar protrusion that may result in an edge-to-edge bite. Dental radiographs may show large pulp chambers (taurodontism) and excessive deposition of cementum on the roots resulting in hypercementosis [30, 33, 34]. The associated soft tissue changes such as macroglossia and hypertrophy of the soft palate may cause or exacerbate sleep apnea.

Treatment Recommendations

Craniofacial changes may be a preliminary sign of hyperpituitarism. Orofacial manifestations should prompt the oral health care provider to further evaluate. Resultant malocclusion can be

Table 4.5 Clinical features of hyperpituitarism

Symptoms	Signs	Related diagnostic abnormalities
Prolactinoma Female: Irregular menstrual bleeding, vaginal dryness	Female: Oligomenorrhea Amenorrhea, Galactorrhea Dyspareunia Osteopenia Osteoporosis Prepubertal: menarche	Hypercalciuria
Male: Decreased libido, erectile dysfunction, or infertility	Male: Prepubertal: small testicles gynecomastia in men	
GH-secreting adenomas – acromegaly:	Craniofacial changes- frontal bossing, mandibular prognathism	
Headache	Carpel tunnel syndrome	
Skin thickening	Raynaud's colonic polyps	
Malodorous sweating	Spade-shaped hands	
Joint pain	Enlarged feet	
Deepening of voice	Bony deformation of the spine with upper dorsal kyphosis	
	Compensatory lumbar hyperlordosis. Vertebral enlargement	
	Widened intervertebral spaces osteophyte formation	
	Atrial hypertension	
	Cardiomyopathy	
	Neuropathy	
	Sleep apnea 60–80%	
	Goiter	

Created with data from Refs. [30, 33]

appropriately treated by orthodontic or orthognathic procedures to improve patients' symptoms and restore function.

Hyperparathyroidism

Hyperparathyroidism is often an incidental finding during routine blood chemistry assessments. It is characterized by an increase in parathyroid hormone (PTH) resulting in hypercalcemia.

Epidemiology

Primary hyperparathyroidism presents as a single adenoma in approximately 85% of patients but may be asymptomatic in 75–80% of cases. Risk factors for primary hyperparathyroidism include a history of neck radiation, age (older than 50 years), and female gender, as women are twice as likely to develop primary hyperparathyroidism. Multiglandular hyperplasia accounts for 10–15% of the cases, while glandular carcinoma accounts for <1%. Other uncommon familial causes include MEN-1 and MEN-2A, which can be associated with parathyroid adenomas or asymmetric hyperplasia [35, 36].

Etiopathogenesis

Primary hyperparathyroidism results from hyperfunction of the parathyroid glands due to a parathyroid adenoma, parathyroid hyperplasia or, rarely, a parathyroid carcinoma. Secondary hyperparathyroidism is due to physiological secretion of parathyroid hormone (PTH) by the parathyroid glands in response to hypocalcemia secondary to factors such as vitamin D deficiency and chronic renal failure. Tertiary hyperparathyroidism is seen in patients with long-standing secondary hyperparathyroidism resulting in hyperplasia of the parathyroid glands and a loss of feedback response to serum calcium levels [35, 36].

Table 4.6 Clinical features of hyperparathyroidism

System	Symptoms	Signs	Related diagnostic abnormalities
General	Fatigue Generalized weakness	Delirium, mild cognitive impairment	Hypercalcemia
Cardiovascular/ respiratory	Angina, dyspnea, palpitations, syncope	Diastolic dysfunction, dysrhythmias, hypertension, left ventricular hypertrophy, vascular calcification	High PTH levels Bone densitometry- osteoporosis, minute bone density variation that may not be evident in conventional radiographs [37, 38]
Skeletal	Arthralgia, bone pain	Insufficiency fractures, osteomalacia, osteoporosis	
Neuromuscular	Anxiety, confusion, depression forgetfulness, impaired vision, insomnia, lethargy		24-h collection of urine for kidney function-elevated urine calcium levels
Gastrointestinal	Anorexia, constipation, epigastric pain, nausea, vomiting		
Renal	Polydipsia, polyuria, renal colic	Nephrocalcinosis, nephrolithiasis	

Created with data from Refs. [26, 35]

Clinical Manifestations

Hyperparathyroidism is most common in postmenopausal women, although it can occur in persons of all ages, including pregnant women. It can be asymptomatic, and often hypercalcemia presents as an incidental finding, which upon further diagnostic testing may be associated with elevated serum PTH levels [35, 37] (Table 4.6).

Oral Signs and Symptoms

Oral manifestations may include bony changes resulting in jaw expansion and/or extraoral or intraoral soft tissue swelling due to dentoalveolar pathology. Dental changes associated with hyperparathyroidism include abnormally narrow dental pulp chambers, generalized loss of the lamina dura of the roots of teeth, and generalized demineralization of medullary bones causing the characteristic "ground glass appearance" radiographically. Brown tumors are osseous lesions that develop in maxillofacial and mandibular bones in both primary (4.5%) and secondary (1.5%) hyperparathyroidism as a component of a metabolic bone disease known as osteitis fibrosa cystica. Brown tumors are considered a reparative cellular process rather than a true neoplasm. These tumors have been reported in both the maxilla and mandible. This phenomenon is considered pathognomonic of hyperparathyroidism secondary to chronic renal disease [39].

Histopathological examination of brown tumors is characterized by vascular fibroblastic stroma with numerous osteoclast-like multinucleated giant cells. The presence of hemorrhage, hemosiderin, and hypervascularity leads to the brown color [39, 40].

Differential Diagnosis

The differential diagnosis for brown tumor should include central giant cell granuloma, ameloblastoma, aneurysmal bone cyst, cherubism, reparative granuloma, fibrous dysplasia, and giant cell tumors.

Treatment Recommendations

Treatment for hyperparathyroidism-related manifestations involves surgical excision of bony lesions and managing the underlying hyperparathyroidism and associated systemic complications which can best be achieved with an interdisciplinary approach. Bone healing in these patients may be compromised. Thus, parathyroid levels must be controlled prior to surgical bone reconstruction for improved outcomes.

Amyloidosis

Amyloidosis is a rare clinical disorder caused by extracellular and/or intracellular deposition of insoluble amyloid fibrils that alter the normal function of tissues. Amyloidosis was formerly, broadly categorized as primary systemic amyloidosis, secondary systemic amyloidosis, hereditary systemic amyloidosis, and localized amyloidosis. Amyloidosis is also classified as amyloid associated amyloidosis (AA) and amyloid light chain (AL) amyloidosis [41].

Epidemiology

AL amyloidosis is the most common type of systemic amyloidosis in developed countries with an estimated incidence of nine cases per million per year. The average age of diagnosis is 65 years. Less than 10% of patients are under 50. Approximately, 73% of the reported cases comprise primary AL, 3% secondary AA, and the remainder familial amyloidoses due to gene mutation and localized amyloidosis [42, 43]. Familial Mediterranean fever can be associated with the secondary type [43].

Etiopathogenesis

About 90% of amyloid is comprised of amyloid fibrils formed by the aggregation of misfolded proteins, while 10% is comprised of glycosaminoglycans (GAGs), apolipoprotein-E (apoE), and serum amyloid P-component (SAP). In immunoglobulin light chain (AL) amyloidosis (previously referred to as primary amyloidosis), the fibrils are composed of fragments of monoclonal light chains. Amyloidosis is often associated with plasma cell dyscrasias such as multiple myeloma and monoclonal gammopathy of undetermined significance (MGUS). AA amyloidosis, in which the fibrils are composed of fragments of the acute-phase reactant serum amyloid A, is typically reactive secondary to chronic inflammation [41].

Clinical Manifestations

Amyloidosis is a condition that can be clinically asymptomatic for a very long time. Amyloid deposits can occur locally in any tissue or may involve several organs in multisystem amyloidosis, therefore resulting in a wide range of clinical manifestations. Progressive nephropathy leading to renal failure including heavy proteinuria (usually in the nephrotic range) is seen in these patients. Other signs and symptoms include edema, hepatosplenomegaly, heart failure, polyneuropathy, carpal tunnel syndrome, malabsorption of unknown cause, and orthostatic hypotension. Rare occasions of primary cutaneous nodular amyloidosis have also been reported [41].

Oral Signs and Symptoms

Amyloid involvement of the tongue in systemic amyloidosis manifests as firm or rubbery macroglossia due to extracellular deposition of amyloid within the muscle. Macroglossia is a pathognomonic sign of the disease, which can significantly impact speech, swallowing, and breathing and in some cases cause obstructive sleep apnea (Fig. 4.3) [44]. Cases of gingival involvement and exophytic changes in the oral mucosa have also been reported [45]. Localized oral amyloido-

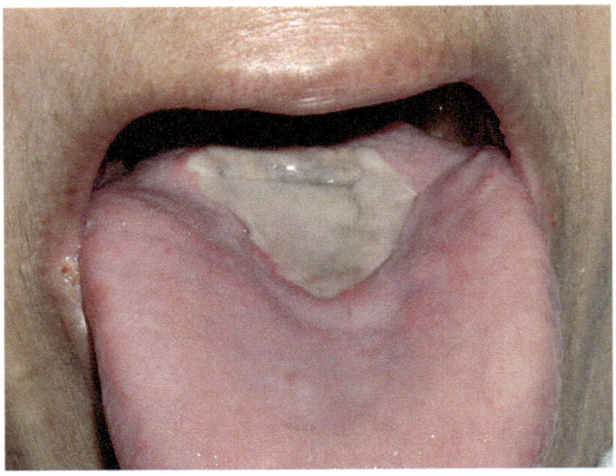

Fig. 4.3 Chronic ulceration and macroglossia in amyloidosis

sis AA can be associated with metabolic syndrome and periodontal disease. Amyloidosis rarely occurs in the sublingual gland [46, 47].

Differential Diagnosis

Macroglossia may be due to various causes that should be considered in the differential diagnosis other than amyloidosis. Macroglossia can be congenital as seen in Down's syndrome, Beckwith-Wiedemann syndrome, and mucopolysaccharidoses. Acquired macroglossia can occur as a result of carcinoma, hemangioma, plasmocytoma, lymphangioma, acromegaly, Ludwig's angina, sarcoidosis, intubation injury, and rarely nutritional deficiencies. Pseudomacroglossia is caused by abnormal positioning and displacement of the tongue due to enlarged tonsils/adenoids, low palate, abnormalities in the maxillary or mandibular arches, oral cavity neoplasms, and occasionally habitual posturing [44, 45].

Treatment Recommendations

Amyloidosis is diagnosed by identifying amyloid on histopathologic examination of oral mucosa and/or skin. In cases of progressive macroglossia, surgical reduction can be considered to improve complications associated with swallowing, respiration, cosmetic appearance, and patient comfort [44]. Accurate diagnosis is essential for the treatment of this condition disease. A poor prognosis is associated with the AL type, especially when accompanied by multiple myeloma and in the setting of cardiac amyloidosis.

Porphyrias

Porphyrias are a group of rare, genetically related metabolic disorders. At least eight different variations can affect the nervous system, skin, and occasionally other organs. These include acute intermittent porphyria (AIP), ALAD porphyria (ADP), variegate porphyria (VP), hereditary coproporphyria (HCP), porphyria cutenea tarda (PCT), erythropoietic protoporphyria (EPP), congenital erythropoietic porphyria (CEP), and hepatoerythropoietic porphyria (HEP). Porphyria cutanea tarda is the most common type of porphyria. Porphyria is caused by a genetic defect leading to dysfunction of various enzymes in the heme biosynthetic pathway leading to insufficient production of heme and accumulation of porphyrins (heme precursors), which can be toxic in high concentrations [48].

Epidemiology

The exact prevalence of porphyria is unknown ranging from 1 in 500 to 1 in 50,000 worldwide. The prevalence of some forms of porphyria is unknown because the genetic mutation associated with the disease may not cause signs or symptoms [49].

Etiopathogenesis

Porphyrias result from a deficiency of any of the last seven enzymes of the heme biosynthetic pathway or from increased activity of the first enzyme ALA synthase-2 (ALAS 2) in the pathway. When an enzyme of heme synthesis is deficient or defective, any other heme precursors or their substrates normally modified by that enzyme may accumulate in the bone marrow, liver, skin, or other tissues and can have neurotoxic effects. These precursors may be elevated in the blood and be excreted in urine, bile, or stool [49]. Porphyria cutanea tarda (PCT) is the most common of the porphyrias and results from a deficiency of the enzyme uroporphyrinogen decarboxylase (UROD). PCT is essentially an acquired disease, but some individuals have a genetic (autosomal dominant) deficiency of UROD that contributes to the development of PCT [48].

Clinical Manifestations

Acute intermittent porphyria generally involves the nervous system. VP, HCP, ALAD porphyria types though acute may or may not involve neuro visceral symptoms. Cutaneous porphyrias may have triggers and may manifest as itching or bullae that can heal with scarring. The clinical manifestations are listed in the Table 4.7.

Table 4.7 Clinical features of porphyrias

System	Symptoms	Signs	Related diagnostic abnormalities
Cardiovascular/ respiratory	Palpitations	Hypertension	Elevated porphobilinogen (PBG) – diagnostic screening
Dermatological (seen in cutaneous porphyrias)	Photosensitivity causing burning pain, itching	Erythema, edema of skin	
		Fragile skin	Neurological symptoms: with urinary delta-aminolevulinic acid (ALA) levels
	Hypertrichosis, pigment, and sclerodermoid changes	Blistering with scarring	
		Hirsutism	
Neuromuscular	Pain in the chest, legs, or back	Seizures	Skin hypersensitivity -total plasma porphyrins
	Insomnia	Muscle pain, tingling, numbness, weakness, or paralysis	
Gastrointestinal	Severe abdominal pain	Abdominal distention	
	Constipation or diarrhea		
	Nausea		
	Vomiting		
Psych	Anxiety	Mental changes, such as confusion, hallucinations, disorientation, or paranoia	
	Restlessness		
Urinary		Discoloration of the urine	

Created with data from Refs. [48, 49]

Oral Signs and Symptoms

Congenital erythropoietic porphyria (CEP) is one of the rarest types of porphyrias. It may present with reddish or purple-colored teeth termed erythrodontia, while delayed eruption of the dentition may also be seen. The discoloration is due to intrinsic heme product accumulation within the pulp chambers causing the characteristic appearance of the teeth [50]. Skeletal class III malocclusion has been reported in patients with erythropoietic protoporphyria (EPP), but the precise etiology or association is unknown [51].

Differential Diagnosis

Differential diagnosis includes dentinogenesis imperfecta, tetracycline-induced staining, or extrinsic causes of staining such as tobacco.

Treatment Recommendations

Patients with porphyria pose unique challenges with regards to treatment planning. Specific modifications should be made according to the type of porphyrias and the clinical manifestations. The safe prescribing of medications, consideration for antibiotic prophylaxis, complications related to local anesthetics, and prolonged bleeding are the main concerns. Patient education is extremely important in these patients as they may have a certain degree of anxiety and nervousness. The use of nitrous oxide is favored over intravenous sedation, but nitrous oxide should be used cautiously and titrated slowly [52].

Hemochromatosis

Hemochromatosis is a common form of iron overload disease, due to altered iron metabolism.

Epidemiology

Hemochromatosis is one of the most common genetic disorders in the USA, affecting about 1 million people, mostly Caucasians.

Etiopathogenesis

Primary hemochromatosis is due to various genetic mutations in the hereditary hemochromatosis (HFE) gene. In most cases of hereditary hemochromatosis, about 80–90% are caused by two copies of a C282Y mutation in the HFE gene. The probability of developing iron overload depends on the combination of genes inherited and encompasses a wide continuum of hepcidin deficiency states. Hepcidin is an important regulator of the entry of iron into the circulation. Secondary hemochromatosis may be due to systemic conditions such as chronic liver disease including hepatitis C, chemotherapy, anemia, alcohol abuse, recurrent blood transfusions, or excessive oral iron supplementation [53].

Clinical Manifestations

Clinical features of hereditary hemochromatosis are diverse and can include constitutional complaints. They are listed in the Table 4.8.

Oral Signs and Symptoms

The primary oral manifestation of hereditary hemochromatosis is areas of blue-gray to brown hyperpigmentation of the palate, buccal mucosa, and gingival tissues irrespective of the severity of iron overload. The pigmentation may be due to the iron deposits in the mucosal layer [56]. Iron deposits may also be identified in minor salivary glands including intracellular hemosiderin deposits. The salivary glands are an appropriate site for diagnostic biopsy as it is the most clinically accessible area and the most consistently involved extrahepatic site. Though minor salivary gland biopsy can be considered, it may not be feasible in infants and neonates and, moreover, the iron deposits may not be microscopically evident in early stages of the disease [57].

Differential Diagnosis

The differential diagnosis may include iron overload due to chronic transfusion, excessive iron supplementation, dysmetabolic hyperferritinemia, hereditary aceruloplasminemia, or chronic hepatitis.

Treatment Recommendations

Early diagnosis of this condition often has a good prognosis. However, a delay in diagnosis can be fatal. A thorough history and laboratory evalua-

Table 4.8 Clinical features of hemochromatosis

System	Symptoms	Signs	Related diagnostic abnormalities
General	Fatigue, weakness	Weakness and lethargy	Hyperglycemia Abnormal liver blood tests
Skeletal	Joint pain	Arthropathy, osteoporosis,	Hypothyroidism
Hematological			Genetic testing can be used to help confirm a diagnosis of hereditary hemochromatosis [HH]
Cardiovascular/ respiratory		Cardiomyopathy	Elevated serum ferritin level,
Dermatological	Changes in skin color, turning gray or bronze	Skin hyperpigmentation	ECG abnormalities
Neuromuscular			
Gastrointestinal	Abdominal pain	Hepatomegaly Hepatocellular carcinoma	
Reproductive	Increased or decreased libido (men)	Amenorrhea Impotence	

Created with data from Refs. [53–55]

tion prior to dentoalveolar procedures may reduce the risk of complications associated with existent liver dysfunction. Furthermore, drugs that are metabolized by the liver should be used with caution in these patients [55, 56].

References

1. Brandão Neto RA, Carvalho JF. Diagnosis and classification of Addison's disease (autoimmune adrenalitis). Autoimmun Rev. 2014;13(4–5):408–11.
2. Tucci V, Sokari T. The clinical manifestations, diagnosis, and treatment of adrenal emergencies. Emerg Med Clin North Am. 2014;32(2):465–84.
3. Charmandari E, Nicolaides NC, Chrousos GP. Adrenal insufficiency. Lancet. 2014;383(9935):2152–67.
4. Brooke AM, Monson JP. Addison's disease. Medicine. 2005;33(11):20–2.
5. Løvås K, Husebye ES. Addison's disease. Lancet. 2005;365(9476):2058–61.
6. Tiemensma J, Andela CD, Kaptein AA, Romijn JA, van der Mast RC, Biermasz NR, et al. Psychological morbidity and impaired quality of life in patients with stable treatment for primary adrenal insufficiency: cross-sectional study and review of the literature. Eur J Endocrinol. 2014;171(2):171–82.
7. Nieman LK, Chanco Turner ML. Addison's disease. Clin Dermatol. 2006;24(4):276–80.
8. Meleti M, Vescovi P, Mooi WJ, van der Waal I. Pigmented lesions of the oral mucosa and perioral tissues: a flow-chart for the diagnosis and some recommendations for the management. Oral Surg Oral Med Oral Pathol Oral Radiol Endod. 2008;105(5):606–16.
9. Böckle BC, Wilhelm M, Müller H, Götsch C, Sepp NT. Oral mucous squamous cell carcinoma – an anticipated consequence of autoimmune polyendocrinopathy-candidiasis-ectodermal dystrophy (APECED). J Am Acad Dermatol. 2010;62(5):864–8.
10. Almandoz JP, Gharib H. Hypothyroidism: etiology, diagnosis, and management. Med Clin N Am. 2012;96(2):203–21.
11. Golden SH, Robinson KA, Saldanha I, Anton B, Ladenson PW. Prevalence and incidence of endocrine and metabolic disorders in the United States: a comprehensive review. J Clin Endocrinol Metab. 2009;94(6):1853–78.
12. Franklyn JA. Hypothyroidism. Medicine. 2009;37(8):426–9.
13. Roberts CG, Ladenson PW. Hypothyroidism. Lancet. 2004;363(9411):793–803.
14. Caturegli P, De Remigis A, Rose NR. Hashimoto thyroiditis: clinical and diagnostic criteria. Autoimmun Rev. 2014;13(4–5):391–7.
15. Chandna S, Bathla M. Oral manifestations of thyroid disorders and its management. Indian J Endocrinol Metab. 2011;12(suppl2):s113–6.
16. Loevy HT, Aduss H, Rosenthal IM. Tooth eruption and craniofacial development in congenital hypothyroidism: report of case. J Am Dent Assoc. 1987;115(3):429.
17. Young ER. The thyroid gland and the dental practitioner. J Can Dent Assoc. 1989;55(11):903–7.
18. Gupta R, Goel K, Solanki J, Gupta S. Oral manifestations of hypothyroidism: a case report. J Clin Diagn Res. 2014;8(5):ZD20–2.
19. Kumar LK, Kurien NM, Jacob MM, Menon PV, Khalam SA. Lingual thyroid. Ann Maxillofac Surg. 2015;5(1):104–7.
20. Santangelo G, Pellino G, De Falco N, Colella G, D'Amato S, Maglione MG, et al. Prevalence, diagnosis and management of ectopic thyroid glands. Int J Surg. 2015;28:S1–6.
21. Femiano F, Gombos F, Esposito V, Nunziata M, Scully C. Burning mouth syndrome (BMS): evaluation of thyroid and taste. Med Oral Patol Oral Cir Bucal. 2006;11(1):E22–5.
22. Pinto A, Glick M. Management of patients with thyroid disease: oral health considerations. J Am Dent Assoc. 2002;133(7):849–58.
23. Ekmektzoglou KA, Zografos GC. A concomitant review of the effects of diabetes mellitus and hypothyroidism in wound healing. World J Gastroenterol. 2006;12(17):2721–9.
24. Menconi F, Marcocci C, Marinò M. Diagnosis and classification of Graves' disease. Autoimmun Rev. 2014;13(4–5):398–402.
25. Devereaux D, Tewelde SZ. Hyperthyroidism and thyrotoxicosis. Emerg Med Clin North Am. 2014;32(2):277–92.
26. Poumpros E, Loberg E, Engstrom C. Thyroid function and root resorption. Angle Orthod. 1994;64(5):389–93; discussion 394.
27. Zahid TM, Wang BY, Cohen RE. The effects of thyroid hormone abnormalities on periodontal disease status. J Int Acad Periodontol. 2011;13(3):80.
28. Guerra G, Cinelli M, Mesolella M, Tafuri D, Rocca A, Amato B, et al. Morphological, diagnostic and surgical features of ectopic thyroid gland: a review of literature. Int J Surg. 2014;12(Supplement 1(0)):S3–S11.
29. Huber MA, Terezhalmy GT. Risk stratification and dental management of the patient with thyroid dysfunction. Quintessence Int. 2008;39(2):139–50.
30. Samarasinghe S, Emanuele MA, Mazhari A. Chapter 47 – Neurology of the pituitary. In: Handbook of Clinical Neurology. Philadelphia: Elsevier; 2012. p. 685–701.
31. Arafah BM, Nasrallah MP. Pituitary tumors: pathophysiology, clinical manifestations and management. Endocr Relat Cancer. 2001;8(4):287–305.
32. Lania A, Spada A. G-protein and signalling in pituitary tumours. Horm Res. 2009;71(2):95–100.
33. Chanson P, Salenave S, Kamenicky P. Chapter 14 – Acromegaly. In: Handbook of Clinical Neurology. Philadelphia: Elsevier; 2012. p. 197–219.
34. Ayuk J, Sheppard MC. Growth hormone and its disorders. Postgrad Med J. 2006;82(963):24–30.

35. Pallan S, Khan A. Primary hyperparathyroidism: update on presentation, diagnosis, and management in primary care. Can Fam Physician. 2011;57(2):184–9.
36. Taniegra ED. Hyperparathyroidism. Am Fam Physician. 2004;69(2):333–9.
37. Sharma J, Itum DS, Moss L, Li C, Weber C. Predictors of bone mineral density improvement in patients undergoing parathyroidectomy for primary hyperparathyroidism. World J Surg. 2014;38(6):1268–73.
38. Miller PD, Bilezikian JP. Bone densitometry in asymptomatic primary hyperparathyroidism. J Bone Miner Res. 2002;17(Suppl 2):N98–102.
39. Verma P, Verma KG, Verma D, Patwardhan N. Craniofacial brown tumor as a result of secondary hyperparathyroidism in chronic renal disease patient: a rare entity. J Oral Maxillofac Pathol. 2014;18(2):267–70.
40. Pati AR, Mubeen KV, Singh C. Diagnosis and clinicoradiological presentation in an aggressive maxillary brown tumour. J Clin Diagn Res. 2014;8(5):ZD13–5.
41. Pinney JH, Hawkins P. Amyloidosis. Ann Clin Biochem. 2012;49(3):229–41.
42. Simms RW, Prout MN, Cohen AS. The epidemiology of AL and AA amyloidosis. Baillieres Clin Rheumatol. 1994;8(3):627–34.
43. Pinney JH, Smith CJ, Taube JB, Lachmann HJ, Venner CP, Gibbs SD, et al. Systemic amyloidosis in England: an epidemiological study. Br J Haematol. 2013;161(4):525–32.
44. Dendy RA, Davies JR, Gorst DW. A tongue resection in macroglossia due to primary amyloidosis. Br J Oral Maxillofac Surg. 1989;27(4):329–33.
45. Bucci T, Bucci E, Rullan AM, Bucci P, Nuzzolo P. Localized amyloidosis of the upper gingiva: a case report. J Med Case Rep. 2014;8:198. https://doi.org/10.1186/1752-1947-8-198.
46. Hu F, Dai AG, Zhu LM. Sublingual gland amyloidosis causing obstructive sleep apnea hypopnea syndrome: a case report and review of the literatures. Zhonghua Jie He He Hu Xi Za Zhi. 2013;36(7):485–9.
47. O'Reilly A, D'Souza A, Lust J, Price D. Localized tongue amyloidosis: a single institutional case series. Otolaryngol Head Neck Surg. 2013;149(2):240–4.
48. Horner ME, Alikhan A, Tintle S, Tortorelli S, Davis DM, Hand JL. Cutaneous porphyrias part I: epidemiology, pathogenesis, presentation, diagnosis, and histopathology. Int J Dermatol. 2013;52(12): 1464–80.
49. Tracy JA, Dyck PJB. Chapter 56 – Porphyria and its neurologic manifestations. In: Handbook of Clinical Neurology. Philadelphia: Elsevier; 2012. p. 839–49.
50. Bhavasar R, Santoshkumar G, Prakash BR. Erythrodontia in congenital erythropoietic porphyria. J Oral Maxillofac Pathol. 2011;15(1): 69–73.
51. Standerwick RG, Yen EHK, Pliska B. Orthodontic treatment considerations for a patient with erythropoietic protoporphyria. Am J Orthod Dentofac Orthop. 2013;144(6):899–908.
52. Brown GJ, Welbury RR. The management of porphyria in dental practice. Br Dent J. 2002;193(3):145–6.
53. Bardou-Jacquet E, Brissot P. Diagnostic evaluation of hereditary hemochromatosis (HFE and non-HFE). Hematol Oncol Clin North Am. 2014;28(4):625–35.
54. Niederau C, Strohmeyer G, Stremmel W. Epidemiology, clinical spectrum and prognosis of hemochromatosis. Adv Exp Med Biol. 1994;356:293–302.
55. Golla K, Epstein JB, Cabay RJ. Liver disease: current perspectives on medical and dental management. Oral Surg Oral Med Oral Pathol Oral Radiol Endod. 2004;98(5):516–21.
56. Schlosser BJ, Pirigyi M, Mirowski GW. Oral manifestations of hematologic and nutritional diseases. Otolaryngol Clin N Am. 2011;44(1):183–203.
57. Chan KC, Edelman M, Fantasia JE. Labial salivary gland involvement in neonatal hemochromatosis: a report of 2 cases and review of literature. Oral Surg Oral Med Oral Pathol Oral Radiol Endod. 2008;106(1):e27–30.

Oral Signs of Nutritional Disease

5

Stanislav N. Tolkachjov and Alison J. Bruce

Introduction

Homeostasis in the human body is dependent on a functioning equilibrium of energy-dependent metabolic pathways. Nutritional elements, typically derived from oral intake, must match the body's needs. With deficiency of a particular nutrient, or overall malnutrition, the metabolic supply and demand are disparate, and this mismatch may manifest phenotypically. Economic, social, medical, and psychosocial circumstances all affect the nutritional status of an individual. Owing to the unique physiologic environment of the oral cavity, manifestations of deficiency states may first become apparent in the mouth.

Mucous membranes have a significantly higher rate of epithelial cell turnover than cutaneous surfaces, 3–7 days as compared to 28 days, respectively [1–3]. Additionally, chronic stressors in the mouth, such as mechanical, thermal, or chemical insults, induce epithelial cell proliferation [4, 5]. The dorsal tongue, representing the highest degree of epithelial cell turnover in the oral cavity, is typically first to manifest signs of nutritional deficiencies [5, 6].

The dentition also provides a reflection of malnutrition, particularly deficiencies of vitamins A, D, and C, while integrity of the oral mucosal lining may be impaired with deficiencies of riboflavin, niacin, folic acid, pyridoxine, cyanocobalamin, biotin, iron, and vitamins C and K [7]. Overall, it must be recognized that not all periorificial cutaneous, mucosal, and lingual changes described in this text in association with nutritional disorders are specific for a particular deficiency; however, correlation of oral findings to an overall clinical presentation helps narrow the differential diagnosis (Table 5.1). Knowledge and early recognition of these manifestations should enhance clinical suspicion for these deficiencies and lead to prompt initiation of therapy.

Iron Deficiency Anemia

A strong epidemiological association has been shown between iron deficiency anemia (IDA) and increasing age. Anemia prevalence increases with age, rising sharply after the age of 80, and may be even higher depending on the study population and comorbid conditions [8–10]. Hospitalized and elderly populations typically have higher rates of anemia, and iron deficiency is the prevailing etiology in roughly 15% of anemic patients in whom causes of anemia are identified [8, 9]. In a population-based study of 16,600 Taiwanese female subjects screened for IDA, the prevalence was 4.9% [11].

S. N. Tolkachjov
Surgical Dermatology Group, Birmingham, AL, USA

A. J. Bruce (✉)
Department of Dermatology, Mayo Clinic, Jacksonville, FL, USA
e-mail: Bruce.Alison@Mayo.edu

N. Fazel (ed.), *Oral Signs of Systemic Disease*, https://doi.org/10.1007/978-3-030-10863-2_5

Table 5.1 Clinical and oral manifestations, workup, and treatment of nutritional deficiencies

Deficiency	Clinical findings	Oral findings	Testing	Treatment[a]
Iron	Pallor Weakness Fatigue	Mucosal pallor Angular stomatitis Glossitis	Hemoglobin (low) Hematocrit (low) MCV (low) Ferritin (low) Iron level (low) TIBC (high)	Oral ferrous sulfate 300 mg BID Parenteral available
Thiamine (B1)	Tachycardia Hypotension Nystagmus Ophthalmoplegia Ataxia Memory abnormalities Confabulation	Painful vesicular mucosal eruption Ulceration of the buccal mucosa, mouth floor, palate Hyperesthesia Burning tongue	Test for signs of alcohol abuse Electrolytes CBC and smear Liver function tests Blood sugar level Magnesium B12 Folate Calcium Phosphate Blood alcohol concentrations MRI or CT head	IV thiamine 200–500 mg TID for 5–7 days followed by oral thiamine 100 mg TID for 1–2 weeks then 100 mg daily Laboratory testing should not delay therapy
Riboflavin (B2)	Oro-oculo-genital syndrome Conjunctivitis Angular palpebritis Photophobia Pruritic scaling Perineal rash Seborrheic dermatitis-like rash	Glossitis (magenta) Cheilitis Angular stomatitis Edema of oropharyngeal mucosa	Plasma erythrocyte glutathione reductase activation coefficient (high) Pyridoxamine phosphate oxidase activity (low)	Oral riboflavin 1–3 mg/day for children 10–20 mg/day for adults
Pyridoxine (B6)	Seborrheic dermatitis-like rash Intertrigo Neuropathy Paresthesias Dysesthesias	Angular stomatitis Gingival erythema Small aphthous ulcerations Atrophic glossitis Burning tongue	Plasma pyridoxal-5-phosphate level (low) Urine 4-pyridoxic acid (low)	Oral pyridoxine 30 mg/day
Cyanocobalamin (B12)	Pallor Weakness Fatigue Ataxia Psychological disturbances	Angular cheilitis Painful glossitis Recurrent aphthous ulcers Diffuse erythematous mucositis Mucosal pallor Burning tongue	Serum vitamin B12 (low) Methylmalonic acid (high) Homocysteine (high) MCV (high) CBC and smear Antiparietal cell Ab Anti-IF Ab	Oral B12, 1000 mcg/day OR IM or subcutaneous 1000 mcg weekly IM until normalization of serum B12 levels or for 8 weeks empirically
Folate (B9)	Pallor Weakness Fatigue	Diffuse stomatitis Angular cheilitis Atrophic glossitis Small lingual ulcers with "fiery red borders" Burning tongue	Serum folate level Serum vitamin B12 CBC and smear	Folic acid 1 mg/day Confirm B12 WNL

Table 5.1 (continued)

Deficiency	Clinical findings	Oral findings	Testing	Treatment[a]
Biotin (B7)	Alopecia Hair brittleness Easy hair plucking Seborrheic dermatitis-like intertriginous rash	Perioral dermatitis Atrophy patches of lingual papillae Generalized mucosal erythema Dry crusted lips	Serum biotin Urinary biotin catabolites and 3-hydroxyisovaleric acid (high)	Biotin 150 mcg daily Supplements available in doses of 2500 or 5000 mcg
Vitamin C	Perifollicular hyperkeratosis Hemorrhage Petechia or ecchymoses Arthralgia Corkscrew hairs Osteopenia	Signs in dentulous patients Gingival swelling Bleeding Ecchymoses Loose teeth	CBC with smear Serum ascorbic acid Iron studies	Oral ascorbic acid 250 mg daily OR 100 mg TID OR 1000 mg split over 4 daily doses If severe: 1000 mg daily for 2 weeks Maintenance therapy 250 mg weekly Replace iron, if low
Vitamin A	Ophthalmopathy Night blindness Bitot's spots Xerosis Acneiform papules Follicular keratosis Corkscrew hairs Easy hair plucking Petechia Phrynoderma	Salivary hypofunction Xerostomia Keratinization of salivary glands Enamel fissures and pits Oral leukoplakia Hypervitaminosis A Dry, scaly, fissured lips, gingival erythema, gingivitis, exfoliative angular cheilitis	Serum retinol Zinc and iron levels Ophthalmology consultation	If night blindness is present: IM vitamin A 100,000 IU single dose If chronic vitamin A deficiency is present: vitamin A 50,000 IU until retinol levels normalize
Vitamin D	Rickets or osteomalacia Diffuse osteopenia Enlarged metaphyses Long bone bowing Rachitic rosary	Typically seen in rickets Loss of periodontal attachment Enamel pitting and hypoplasia	Serum 25-hydroxyvitamin D Calcium Ionized calcium Phosphate Parathyroid hormone	Treatment depends on age, sex, comorbid conditions 600 IU for age 1–70 or pregnant or breastfeeding 800 IU for age >71
Vitamin K	Ecchymoses Petechia	Gingival erythema and bleeding Petechia Ecchymoses Hematomas of oral mucosa	Prothrombin time (high) Serum vitamin K Serum uncarboxylated osteocalcin (high)	Oral phytonadione (K1) 2.5–25 mg daily OR IM/IV/SC 10 mg once

(continued)

Table 5.1 (continued)

Deficiency	Clinical findings	Oral findings	Testing	Treatment[a]
Zinc	Eczematous, erythematous, vesiculobullous, or pustular acrofacial and intertriginous dermatitis	Perioral dermatitis sparing upper lip	Serum zinc level	Oral zinc sulfate 50 mg/day for 6 months
		Angular cheilitis		OR
		Oral ulcerations		15–30 mg/kg/day for adults
	Diarrhea	Flattening of filiform papillae		
	Pneumonia	Hypogeusia		0.5–1.0 mg/kg/day for children
	Poor wound healing			
	Growth delay	Xerostomia	Hair zinc level	
			Zinc-dependent enzymes activities	
Niacin (B3)	3 Ds: dementia, dermatitis, and diarrhea	Prodromal burning of mucosa	Serum niacin	Oral nicotinamide 100 mg TID for 3–4 weeks
			Serum tryptophan	
	Photosensitivity	Erythema of the lingual tip (early)	Whole blood nicotinamide adenine dinucleotide (NAD) and nicotinamide adenine dinucleotide (NADP) levels and NAD/NADP ratio (low)	
	Dyspigmentation			OR
	Cracking and crusting of skin	Tongue swelling and burning		500 mg daily for 1 week with transition to 100–300 mg daily for 3–4 weeks
	Depression	"Fiery scarlet hue" of tongue		
	Anxiety			
	Hallucinations	Smooth erythematous tongue		
	Casal's necklace: photosensitive erythema and dyschromia around the neck			Adults: 100 mg every 6 h until CNS and GI symptoms resolve
		Pseudomembrane		
		Patchy inflammation mucosa	Urinary 1-methyl-2-pyridone-5-carboxamide (2-PYR) and 1-methylnicotinamide (1-MN) (more sensitive)	
		Ulceration of lingual margin and buccal mucosa		Maintenance therapy with 50 mg every 8–12 h until cutaneous symptoms resolve
		Angular cheilitis		
		Gingival erythema		
		Dental caries		Children: 10–50 mg every 6 h

MCV mean corpuscular volume, *BID* twice daily, *TIBC* total iron biding capacity, *IV* intravenous, *TID* three times daily, *CBC* complete blood count, *MRI* magnetic resonance imaging, *CT* computerized tomography, *Ab* antibody, *IF* intrinsic factor, *WNL* within normal limits, *IU* international units, *SC* subcutaneously

[a]Treatment course are suggestions, and each patient should be clinically evaluated for comorbidities affecting absorption and metabolism of each vitamin and mineral

IDA may occur secondary to malabsorption states, abnormal bleeding, as well as diets high in oxalates, coffee, tea, and phytate [10, 12, 13]. Ascorbic acid deficiency may also decrease iron absorption [14].

Clinical manifestations of IDA include generalized pallor, weakness, and fatigue. Central nervous system (CNS) changes such as dementia have also been associated with anemia [11].

In the oral cavity, oral mucosal pallor is the characteristic sign of IDA, but this may be associated with angular stomatitis and lingual changes [15, 16]. Specifically, the lingual changes are manifest as a glossitis with atrophy of the papillae resulting in swelling and complaints of soreness and a burning sensation [17, 18] (Fig. 5.1). Continued atrophy and eventual balding of the dorsal tongue is secondary to a decrease in lingual epithelial keratinization and eventual loss of papillae [17]. Atrophy of the tongue and angular stomatitis are not specific for IDA, however, and may be seen in other B-complex vitamin deficiencies. The glossitis of vitamin B12 deficiency and IDA can be exacerbated by candidiasis [18].

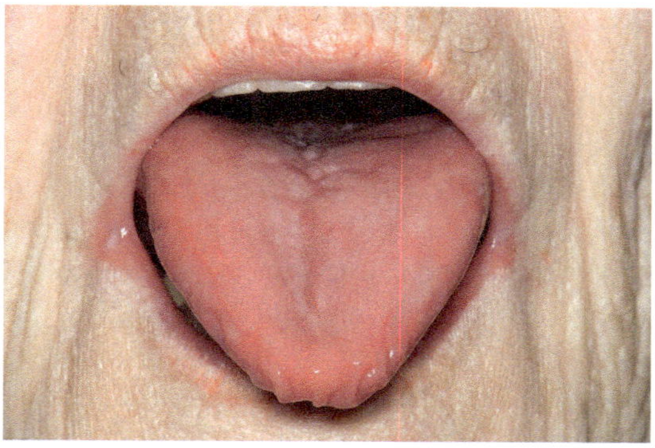

Fig. 5.1 Erosive glossitis and mucosal pallor associated with iron deficiency anemia

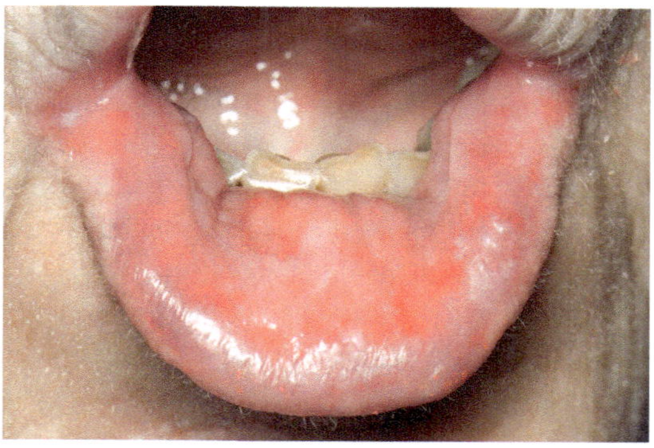

Fig. 5.2 Angular cheilitis and mucosal pallor in a patient with combined vitamins B2 and B6 deficiency

Additionally, since iron absorption depends on adequate vitamin C, the characteristic signs of hemorrhagic gingivitis seen in scurvy may also occur in IDA secondary to ascorbic acid deficiency [14, 19].

Importantly, an association between Plummer-Vinson syndrome (PVS), with its concomitant anemia, and increased risk of oral and hypopharyngeal carcinoma has been proposed [20–22]. PVS is a triad of angular stomatitis, glossitis, and dysphagia, seen with IDA and esophageal webs, which consistently respond to iron therapy [22]. In patients with PVS, a detailed oral cavity examination and review of systems is prudent in order to assess for possible malignant transformation.

The differential diagnosis of IDA and its oral manifestations includes vitamin B12 deficiency, folate deficiency, and other causes of anemia such as anemia of chronic disease.

The treatment of anemia depends on its etiology, and the treatment of IDA specifically is contingent upon absorption status. In the case of normal vitamin C levels and normal gastrointestinal (GI) function, oral ferrous sulfate 300 mg twice daily may be used. Parenteral iron may also be administered, if the GI system is compromised.

Water-Soluble Vitamin Deficiencies

Vitamin B Deficiencies

B-complex vitamin deficiencies have overlapping clinical and sometimes indistinguishable oral findings. Furthermore, multiple vitamins may be deficient in the same patient. Studies assessing nutritional status in women of low socioeconomic groups showed that a majority of this population had vitamin B6 and vitamin B2 deficiencies (Fig. 5.2) [23, 24]. Glossitis and angular stomatitis, formerly thought to be pathognomonic for riboflavin deficiency, may be seen in any of the B-vitamin disorders, as well as previously mentioned IDA. Nonetheless, glossitis, with an associated burning sensation, is the hallmark finding in B-complex vitamin deficiencies [23, 24]. Initially noted as hypertrophy, erythema, and inflammation of the lingual papillae, the fissured appearance of early glossitis eventually evolves to a smooth glazed appearance from papillary atrophy [23]. This atrophy may be further exacerbated, if elderly patients have concomitant sarcopenia (loss of skeletal muscle secondary to malnutrition and age), affecting the tongue [25]. While not specific for these deficiencies, a constellation of glossitis and angular stomatitis should raise suspicion for a vitamin deficit.

Thiamine (Vitamin B1, Aneurin)

Thiamine is a coenzyme of biochemical pathways required for appropriate neurological and cardiac function [26–28]. The true worldwide incidence of thiamine deficiency is undetermined. However, population studies of refugee camps or suspected "thiamine deficiency outbreaks" have been done [29–32]. A recent study showed the prevalence of thiamine deficiency to be 10.5% in Yunnan province in China [33]. While malnutrition and polished rice diet are typically associated with thiamine deficiency, a study of 118 elderly hospitalized patients in a geriatric ward showed moderate thiamine deficiency in up to 40% of patients [34].

Thiamine deficiency produces a group of disorders manifest with neurologic and/or cardiac dysfunction. "Wet beriberi" is a cardiovascular dysfunction characterized by tachycardia and hypotension, mimicking acute coronary syndrome and shock [27]. "Dry beriberi" usually refers to the effects of thiamine deficiency on the peripheral nervous system causing wasting and partial paralysis. Lower extremity weakness, calf pain, edema, and foot drop may be seen [35]. This often occurs in tandem with central nervous system abnormalities due to thiamine deficiency manifesting as Wernicke's encephalopathy (WE), which is the constellation of acute ophthalmoplegia, gait ataxia, and an abnormal mental state [36]. The classic triad, however, is only seen in 16% of patients in whom necropsy studies were confirmatory of WE [36]. Korsakoff's psychosis is another presentation of thiamine deficiency affecting the CNS, characterized by memory abnormalities, anterograde and variable retrograde, as well as confabulation [37]. Neurologic symptoms of thiamine deficiency therefore manifest as "dry beriberi," WE (the aforementioned triad of nystagmus, ophthalmoplegia, and ataxia), and Wernicke-Korsakoff syndrome (WKS – the latter encompassing WE and Korsakoff's psychosis). MRI visualization and postmortem biopsy demonstrating atrophy of the mammillary bodies, thalamus, or the periaqueductal gray matter are consistent with WKS [37].

Sechi and Serra reviewed previous population studies of WE prevalence, citing a 0–2.2% prevalence in the US population and a 1.7–2.8% prevalence in Australia. While the authors considered alcohol abuse as a common etiological factor for WE, they were not able to find a correlation between the prevalence of WE and national alcohol consumption data. Therefore, national thiamine supplementation and dietary habits are also thought to contribute to national prevalence differences in WE [38].

Traditionally, hypermetabolic states, such as pregnancy, fevers, exercise, and diets high in milled (polished) rice, have been risk factors for thiamine deficiency [39]. Alcohol abuse, chronic disability, and poor access to nutritional food also negatively impact thiamine levels [39, 40]. Additionally patients with cyclic vomiting, anorexia, bulimia, and hyperemesis gravidarum may also be at risk.

Thiamine deficiency is typically not associated with oral manifestations and when reported is rare and non-specific [41]. Notwithstanding, however, painful vesicular eruptions and eventual ulceration affecting the buccal mucosa, floor of the mouth, and occasionally palate have rarely been reported [42]. Recurrent aphthous stomatitis (RAS) has also been shown to be associated with low vitamin B1 levels [43, 44]. Glossitis was also noted in a patient with thiamine-responsive wet beriberi [45]. Hyperesthesia and a burning tongue sensation have also been reported [4]. In infants with vitamin B1 deficiency, erythema of the papillae over the anterior third or apex of the tongue has been shown to precede glossitis. Additionally, pinpoint herpetiform vesicles on the buccal mucosa, ventral tongue, and palate have been described [4, 46, 47].

Since oral signs are often absent or non-specific, correlation between neurologic, cardiac, and autonomic findings is necessary, if a thiamine deficiency is suspected. Additional signs of poor hygiene, alcohol use, or malnutrition such as cheilitis, glossitis, and bleeding gums can be helpful clues [48]. Most patients with WKS have a history of alcohol abuse and present in acute settings and are therefore unlikely to be initially seen by an outpatient dermatologist or dentist.

Treatment of patients with WE or WKS will depend on the patient's state of malnutrition. Recommendations also change depending on whether prophylactic dosing or treatment dosing are needed. IV thiamine 200–500 mg three times daily for 5–7 days followed by oral thiamine 100 mg three times daily for 1–2 weeks, then 100 mg daily thereafter, is a reasonable regimen for patients with severe WKS and thiamine deficiency [48].

Riboflavin (Vitamin B2)

Riboflavin and its derivatives are found in multiple food groups including dairy products, meat, and dark green vegetables. Milk is a particularly important source of riboflavin, and poor riboflavin status has been documented in populations lacking dairy products and meats [49–52]. A 2009 study of 179,172 screened individuals in Uganda showed around 90% of patients had evidence of riboflavin deficiency [53]. While nutrient deficiencies are often studied and demonstrated in socioeconomic emergency settings such as refugee camps, other groups with documented low levels of riboflavin or low riboflavin dietary intake are the elderly, as well as schoolchildren and adolescent girls in Western European settings [49, 50, 54]. Additionally, alcoholics, patients taking chlorpromazine, and those with malabsorption syndromes are at risk for riboflavin deficiency [55, 56]. Patients with schizophrenia taking chlorpromazine have depleted levels of flavin adenine dinucleotide (FAD), a coenzyme with riboflavin as its central component.

The classic, yet uncommon, clinical presentation of riboflavin deficiency is an oro-oculo-genital syndrome. Conjunctivitis, photophobia, and a pruritic scaling perineal and scrotal dermatitis may be associated with oral signs [57]. A seborrheic dermatitis-like rash may also be present around the nasolabial folds, nasal ala, forehead, cheeks, and retroauricular areas [47, 58–61]. Cardiovascular disease, mediated by increased levels of homocysteine, and vision deficits with angular palpebritis have been associated with riboflavin deficiency and may necessitate evaluation, if an insufficiency is confirmed [35, 49, 62].

Oral findings of patients deficient in riboflavin include glossitis, cheilitis, stomatitis, and edema of the oral and pharyngeal mucous membranes [1, 3, 60, 63–65]. Angular stomatitis, once thought to be pathognomonic for vitamin B2 deficiency, has been shown to be ameliorated in schoolchildren in India, 21% of whom had stomatitis at baseline, when fortification with riboflavin was instituted [66]. Additionally, when evaluating 1313 adolescents in China, signs of riboflavin deficiency were angular stomatitis, cheilosis, and magenta tongue. Magenta tongue was found in 36% of boys and 40.8% of girls, while angular stomatitis was found in 5.8% and 2.7%, respectively. Cheilosis was present in 8% of boys and 5.6% of girls [61]. Magenta tongue is often used to refer to glossitis of riboflavin deficiency; however, the description is non-specific. On the dorsal tongue, fungiform papillae may expand and overlie the atrophied filiform papillae [42]. A "pebbly" or "granular" appearance of the lingual dorsum may be visualized [5]. A distinct purple discoloration, associated with vascular engorgement, may also be noted, but eventual atrophy of the papillae leads to a smooth and shiny appearance [4]. Patients may complain of a burning mouth sensation and glossodynia; however, this is typically less symptomatic than with pernicious anemia or pellagra [5, 67]. Analogous to studies paralleling low iron levels and oral carcinoma risk, inadequate levels of riboflavin have been evaluated as a risk factor for oral cancer, further emphasizing the importance of a thorough oral examination in patients with suspected vitamin B2 deficiency [68–70].

The differential diagnosis of patients with riboflavin deficiency includes other B-vitamin deficiencies associated with glossitis such as pellagra, vitamin B6, and vitamin B12 deficiencies. Additionally, similar cutaneous findings of perineal and a seborrheic dermatitis-like rash can be seen in zinc deficiency. Concomitant vitamin and/or mineral deficiencies may also be present. If the dietary intake of a patient is balanced, evaluation for a malabsorption disorder may be necessary.

Treatment of riboflavin deficiency, until the resolution of cutaneous signs, can be done with 1–3 mg/day for children or 10–20 mg/day for adults [41, 61]. Perineal and scrotal dermatitis should resolve within several days; however, tongue and lip involvement may be more recalcitrant [61].

Pyridoxine (Vitamin B6)

Pyridoxine deficiency is often present concurrently with overall malnutrition. The documented prevalence of pyridoxine deficiency in the European institutionalized elderly varies broadly, and differences exist between hospitalized and healthy elderly individuals (51% and 9%, respectively) [71]. Additionally, in a study of 61 residents in Norwegian nursing homes, half of the patients had vitamin B6 deficiency [72]. The data on the epidemiology of pyridoxine deficiency is inconsistent, however, and vitamin B6 deficiency was only found in 1 out of 218 institutionalized elderly patients in Spain [73]. Some of these differences may be due to ethnic and geographical population variations or be secondary to the unreliability of serum vitamin levels and discrepancies in laboratory reference ranges.

Vitamin B6 is found in whole grains, meat, poultry, nuts, eggs, vegetables, and non-citrus fruits such as bananas [41, 74]. Cooking, processing, and storage may decrease available pyridoxine in foods [74]. Analogous to riboflavin, pyridoxine is associated with general malnutrition, and indeed, both deficiencies can be seen simultaneously. As previously mentioned, a study assessing nutrition in a low-income female population found both vitamin B2 and B6 to be deficient in this population [23]. Other patients at risk for pyridoxine deficiency are those with systemic inflammatory states such as rheumatoid arthritis (RA), immune system dysfunction and human immunodeficiency virus (HIV) infection, type 1 diabetes mellitus, dialyzed patients, and those taking certain medications [75–79]. Of note, medications that may alter levels of pyridoxine should be considered in the assessment including oral contraceptives (OCP) and isoniazid [80]. Conversely, pyridoxine supplementation has also been shown to decrease isoniazid absorption in animal models [81]. Pyridoxine is often used in combination with isoniazid for the prevention of isoniazid-induced peripheral neuropathy, thought to be secondary to decreased vitamin B6 levels, during tuberculosis therapy [82].

Similar to the aforementioned vitamin deficiencies, a seborrheic dermatitis-like eruption, intertrigo, and neuropathy, along with other non-specific neurologic symptoms such as paresthesias and dysesthesias, can also be clinical manifestations of pyridoxine deficiency [77, 83].

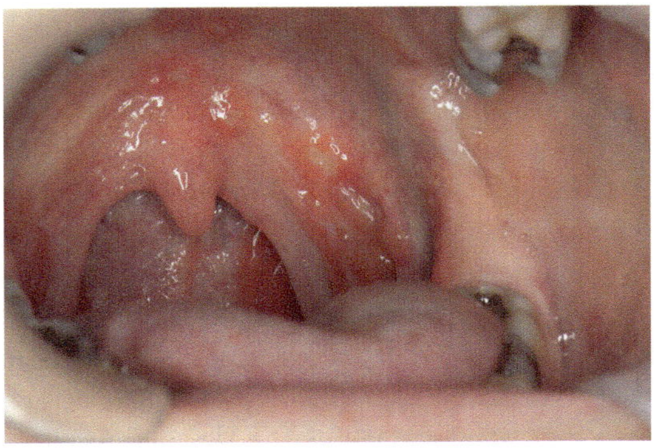

Fig. 5.3 Aphthous ulcers presenting as shallow white to yellow ulcerations with bright erythematous halos

Oral signs of vitamin B6 deficiency include angular stomatitis, gingival erythema, small aphthous ulcerations (Fig. 5.3), and atrophic glossitis [1, 41, 42, 58]. Patients may also give a history of burning tongue with significant erythema demonstrated on examination [5, 42]. "Hypertrophied red knobs" is the term used to describe the flattening of the filiform papillae of the tongue [5].

The differential diagnosis is similar to that of vitamin B2 deficiency. Pellagra, vitamin B12 and folate deficiency, and iron deficiency anemia may present with similar oral and sensory findings. A peripheral smear, demonstrating sideroblasts with vitamin B6 deficiency, and hypersegmented neutrophils with both vitamin B12 and folate deficiencies and mean corpuscular volume (high in B12 and folate deficiencies and low in IDA) may be used to differentiate these disorders [84].

Treatment recommendations vary depending on the etiology and severity of the disease. Prophylaxis for patients taking isoniazid may be done with 50–100 mg daily [85]. The recommended dietary dose is usually below 100 mg/day, while 30 mg/day orally is the suggested dose for correction of pyridoxine deficiency [85]. Excessive supplementation with vitamin B6 may lead to sensory neuropathy [86, 87].

Cyanocobalamin (Vitamin B12)

The prevalence of vitamin B12 deficiency varies among age groups and geographic locations. In the general population, prevalence varies between 3% and 5% and may be as high as 20% in people older than 65 years [88, 89]. In the United Kingdom (UK) and the USA, vitamin B12 deficiency is 6% in patients below 60 years of age and approaches 20% in people older than 60 [90, 91]. Certain populations of African children and Indian adults have significantly higher rates of vitamin B12 deficiency [91]. Malnutrition and ethnic dietary variations may explain these differences. Since vitamin B12 is almost exclusively found in animal products, vegans and strict vegetarians are at risk of deficiency. Studies following Bhutanese refugees resettled in the USA in 2008 confirmed a vitamin B12 deficiency prevalence drop from 64% to 27% [92]. Furthermore, patients with malabsorption and terminal ileum abnormalities, such as those with Crohn's disease (CD), may be deficient in vitamin B12. Pernicious anemia is an autoimmune megaloblastic anemia secondary to the destruction of gastric parietal cells or intrinsic factor released by these cells. Antiparietal cell antibodies and antibodies against intrinsic factor, a glycoprotein required for vitamin B12 absorption on the surface of ileal enterocytes, are usually implicated in the etiology of pernicious anemia [93, 94]. Less commonly discussed causes of vitamin B12 deficiency are gastric bypass surgery, pancreatic insufficiency, bacterial overgrowth, and fish tapeworm infestation [93].

Significant vitamin B12 deficiency may manifest with a combination of anemia and ataxia. The typical pallor of anemia may be present, and a peripheral blood smear will show macrocytosis, hypersegmented neutrophils, and, potentially, depression of all cell lines [91]. CNS involvement includes motor and sensory disturbances, cognitive impairment, and memory alterations. Decrease in vibratory sense, proprioception, and areflexia may be accompanied by motor deficits, ranging from clumsiness to difficulty walking due to poor coordination [91]. Psychological disturbances associated with B12 deficiency may present as stupor or frank psychosis with hallucinations and paranoia [91]. Osteoporosis and alopecia have also been associated with cobalamin deficiency [35, 91].

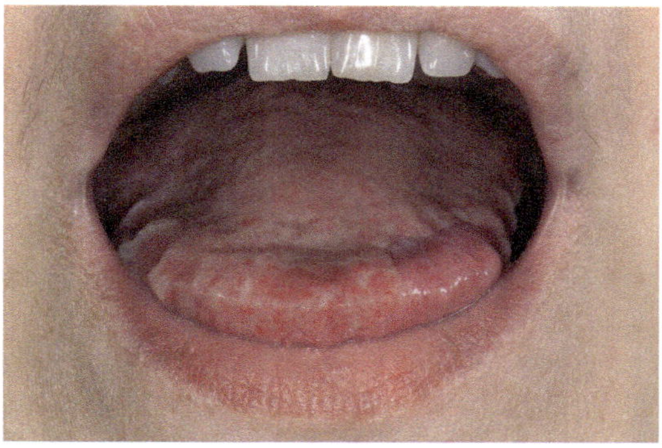

Fig. 5.4 Glossitis secondary to vitamin B12 deficiency

An early diagnosis of oral signs may prevent the development of neurological symptoms [95]. Additionally, in a review of 14 patients, it was noted that the oral signs of low vitamin B12 may occur even in the absence of measurable anemia [96]. Oral manifestations of vitamin B12 deficiency included angular cheilitis, glossitis, recurrent aphthous ulcers, diffuse erythematous mucositis, mucosal pallor, and possible superimposed candidiasis [95, 96]. Eighteen percent to 28% of patients with anemia secondary to vitamin B12, folate, or iron deficiencies may develop RAS, and hence aphthous ulcers may also be one manifestation of vitamin B12 deficiency [3, 97–99]. Hunter's glossitis describes the atrophic, erythematous, and painful tongue of cyanocobalamin deficiency (Fig. 5.4) [100]. The atrophy is accompanied by fissuring and possible loss of the circumvallate papillae. These physical findings are associated with sensory alterations including a prodrome of burning and soreness. Patients may also complain of diminished taste sensation, likely secondary to the atrophy of circumvallate papillae [5]. As with other causes of glossitis, candidiasis should be ruled out by culturing the dorsal tongue [99].

Hypersegmented neutrophils and megaloblasts on peripheral blood smear may be seen with both cyanocobalamin and folate deficiencies, but elevated methylmalonic acid and homocysteine levels, seen exclusively in vitamin B12 deficiency, can differentiate the two entities. Riboflavin and pyridoxine deficiencies should also be considered. Additionally, neurologic symptoms and anemia may be secondary to other etiologies such medication use or illicit drug effects. Ataxia and loss of vibration and proprioception should also alert a clinician to the possibility of tertiary syphilis or other neurologic diseases.

The replacement route of vitamin B12 deficiency depends on the absorption status of the patient. If enteral absorption is possible, oral replacement with 1000 mcg/day may be given [101, 102]. If parietal cells and the terminal ileum are destroyed or absent or the patient is deficient in intrinsic factor, intramuscular (IM) monthly vitamin B12 injections may be given [85, 102]. One thousand micrograms weekly IM or subcutaneously have been suggested until the normalization of serum vitamin B12 levels, or for 8 weeks, if used empirically. Levels of cyanocobalamin after an IM injection may be exhausted within 3 weeks; therefore, ongoing monthly supplementation is recommended in patients with pernicious anemia, if parenteral supplementation is required [85].

Folic Acid

With the fortification of cereal and other foods, folate deficiency is almost nonexistent in the USA. In a recent study of 2563 red blood cell folate samples in a large urban inpatient hospital, only 4 samples (0.16%) were found to be in the deficient range [89]. But this low prevalence is not ubiquitous. In a Swiss population of pregnant women, 4% had low serum folate levels and 63% of women were taking folate supplementation [103]. In Jordan, a study of pregnant women in 2010 demonstrated the prevalence of folate deficiency and insufficiency to be 13.6% and 82.9%, respectively [104]. Multiple nutrients, including folate, were measured in 1163 Chinese pregnant women. In the cohort with anemia – 44% of the overall study population – folate deficiency was found in 22.7% [105]. In older Belgian patients diagnosed with all forms of anemia, folate deficiency typically makes up 5.5% of the etiologies [8, 9].

Folate is present in fruits, grains, nuts, poultry, and dark green leafy vegetables. Alcoholics and the elderly, as well as patients taking medications interfering with folate metabolism, such as methotrexate or antipsychotics, are at risk of folic acid deficiency [3]. In the aforementioned study on 2563 folate samples with 4 demonstrating deficiency, 1 patient had a malabsorption syndrome, 1 was an alcoholic, 1 had schizophrenia, and in the last patient, no obvious etiologic factor was identified [89]. Biliary stasis can also cause an immediate drop in serum folate levels [93, 106]. Physiologic and pathologic states with hyperproliferation or growth of tissues, such as pregnancy, hemolysis, leukemia, and exfoliative dermatitis, may also lower serum folate concentration [93].

Megaloblastic anemia is the typical measurable hematologic presentation of folate deficiency. Homocysteine levels alone would be elevated in folate deficiency, as opposed to both methylmalonic acid and homocysteine elevations in vitamin B12 deficiency. Clinically, CNS signs are more closely associated with vitamin B12 deficiency and will progress in the absence of supplementation. No other consistent clinical findings are noted with folate-deficient patients. It is important to remember, however, that folate deficiency in pregnant women is associated with fetal neural tube defects.

While most general signs of folate deficiency are unremarkable, the oral cavity can be significantly involved and symptomatic in affected individuals. The earliest complaints may be significant burning and soreness, and these sensations may persist throughout the clinical course until the patient is appropriately treated [1, 3, 5, 41]. The burning sensation of the tongue can be quite severe. Diffuse stomatitis and angular cheilitis may also be present. Atrophic glossitis with small lingual ulcers with "fiery red borders" have also been described [5, 42].

Since folate therapy may mask a vitamin B12 deficiency, checking vitamin B12 levels and performing a CNS examination prior to treating with folate is recommended [93, 107]. Multiple folate dosing regimens, ranging from 400 mcg to 5 g, have been proposed, depending on pregnancy status, risk for neural tube defects, and concurrent medication use. A dose of 1 mg/day is an appropriate therapy for chronic deficiency [85].

Biotin

Biotin is sometimes called vitamin B7 or vitamin H. It may be found in nuts, legumes, and cooked egg yolks. Biotin supplements are also quite popular due to anecdotal efficacy in various forms of alopecia. Biotin deficiency may be acquired due to anticonvulsant therapy or excess ingestion of raw eggs. Avidin, a glycoprotein in raw eggs, binds to biotin, making it unavailable in tissues [108, 109]. Anticonvulsants, on the other hand, increase biotin breakdown [110, 111]. Biotin deficiency may also be seen when infants are weaned from breastfeeding [112]. Genetic or inborn forms of biotin deficiency include biotinidase deficiency and holocarboxylase deficiency [113, 114]. In the general population, the highest estimated incidence of biotinidase deficiency is 1:35,000 [115].

Alopecia, brittleness, and easy plucking of hair may clinically present in patients with a biotin deficiency [35]. A seborrheic dermatitis-like rash in the intertriginous areas may be noted, in association with periorificial dermatitis [58].

Intraoral signs of biotin deficiency are extremely rare. These may include patches of atrophy of the lingual papillae and generalized mucosal erythema [42]. Dry crusted lips and periorificial dermatitis are more common [42].

Zinc deficiency, pellagra, and other eczematoid dermatitides should be considered in the differential diagnosis of biotin deficiency. Since many of these signs and symptoms are nonspecific, urinary testing with excreted 3-methylcrotonylglycine, 3-hydroxyisovaleric acid, and methylcitric acid can be done, showing significant elevation in patients with biotin deficiency [112]. Serum biotin can be measured but is a less sensitive marker of tissue levels, as compared with the urinary biotin catabolites [110].

Biotin has been described as a "nontoxic" supplement. Toxicity has not been documented in humans, and doses as high as 200 mg orally and 20 mg intravenously have been used [116, 117]. For biotin replacement, 150 mcg daily is recommended [58]. Supplements on the market, however, may come in doses of 2500 or 5000 mcg and often combined with B-complex vitamins and vitamin C.

Vitamin C Deficiency (Scurvy)

Vitamin C (aka ascorbic acid) deficiency has been studied extensively in multiple population studies. Most authors have focused on lower socioeconomic groups, and indeed, studies from the UK and North America have estimated one in five men and one in nine women being deficient in vitamin C [118]. In the US population, 13% were deficient in vitamin C from 1988 to 1994, but this prevalence decreased to 7.1% in a 2009 follow-up study [119, 120]. The groups that were found to be most at risk were smokers, those who did not use vitamin C supplements, and non-Hispanic Black males [119]. Low socioeconomic status was consistently associated with risk for deficiency [120]. When looking at gender in the lower income groups in Glasgow, 26% of men and 14% of women, ages 25–74, had insufficient serum vitamin C levels [121]. Additionally, in the UK, 25% of men and 16% of women over 19 years of age had low vitamin C levels [122]. In Toronto, 14% of non-smoking women ages 20–29 had vitamin C deficiency [123]. In a 2003 Mexican study, Villalpando et al. found that 40% of women between 12 and 49 years of age were deficient [124]. Additionally, in 5638 randomly selected people in India, 45.7% of individuals from southern India and 73.9% of individuals from northern India were vitamin C deficient. Male sex, tobacco use, and older age were all considered risk factors for vitamin C deficiency in this population, most of whom had poor nutrition at baseline [118]. Another study from western India showed that only 9.6% and 13% of men and women, respectively, were deficient; however, over half had suboptimal vitamin C levels [125].

The elderly and patients with Roux-en-Y gastric bypass, in addition to tobacco users and lower income groups, are at risk of vitamin C deficiency. From 145 consecutive patients admitted to an acute geriatric ward in France, 12% had clinical symptoms and signs of scurvy, such as perifollicular hyperkeratosis, bruising, easy bleeding, and gingivitis [126]. In 1163 pregnant Chinese women, in the anemia cohort, 64% were also deficient in ascorbic acid [105]. 32.9% of patients having undergone a Roux-en-Y gastric bypass surgery in Brazil demonstrated a significant reduction in vitamin C levels [127]. Since vitamin C is found in fresh fruits, vegetables, and semi-skimmed milk, patients on strictly fast food diets without supplementation are also at risk [128]. Furthermore, cooking or prolonged storage of food may also decrease the available vitamin C [129].

Since ascorbic acid is a necessary cofactor for collagen biosynthesis, including pericapillary collagen, bleeding is the cardinal clinical sign of vitamin C deficiency, secondary to weakened vascular walls and capillary fragility [128, 129]. Additionally, anemia is also a hallmark of scurvy, since ascorbic acid aids iron absorption by reducing it to a ferrous state [128]. Symptoms similar to those in patients with IDA may manifest. Scurvy, the symptomatic form of severe vitamin C deficiency, is manifest by perifollicular hyperkeratosis and hemorrhage, petechia or ecchymoses, arthralgia, corkscrew hairs, and osteopenia [35, 126, 128]. Signs of easy bleeding from venous puncture sites may also be seen.

Oral signs of scurvy are typically only seen in patients with teeth [5, 63, 128, 130]. Oral manifestations and an accurate history may be the only clues to a diagnosis of vitamin C deficiency [131]. These manifestations include extensive gingival swelling, bleeding, petechia, and loose teeth (Fig. 5.5) [63, 131]. Erythema may involve the labial-free gingival margins adjacent to the teeth, and spontaneous hemorrhage can occur due to vascular instability [128, 131]. Edentulous areas of the mucosa and gingiva may demonstrate pallor secondary to anemia [129]. Halitosis may also be noted [131]. A study of gingivitis and periodontitis in healthy and diabetic patients demonstrated low levels of ascorbic acid in healthy subjects with gingivitis and diabetics with periodontitis. Supplementation with ascorbic acid improved these symptoms [132].

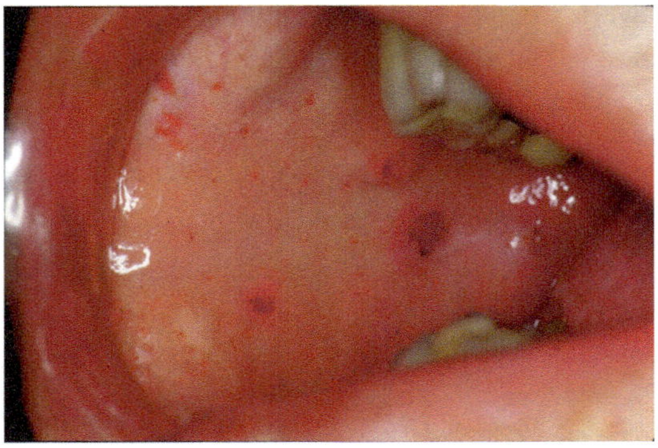

Fig. 5.5 Mucosal petechia and hemorrhage seen in scurvy

Scurvy should be considered, if a patient presents with the "four Hs" including hemorrhagic signs, hyperkeratosis, hematologic abnormalities, and hypochondriasis [128, 133]. Other differential diagnoses include leukemia, musculoskeletal infections, bleeding diatheses, vasculitides, and vitamin K deficiency [128]. Although iron deficiency may be concomitant with vitamin C deficiency, patients may have a slightly elevated mean corpuscular volume (MCV) or microcytosis and a reduced serum ascorbic acid level upon laboratory assessment [129].

Treatment with 250 mg of ascorbic acid orally twice daily, 100 mg three times daily, or 1000 mg daily split over four doses, depending on dosing preference, are all recommended treatment options [41, 131, 134]. Patients with severe deficiency may benefit from the 1000 mg regimen for 2 weeks followed by maintenance therapy with 250 mg weekly [134]. If iron replacement is needed, a supplement of iron and vitamin C is also available in a combination form of ferrous fumarate and ascorbic acid [135].

Fat-Soluble Vitamin Deficiencies

Vitamin A

Vitamin A, typically measured as retinol in the serum, is required for proper epithelial cell turnover and vision development. Most studies regarding the prevalence of vitamin A deficiency (VAD) are done in children in order to assess for night blindness. In fact, several studies use night blindness as a screening tool to identify cases of VAD. Additionally, the normal values of retinol vary among studies; however, subclinical VAD is usually defined as <20 or <30 µg/dl. As with most studies on nutritional deficiencies, lower income groups are typically investigated. By 2009, the prevalence of VAD in China was 10%. No gender differences existed, but prevalence increased with age [33]. In Brazil, 546 schoolchildren between 7 and 14 years of age demonstrated a 27.5% prevalence of VAD, as demonstrated by retinol values <30 μg/dL. Lower weight and younger age were thought to be variables predisposing children to VAD [136]. In Panama and El Salvador, as defined by serum retinol <20 μg/dL, the prevalence of VAD in children less than 5 years of age was 6 and 36%, respectively [137]. In Bangladesh, severe VAD in preschool children, demonstrated by night blindness, was 0.6% by 1996; however, subclinical VAD was high [138]. In the same study, the prevalence of night blindness in rural mothers was 1.4% [138]. Similarly, in Nepal, the prevalence of night blindness was 5% in women and 1% among school-aged children. Low serum retinol levels were found in 32.3% of children and 16.6% of women [139]. In Ethiopia, 37.7% of children had VAD and 0.8% had night blindness [140].

Risk factors for VAD, as suggested by these studies, are male gender, older age in children, wasting or low body weight, and living in a rural setting [33, 139, 140]. However, the Brazilian study showed that younger age groups and lower body weight were associated with VAD risk as opposed to heavier and older patients tested in the study population [136]. Nevertheless, children in general are an at-risk group for VAD and the associated sequelae. In women, risks for VAD include age less than 20 years, pregnancy, and a rural setting [139]. Other groups at risk for VAD are patients with short bowel syndrome, of whom 5% have been shown to have VAD in a prospective US study [141]. Additionally, in an Australian study, 13% of patients with cystic fibrosis (CF) were deficient in vitamin A [142]. Patients with CF, exocrine pancreatic insufficiency, and biliary stasis often have vitamin A and other fat-soluble vitamin deficiencies, due to malabsorption. Another unique patient population shown to have acute VAD is children with measles [143].

Clinical manifestations of VAD include ophthalmopathy with night blindness and Bitot's spots – areas of keratin deposition on the conjunctiva. Bitot's spots were found in 1.7% of all children in Ethiopia [140]. Cutaneous signs of VAD are xerosis, acneiform papules, follicular keratosis, corkscrew hairs similar to those of vitamin C deficiency, easy hair plucking, and petechia [35]. Phrynoderma, "frog skin," is also seen in chronic VAD [144, 145]. The xerophthalmia of VAD is a common cause of blindness in childhood [146].

Salivary hypofunction, as manifested by xerostomia, is frequently associated with VAD. Patients complain of dry mouth and are at increased risk of oral infections such as candidiasis due to lower levels of protective enzymes and an altered mucosal barrier [147]. The teeth of patients with VAD may demonstrate alterations of enamel including fissures and pits [4]. The teeth may also appear to be white and "unglazed" [4]. Oral leukoplakia may be seen and has been demonstrated to respond to vitamin A therapy in these cases [148].

In an era of systemic retinoid use, it is important to also be familiar with the potential risk of hypervitaminosis A. Oral manifestations of this excess are dry, scaly, fissured lips, gingival erythema, gingivitis, and exfoliative angular cheilitis [3, 4, 41].

The differential diagnosis of VAD includes scurvy, ichthyosis vulgaris or other ichthyotic conditions, and asteatotic dermatitis.

Treatment of VAD deficiency depends on the severity of symptoms and etiology of the deficiency. For xerostomia, artificial saliva and soft, nonirritating foods, such as soup, may be used [149]. For VAD associated with night blindness and a clear diagnosis of low retinol levels, an IM injection of 100,000 international units (IU) of vitamin A may be given as a single dose [150]. In cases of chronic vitamin A deficiency, such as patients with bariatric surgery, a daily dose of 50,000 IU of vitamin A may be used until retinol levels normalize. However, treatment should be undertaken on a case-by-case basis, and patients should be monitored for signs of vitamin A excess.

Vitamin D

Vitamin D has been a popular topic of investigation in recent years. Its importance in calcium absorption and homeostasis is well established; however, vitamin D levels and clinical correlations are being investigated in almost all fields of medicine. Among population studies, addressing the epidemiology of vitamin D deficiency varies with season of the year, level of ultraviolet light exposure, and ethnicity. 25-Hydroxyvitamin D2 and sometimes 25-hydroxyvitamin D3 – 25(OH) D – are the vitamin D metabolites used for screening patients' sera in order to assess for deficiency. Blood levels of vitamin D metabolites with deficiency and insufficiency vary for each study, depending on selected laboratory ranges and cutoffs. Patients with insufficiency have higher levels of vitamin D than those with a deficiency. In the USA, Whites have higher vitamin D levels than Blacks and Hispanics [151]. In the month of January, 65.4% of non-Hispanic Blacks are estimated to be deficient versus 28.9% of Hispanics and 14% of Whites. Insufficiency rates in these groups are 84.2%, 56.3%, and 34.8%, respectively [152]. In Ireland, 40.1% of adult individuals had 25(OH)D levels inadequate for bone health at the level of <50 nmol/L [153]. Vitamin D deficiency, defined as <30 nmol/L in this study, was prevalent in 6.7% of this population [153]. In a large national study in Mexico, the prevalence of vitamin D insufficiency, as defined by 25(OH)D <50 nmol/L, was 24%, 10%, 8%, and 10% for preschoolers, school-aged children, adolescents, and adults, respectively. The overall deficiency prevalence, defined by 25(OH)D <20 nmol/L, was actually less than 1% in all age groups [154]. When evaluating the presence of chronic kidney disease (CKD) in association with vitamin D deficiency, in a cohort of 1145 patients, vitamin D concentrations and deficiency status were similar in the CKD and healthy groups. In this study 11.8% of patients had CKD without dialysis, and 69.1% had either deficient or insufficient levels of 25(OH)D, as compared to 75.3% of the healthy subjects – hence very similar rates [155].

Typically, children have higher 25(OH)D levels than adults, and males have higher intake and levels of vitamin D than females [151]. Leaner individuals have higher 25(OH)D concentrations and are more likely to use supplements than their heavier counterparts [151]. Other major determinants of vitamin D status were altitude, exercise, and serum albumin-corrected calcium [155]. Deficiency is typically seen in the spring and winter, except for patients in Brazil, who demonstrated lowest concentrations of 25(OH)D in the summer [33, 151, 153, 156]. An evaluation of 635 patients in Sao Paulo, Brazil, identified male sex, high body mass index (BMI), high waist circumference, low physical activity, tobacco and alcohol use, younger age, low family income, darker skin color, and season of the year, as risk factors for vitamin D deficiency [156]. Lastly, patients with fat malabsorption are at risk of deficiency. Notably, 15.5% of CF patients in Australia demonstrated a vitamin D deficiency [142]. Since 25-hydroxyvitamin D3 is synthesized in the liver, patients with cholestasis or liver cirrhosis are prone to deficiency in functional forms of vitamin D. Ultraviolet light (UVB) converts 7-dihydrocholestorol (provitamin D3) in the skin to previtamin D3. Subsequently, this form is converted to vitamin D3 by the keratinocytes and eventually is transferred to the liver and kidneys for conversion to 25-hydroxyvitamin D3 and 1,25-dihydroxyvitamin D3, respectively [157]. This partially explains why patients with darker skin types and those with liver disease have been shown to have lower levels of 25(OH)D [158]. Ergocalciferol (vitamin D2) and cholecalciferol (vitamin D3) can be ingested as supplements; however, only vitamin D3 is also endogenously synthesized with exposure to sunlight [157].

Clinical manifestations of severe vitamin D deficiency are manifest as rickets. Rickets may be secondary to improper intake or malabsorption of vitamin D or due to congenital aberrant homeostasis of phosphorus, calcium, and parathyroid hormone [159–163]. Patients demonstrate diffuse osteopenia and enlarged metaphyses, as evidenced by radiographic films, long bone bowing, and prominent nodules at the costochondral joints, known as rachitic rosary. Patients with genetic vitamin D deficiency or pseudo-vitamin D deficiency rickets (PDDR), secondary to CYP27B1 mutation, may also demonstrate failure to thrive, hypotonia, and growth retardation [163]. The adult equivalent of rickets is termed osteomalacia or thinning of bones. Other manifestations of vitamin D deficiency, such as increased risk for Alzheimer's disease, have been investigated [164].

Oral signs of vitamin D deficiency are typically associated with improper tooth eruption, jaw development, and enamel formation. In patients with rickets, tooth eruption is delayed and enamel hypoplasia is present in the erupted teeth [163]. Inadequate calcification, secondary to lack of proper calcium absorption and homeostasis in the setting of vitamin D deficiency, can lead to hypoplastic defects in the teeth such as fissures, pits, and grooves in the enamel [4]. A dental examination of patients with vitamin D-dependent rickets (VDDR) may demonstrate hypoplastic enamel, with a yellow-to-brown color, malocclusion, and chronic periodontal disease [165]. Dental radiographs may reveal short roots, poorly outlined lamina dura, large quadrangular pulp chambers, and hypoplastic alveolar ridges [161, 165].

Jaw bones and crowns of teeth may also be deformed. The predentin may be wider in severe deficiency, due to lack of dentin matrix mineralization [4]. Patients with PDDR and vitamin D-resistant rickets (VDRR) have abnormal teeth with thin globular dentin and enlarged pulp horns extending into the dentinoenamel junction [161]. On physical examination of patients with VDRR, short stature and a concave facial profile are noted [160]. The mandibular arch may be edentulous, while the maxillary molars may demonstrate root resorption, hypoplasia, and dentin abnormalities [160]. Additionally, spontaneous gingival and dental abscesses may develop in patients with VDDR without a preceding traumatic history [161]. In summary, loss of the periodontal attachment, alterations in the permanent dentition, and enamel pitting are commonly seen in disorders of vitamin D homeostasis [166, 167].

The differential diagnosis of vitamin D deficiency includes overall states of malnutrition, poor hygiene, various forms of rickets, conditions of amelogenesis or dentinogenesis imperfecta, and disorders of dental dysplasia [159–162].

Recommendations for treatment of vitamin D deficiency depend on the severity and etiology of the disease, comorbid conditions, as well as age and pregnancy status of patients. Calcium, phosphate, and parathyroid hormone may also influence the therapeutic regimen. The use of sunscreens has been linked to decreased endogenous vitamin D production [157]. While this topic is controversial, the damaging effects of UVR overshadow the positive benefit of endogenous vitamin D production [168]. Some studies suggest that 15 min of sun exposure daily is enough to achieve appropriate vitamin D levels with minimal UVR-induced damage; however, geographical differences and multiple confounding variables make the determination of appropriate amounts of UV exposure for vitamin D production difficult [169]. Oral supplementation is commonly recommended, often taken in addition to calcium. The appropriate amount of vitamin D supplementation varies due to a lack of guidelines and standardization; however, 400 IU/day is typically recommended for most adults [170]. Additionally, natural sources of vitamin D include fish, liver, eggs, cheese, fortified milk, and other dairy products [168].

Vitamin K

Vitamin K is essential in the formation of clotting factors produced by the liver, in maintaining bone strength, and preventing vascular calcification [171–174]. The prevalence of vitamin K deficiency (VKD) is frequently studied in the newborn population due to the risk of intracranial and systemic hemorrhage in infants with a deficiency of vitamin K-dependent coagulation factors. For this reason, many countries have instituted prophylactic vitamin K injections at birth. In the US state of Tennessee, early VKD bleeding (VKDB) ranges from 0.25% to 1.7% of births. Late bleeding, typically seen between 6 and 15 weeks after birth, occurs in 4.4–7.2 per 100,000 infants. The estimated risk of late VKDB in infants who do not receive prophylaxis was 81 times greater in this US study. In China from 1998 to 2001, the incidence of

VKDB was 3.3%, with rural areas being disproportionately affected [33]. In special populations, such as patients with inflammatory bowel disease (IBD), the prevalence of VKD is 54% and 43% in CD and ulcerative colitis (UC), respectively [175]. In CF children, low vitamin K was demonstrated in 29% of patients, a finding partially explained by the malabsorption of fat-soluble vitamins in this patient population [142]. VKD was seen in 63% of patients with chronic pancreatitis, half of whom had alcohol abuse as the driving etiology [176]. Since vitamin K may be ingested in food and synthesized by gut bacteria, patients with abnormalities in gut flora may also be deficient. Drugs interfering with the action of vitamin K, such as warfarin and fluoroquinolones, may also cause the signs of VKD.

As discussed, bleeding tendencies, evidenced by a prolonged prothrombin time on laboratory evaluation, and osteoporosis clinically are the major clinical and radiological manifestations of VKD.

Oral manifestations of VKD include gingival erythema and bleeding, especially after brushing of teeth. Petechia, ecchymoses, and hematomas of the oral mucosa may also be present. Severely deficient patients may demonstrate constant slow bleeding from the gums [4, 41].

Vitamin C deficiency may mimic VKD. Other differential diagnoses for the oral manifestations of VKD are leukemia and vasculitides.

Oral phytonadione (K1) is typically used in patients with normal absorption and metabolism of vitamin K. If patients have fat malabsorption, such as those with CF or pancreatitis, oral menadione, a synthetic provitamin of vitamin K, may be used. IM or subcutaneous forms of vitamin K are also available.

Zinc Deficiency

Zinc deficiency, termed acrodermatitis enteropathica (AE) when symptomatic, is quite common in subclinical testing. An estimated 20% of the world population is zinc deficient, particularly in low-income settings [177–179]. In a Chinese study from 1995 to 2006, 50–70% of people were found to be zinc deficient [33]. An astounding 90% of women in Malawi were found to be deficient in zinc [180]. The genetic form of AE, typically secondary to SLC39A4 mutations on chromosome 8q24.3, encoding the Zip4 zinc transporter, has an incidence of 1 in 500,000 children [177].

In addition to genetic AE, vegans, alcoholics, as well as patients with HIV, CF, and IBD are at risk for zinc deficiency [181]. Some infants demonstrate zinc deficiency, if the mother's milk has low zinc levels, as seen in mothers with the SLC30A2 mutation [182, 183]. Patients on TPN and some enteral nutrition (EN) formulas may also demonstrate a deficiency [184].

An eczematous, erythematous, vesiculobullous, or pustular acrofacial and intertriginous dermatitis may be seen with AE [35]. Diarrhea and pneumonia are also associated with zinc deficiency. Wound healing and growth may also be impaired [185, 186].

Perioral and periorificial eczematous to pustular dermatitis are characteristically seen in AE. Angular cheilitis with oral ulcerations may also be present [143, 187, 188]. A "U-shaped or horseshoe-shaped configuration" is used to describe perioral dermatitis of zinc deficiency due to sparing of the upper lip [58]. Intraoral findings may include flattening of the filiform papillae, impaired healing, and sensations of hypogeusia and xerostomia [35, 181, 189, 190]. Associated diarrhea and eczematous and bullous dermatitis of acral surfaces may accompany the periorificial and oral findings (Fig. 5.6).

The differential diagnosis of AE includes diaper dermatitis, protein malnutrition, vitamin A deficiency or excess, certain forms of psoriasis, necrolytic migratory erythema, and other causes of periorificial dermatitis, including other vitamin deficiencies.

Therapeutic recommendations are inconsistent. Oral supplementation with zinc sulfate 50 mg daily for 6 months is reasonable. Also, a potential weight-based dosing regimen is 0.5–1.0 mg/kg/day for children and 15–30 mg/kg/day for adults [35, 181, 191].

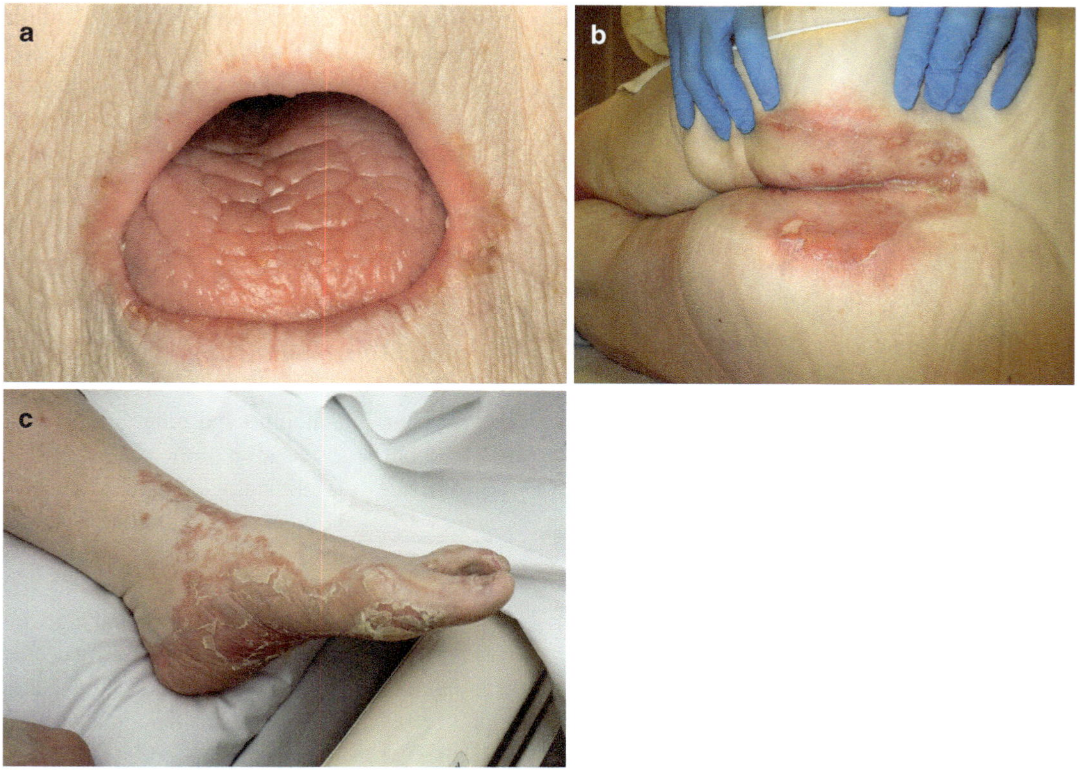

Fig. 5.6 Acrodermatitis enteropathica – zinc deficiency – in a patient with a Roux-en-Y gastric bypass procedure. (**a**) Glossitis and angular cheilitis. (**b**) Eczematous dermatitis and superficial ulcerations of the buttocks and intergluteal cleft. (**c**) Significant acrally distributed desquamation and scaling

Niacin Deficiency (Vitamin B3)

The classic form of niacin deficiency is pellagra, a triad of dermatitis, diarrhea, and dementia [192]. Since this triad is not always present, most studies suggest that pellagra is underdiagnosed [193]. In long-term care patients from Ontario, 37% of patients had niacin deficiency, while in Sweden, 15% of women had suboptimal niacin levels [194, 195]. In a small necropsy study in the alcoholic population, 27% of cases suggested the diagnosis of pellagra [196].

Niacin is ingested from eggs, fish, legumes, cereals, fortified grains, and meats. It is also produced from tryptophan in the human body [41, 191]. Homelessness, chronic alcoholism, and poor nutritional intake associated with these, as well as hypermetabolic states such as acquired immune deficiency syndrome (AIDS) or IBD, are risk factors for niacin deficiency [193]. Additionally, patients with acquired or inherited tryptophan deficiencies, such as carcinoid syndrome or Hartnup disease, may also demonstrate signs of pellagra [197, 198].

All three findings of the aforementioned triad of dementia, dermatitis, and diarrhea is seldom manifested [193]. Photosensitivity, pigment alterations, cracking, and crusting of the skin in a symmetrical distribution may accompany the emotional and psychiatric symptoms of depression, anxiety, and even hallucinations [35]. The characteristic photosensitive erythema and dyschromia around the neck is called Casal's necklace [199].

Prodromal burning of the oral mucosa may precede other oral manifestations [5]. In the early stages of oral involvement, erythema of the lingual tip develops and eventually intensifies to involve the entire dorsal tongue with swelling and a burning sensation [4, 47]. A "fiery scarlet

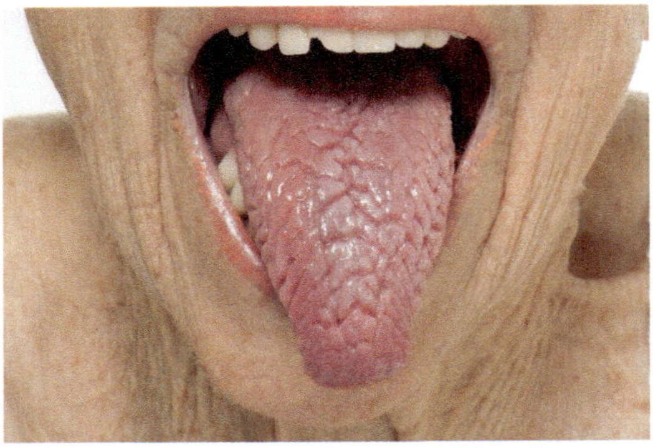

Fig. 5.7 Thick exudative pseudomembrane of the dorsal tongue. Candida superinfection must be ruled out

hue" is used to describe the lingual erythema in pellagra [5, 59]. This erythema and initial swelling may progress to atrophy of the lingual papillae and eventually to a smooth erythematous tongue, secondary to desquamation of the superficial epithelial layers [4, 47]. A thick exudative pseudomembrane, composed of degenerating cells, fibrin, and microorganisms, may form on the dorsal tongue (Fig. 5.7) [5]. Generalized patchy inflammation of the oral mucosa may accompany the lingual changes and sensory complaints [4]. The tongue margins and posterior buccal mucosa may develop ulcerations [5, 42, 59, 192]. Angular cheilitis, gingival erythema and pain, and dental caries may also be present [1, 3, 42, 64].

Niacin deficiency should be considered in states of malnutrition or the aforementioned systemic inflammatory conditions. Protein malnutrition, notably Kwashiorkor, should also be considered. The photosensitivity and dermatitis may also be seen in connective tissue diseases such as lupus. The oral manifestations are nonspecific and may be seen in other B-complex vitamin deficiencies previously discussed. A correlation between the oral signs and neurological, cutaneous, and GI manifestations would suggest pellagra.

Pellagra should be treated, as it may be fatal in severe cases. Oral nicotinamide or niacinamide is the recommended therapy for pellagra. A regimen of 100 mg three times daily for 3–4 weeks is reasonable [193]. Five hundred milligram daily for 1 week with transition to 100–300 mg daily for 3–4 weeks may also be used [40, 199]. Adults may be treated orally with 100 mg every 6 h until acute CNS and GI symptoms resolve. Maintenance therapy with 50 mg every 8–12 h can be given until cutaneous symptoms resolve [41]. Ten to 50 mg every 6 h may be given to children until similar endpoints are reached [41]. Cutaneous signs may resolve rapidly in 2 weeks [199].

Burning Mouth Syndrome

Primary burning mouth syndrome (BMS) presents as a burning sensation of the oral mucosa in the absence of clinically apparent mucosal changes [200]. Middle-aged and elderly women are disproportionally affected. The most commonly involved intraoral anatomic sites are the lingual tip and lateral margins, lips, and hard and soft palate [200]. A 10-year retrospective population-based study from the Mayo Clinic found 169 incident cases with an annual age- and sex-adjusted incidence of 11.4 per 100,000 person years [201]. As expected, women had a significantly higher incidence, 18.8% versus 3.7%, respectively. Demographically, postmenopausal women 50–89 years of age had the highest incidence. Women between 70 and 79 years in particular had the highest incidence [201].

Primary or idiopathic BMS is usually diagnosed upon exclusion of other etiologies. Secondary BMS, on the other hand, may be due to local or systemic factors [202]. Etiopathogenic causes of BMS have not been clearly identified, but investigations into associated nutritional deficiencies have yielded some promise [203]. Nutritional studies are generally ordered when evaluating these patients; however, the literature regarding the efficacy of vitamin replacement in BMS is often contradictory. A large study of 399 patients with BMS identified a significant association between BMS and deficiencies of iron and vitamin B12. Low hemoglobin (Hgb), positivity of serum gastric parietal cell antibodies (GPCA), normal folic acid, and high blood homocysteine were also found to be significant in this population [200]. A follow-up study of the same group of patients evaluated the efficacy of replacement therapy with vitamin BC capsules (containing 10 mg of vitamin B1, 5 mg of vitamin B2, 5 mg of vitamin B6, 5 μg of vitamin B12, 20 mg of calcium pantothenate, 50 mg of nicotinamide, and 60 mg of calcium) and corresponding hematinics, such as vitamin B12, folate, and iron, in which specific cohorts of patients were deficient [202]. One hundred and seventy-seven patients (44%) of the treated patients with primary and secondary BMS with hematinic deficiencies had complete remission of their BMS symptoms [202]. Of the 177 complete responders, 62 patients lacking definite hematinic deficiencies also had a complete remission of their BMS symptoms. A majority of patients with BMS and hematinic deficiencies responded to therapy; however, just under half of patients with IDA and BMS had symptom remission [202].

IDA has often been associated with the symptoms of burning mouth. In an evaluation of 75 patients with IDA and 150 controls, 14 patients had IDA and BMS. It was found that IDA patients had a higher frequency of oral symptoms than their matched controls, and burning oral mucosa was found in 76% of the IDA group [19]. In another population of 276 patients with BMS, it was found that 26.8% had a low serum zinc level [204]. Oral zinc at the dose of 14.1 mg/day was administered to a treatment group with zinc deficiency, and change in pain intensity from baseline was evaluated using a numerical pain scale. The pain scale in the treatment group dropped from 8.1 to 4.1 versus 7.7–6.7 in controls. The authors concluded that zinc replacement may be beneficial for the treatment of BMS in a specific subset of patients with zinc insufficiency [204]. Lastly, an interesting case report of a 46-year-old female with BMS, who failed amitriptyline, gabapentin, and pregabalin, suggested that the addition of 3 g daily of vitamin C completely resolved her symptoms [205]. In this patient, evaluation for deficiency of other vitamins and minerals was negative; however, a vitamin C level was not tested.

These reports allude to potential therapeutic avenues with nutritional supplementation in BMS patients deficient in vitamins and minerals, although other studies refute the etiologic role of hematinic deficiencies and cast doubt on the effectiveness of replacement therapy in symptom resolution [206, 207]. Further investigation is clearly needed. With the current body of evidence, it is prudent to evaluate patients with BMS for nutritional deficiencies including iron, B-vitamins, vitamin C, and zinc (Table 5.2). An empiric therapeutic trial of vitamin BC may be beneficial to patients. Hormonal changes and psychological disorders have also been implicated, but no causality has been established, and a multifactorial origin for BMS is likely [208].

In patients presenting with symptoms of a sore or burning mouth, a broad differential diagnosis must be considered, and secondary etiologies must be ruled out before primary BMS is diagnosed. A complete history and a careful physical exam of the oral cavity should aid in ruling out local or systemic causes. Cultures may be done, as candidiasis and coliform bacterial infections have been associated with a burning sensation [209].

As discussed, hematinic deficiencies should always be considered in patients with symptoms such as dysgeusia, subjective xerostomia, or glossodynia. Abnormalities of the tongue and/or mucosa may be evident, but signs may be subtle and difficult to appreciate, particularly in mild or early stage deficiencies. Therefore, screening tests for nutritional deficiencies, as well as autoimmune conditions, are frequently done when evaluating patients with BMS [208]. While some authors suggest neurological imaging, we recommend that history, physical examination, and review of systems guide clinicians when deciding on the need for imaging.

Recurrent Aphthous Stomatitis

Recurrent aphthous ulcers may be associated with a multitude of systemic diseases, as well as several nutritional deficiencies. Nutritional insufficiencies should be considered in patients with RAS, especially when other aforementioned signs or symptoms are present, concurrently. Specifically, RAS has been commonly associated with IDA, vitamin B12 deficiency, and folate

Table 5.2 Burning mouth syndrome treatment with vitamin replacement

Study	Vitamin intervention	Study parameters	Comments/conclusion
Cho et al. 2010 [204]	Oral zinc 14.1 mg/day	276 patients with BMS 74 (26.8%) low serum zinc Pain intensity 6 months after zinc replacement evaluated using an 11-point numerical scale	Zinc replacement lowered mean numerical pain scale from 8.1 to 4.1 (in zinc-deficient group) From 7.7 to 6.7 (in controls) Zinc deficiency might play a role in some BMS (low zinc) Zinc replacement effective in this group
Sun et al. 2013 [202]	Vitamin BC capsules and appropriate hematinics (B12, folate, iron)	399 patients with primary and secondary BMS Blood homocysteine, vitamin B12, folic acid, iron, and hemoglobin concentrations measured at baseline and after treatment	177 patients (44%) showed complete BMS symptom remission Supplementation with vitamin BC capsules with or without corresponding vitamin B12 and/or folic acid deficiency can reduce high serum homocysteine in BMS patients with or without deficiencies of corresponding hematinics
Lin et al. 2013 [200]	None	399 patients with BMS and 399 controls Blood Hgb, iron, vitamin B12, folic acid, and homocysteine concentrations and the serum GPCA level measured	BMS patients had higher frequency of Hgb, iron, or vitamin B12 deficiency, elevated blood homocysteine level, and serum GPCA positivity than healthy controls
Murray 2014 [205]	Vitamin C 3 gm daily	46-year-old female 4-month history of BMS	Complete symptom resolution
Wu et al. 2014 [19]	None	75 IDA and 150 healthy controls 14 patients with BMS and IDA CBC, iron, vitamin B12, folic acid, and homocysteine measured	IDA patients had significantly higher frequencies of all oral manifestations than healthy controls (burning oral mucosa 76%)

BMS burning mouth syndrome, *IDA* iron deficiency anemia, *CBC* complete blood count, *GPCA* gastric parietal cell antibodies

deficiency [3, 19, 97–99]. Angular cheilitis, glossitis, and mucosal pallor may also be seen in these patients. The ulcerations in folate deficiency may more commonly involve the lingual borders and demonstrate intensely red edges [5, 42]. For these patients, a CBC, iron studies, folate, and vitamin B12 levels may be helpful. Less commonly, RAS has been reported in patients with low serum thiamine, pyridoxine, niacin, or zinc [44]. Appropriate tests for these nutrients may help rule out these etiologies. Aphthous ulcers have been described in pellagra; however, the ulcerations associated with pellagra are generally not recurrent, but persistent. While RAS is a symptom not unique to nutritional deficiencies, a laboratory investigation for these vitamins and minerals is prudent, as replacement of hematinic deficiencies has been shown to aid in alleviating the severity of RAS [44].

Conclusion

Nutritional deficiencies should be considered when patients present with oral symptoms such as pain, burning, or taste disturbance; when the oral cavity displays signs such as glossitis, cheilitis, and stomatitis; or when the history or background indicates potential for a vitamin deficiency. The oral or mucosal findings are not pathognomonic for a specific deficiency, and synchronous deficiencies often occur. But a high index of suspicion can aid in evaluating unusual symptoms, as nutritional deficiencies are frequently overlooked when practicing in developed nations. Also nutritional deficiencies may accompany or complicate other oral diseases such as pemphigus, or pemphigoid, particularly when pain limits oral intake and, unless specifically sought, may be overlooked in the presence of more obvious pathology.

BMS and RAS are two common clinical scenarios where screening for associated nutritional insufficiencies may provide opportunities for helpful therapeutic intervention. Appropriate therapy can lead to resolution of symptoms and confirm the diagnosis. A high index of suspicion is paramount in identifying nutritional insufficiencies, and knowledge of the symptoms and signs that may occur in the oral cavity can lead to prompt diagnosis and therapy.

References

1. Boyd LD, Palmer CA. Nutrition and oral health. Saddle River: Prentice-Hall; 2001.
2. Weinberg MA. Anatomy of the periodontal structures: the healthy state. Saddle River: Pearson Prentice-Hall; 2006.
3. Thomas DM, Mirowski GW. Nutrition and oral mucosal diseases. Clin Dermatol. 2010;28:426–31.
4. Khadim MI. Oral manifestations of malnutrition I. The effect of vitamins. JPMA. 1981;31:44–8.
5. Dreizen S. Oral indications of the deficiency states. Postgrad Med. 1971;49:97–102.
6. Cutright DE, Bauer H. Cell renewal in the oral mucosa and skin of the rat. I. Turnover time. Oral Surg Oral Med Oral Pathol. 1967;23:249–59.
7. Dreizen S. The mouth as an indicator of internal nutritional problems. Pediatrician. 1989;16:139–46.
8. Balducci L, Ershler WB, Krantz S. Anemia in the elderly-clinical findings and impact on health. Crit Rev Oncol Hematol. 2006;58:156–65.
9. Joosten E, Pelemans W, Hiele M, Noyen J, Verhaeghe R, Boogaerts MA. Prevalence and causes of anaemia in a geriatric hospitalized population. Gerontology. 1992;38:111–7.
10. Ania BJ, Suman VJ, Fairbanks VF, Rademacher DM, Melton LJ 3rd. Incidence of anemia in older people: an epidemiologic study in a well defined population. J Am Geriatr Soc. 1997;45:825–31.
11. Chung SD, Sheu JJ, Kao LT, Lin HC, Kang JH. Dementia is associated with iron-deficiency anemia in females: a population-based study. J Neurol Sci. 2014;346(1–2):90–3.
12. Ma G, Li Y, Jin Y, Zhai F, Kok FJ, Yang X. Phytate intake and molar ratios of phytate to zinc, iron and calcium in the diets of people in China. Eur J Clin Nutr. 2007;61:368–74.
13. Zijp IM, Korver O, Tijburg LB. Effect of tea and other dietary factors on iron absorption. Crit Rev Food Sci Nutr. 2000;40:371–98.
14. Lane DJ, Richardson DR. The active role of vitamin C in mammalian iron metabolism: much more than just enhanced iron absorption! Free Radic Biol Med. 2014;75C:69–83.
15. Darby WJ. The oral manifestations of iron deficiency. JAMA. 1946;130:830–5.
16. Jacobs A, Cavill I. The oral lesions of iron deficiency anaemia: pyridoxine and riboflavin status. Br J Haematol. 1968;14:291–5.
17. Monto RW, Rizek RA, Fine G. Observations on the exfolative cytology and histology of the oral mucous membranes in iron deficiency. Oral Surg Oral Med Oral Pathol. 1961;14:965–74.
18. Lu SY, Wu HC. Initial diagnosis of anemia from sore mouth and improved classification of anemias by MCV and RDW in 30 patients. Oral Surg Oral Med Oral Pathol Oral Radiol Endod. 2004;98:679–85.
19. Wu YC, Wang YP, Chang JY, Cheng SJ, Chen HM, Sun A. Oral manifestations and blood profile in patients with iron deficiency anemia. J Formosan Med Assoc. 2014;113:83–7.
20. Larsson LG, Sandstrom A, Westling P. Relationship of Plummer-Vinson disease to cancer of the upper alimentary tract in Sweden. Cancer Res. 1975;35:3308–16.
21. Richie JP Jr, Kleinman W, Marina P, Abraham P, Wynder EL, Muscat JE. Blood iron, glutathione, and micronutrient levels and the risk of oral cancer. Nutr Cancer. 2008;60:474–82.
22. Tahara T, Shibata T, Okubo M, Yoshioka D, Ishizuka T, Sumi K, et al. A case of Plummer-Vinson syndrome showing rapid improvement of Dysphagia and esophageal web after two weeks of iron therapy. Case Rep Gastroenterol. 2014;8:211–5.
23. Prema K, Srikantia SG. Clinical grading of lingual lesions in vitamin B-complex deficiency. Indian J Med Res. 1980;72:537–45.
24. Bamji MS, Prema K, Rama Lakshmi BA, Ahmed F, Jacob CM. Oral contraceptive use and vitamin nutrition status of malnourished women-effects of continuous and intermittent vitamin supplements. J Steroid Biochem. 1979;11:487–91.
25. Tamura F, Kikutani T, Tohara T, Yoshida M, Yaegaki K. Tongue thickness relates to nutritional status in the elderly. Dysphagia. 2012;27:556–61.
26. Manzo L, Locatelli C, Candura SM, Costa LG. Nutrition and alcohol neurotoxicity. Neurotoxicology. 1994;15:555–65.
27. Long L, Cai XD, Bao J, Wu AM, Tian Q, Lu ZQ. Total parenteral nutrition caused Wernicke's encephalopathy accompanied by wet beriberi. Am J Case Rep. 2014;15:52–5.
28. Wooley JA. Characteristics of thiamin and its relevance to the management of heart failure. Nutr Clin Pract. 2008;23:487–93.
29. Aykroyd WR. Nutritional problems of urban communities. Proc Nutr Soc. 1970;29:148–50.
30. Dahlberg K. Medical care of Cambodian refugees. JAMA. 1980;243:1062–5.
31. Thanangkul O, Whitaker JA. Childhood thiamine deficiency in northern Thailand. Am J Clin Nutr. 1966;18:275–7.
32. Tang CM, Rolfe M, Wells JC, Cham K. Outbreak of beriberi in The Gambia. Lancet. 1989;2:206–7.

33. Wong AY, Chan EW, Chui CS, Sutcliffe AG, Wong IC. The phenomenon of micronutrient deficiency among children in China: a systematic review of the literature. Public Health Nutr. 2014;17:2605–18.
34. Pepersack T, Garbusinski J, Robberecht J, Beyer I, Willems D, Fuss M. Clinical relevance of thiamine status amongst hospitalized elderly patients. Gerontology. 1999;45:96–101.
35. Jensen GL, Binkley J. Clinical manifestations of nutrient deficiency. JPEN. 2002;26:S29–33.
36. Harper CG, Giles M, Finlay-Jones R. Clinical signs in the Wernicke-Korsakoff complex: a retrospective analysis of 131 cases diagnosed at necropsy. J Neurol Neurosurg Psychiatry. 1986;49:341–5.
37. Becker DA, Ingala EE, Martinez-Lage M, Price RS, Galetta SL. Dry Beriberi and Wernicke's encephalopathy following gastric lap band surgery. J Clin Neurosci. 2012;19:1050–2.
38. Sechi G, Serra A. Wernicke's encephalopathy: new clinical settings and recent advances in diagnosis and management. Lancet Neurol. 2007;6:442–55.
39. Rolfe M, Walker RW, Samba KN, Cham K. Urban beriberi in The Gambia, West Africa. Trans R Soc Trop Med Hyg. 1993;87:114–5.
40. Johnson KA, Bernard MA, Funderburg K. Vitamin nutrition in older adults. Clin Geriatr Med. 2002;18:773–99.
41. Schlosser BJ, Pirigyi M, Mirowski GW. Oral manifestations of hematologic and nutritional diseases. Otolaryngol Clin N Am. 2011;44:183–203, vii.
42. Eisen D, Lynch DL. The mouth: diagnosis and treatment. St. Louis: Mosby-Year Book; 1998.
43. Haisraeli-Shalish M, Livneh A, Katz J, Doolman R, Sela BA. Recurrent aphthous stomatitis and thiamine deficiency. Oral Surg Oral Med Oral Pathol Oral Radiol Endod. 1996;82:634–6.
44. Nolan A, Mcintosh WB, Allam BF, Lamey PJ. Recurrent aphthous ulceration: vitamin B1, B2 and B6 status and response to replacement therapy. J Oral Pathol Med. 1991;20:389–91.
45. Mendoza CE, Rodriguez F, Rosenberg DG. Reversal of refractory congestive heart failure after thiamine supplementation: report of a case and review of literature. J Cardiovasc Pharmacol Ther. 2003;8:313–6.
46. Weisberger D. Lesions of the oral mucosa treated with special vitamins. Am J Orthod. 1941;27:25.
47. Stones HH. Oral manifestations in systemic diseases; hypervitaminoses and blood dyscrasias. Ann R Coll Surg Engl. 1951;9:234–44.
48. Latt N, Dore G. Thiamine in the treatment of Wernicke encephalopathy in patients with alcohol use disorders. Intern Med J. 2014;44:911–5.
49. Powers HJ. Riboflavin (vitamin B-2) and health. Am J Clin Nutr. 2003;77:1352–60.
50. Oppenheimer SJ, Bull R, Thurnham DI. Riboflavin deficiency in Madang infants. Papua New Guinea Med J. 1983;26:17–20.
51. Boisvert WA, Castaneda C, Mendoza I, Langeloh G, Solomons NW, Gershoff SN, et al. Prevalence of riboflavin deficiency among Guatemalan elderly people and its relationship to milk intake. Am J Clin Nutr. 1993;58:85–90.
52. Wilson JM. Riboflavin deficiency in late pregnancy: a problem in south Asia too? Trans R Soc Trop Med Hyg. 1988;82:656.
53. Nichols EK, Talley LE, Birungi N, McClelland A, Madraa E, Chandia AB, et al. Suspected outbreak of riboflavin deficiency among populations reliant on food assistance: a case study of drought-stricken Karamoja, Uganda, 2009–2010. PLoS One. 2013;8:e62976.
54. Bates CJ, Prentice A, Cole TJ, Van Der Pols JC, Doyle W, Finch S, et al. Micronutrients: highlights and research challenges from the 1994–5 national diet and nutrition survey of people aged 65 years and over. Br J Nutr. 1999;82:7–15.
55. Cimino JA, Epel R, Cooperman JM. Effect of diet on vitamin deficiencies in retarded individuals receiving drugs. Drug Nutr Interact. 1985;3:201–4.
56. Pelliccione N, Pinto J, Huang YP, Rivlin RS. Accelerated development of riboflavin deficiency by treatment with chlorpromazine. Biochem Pharmacol. 1983;32:2949–53.
57. Jacobs EC. Oculo-oro-genital syndrome: a deficiency disease. Ann Intern Med. 1951;35:1049–54.
58. Jen M, Yan AC. Syndromes associated with nutritional deficiency and excess. Clin Dermatol. 2010;28:669–85.
59. Rosenblum IA, Jallaffe N. The oral manifestations of vitamin deficiencies. JAMA. 1941:2245–8.
60. Jolliffe N, Fein HD, Rosenblum IA. Riboflavin deficiency in man. N Engl J Med. 1939;221:921.
61. Lo CS. Riboflavin status of adolescents in southern China. Average intake of riboflavin and clinical findings. Med J Aust. 1984;141:635–7.
62. Tavares NR, Moreira PA, Amaral TF. Riboflavin supplementation and biomarkers of cardiovascular disease in the elderly. J Nutr Health Aging. 2009;13:441–6.
63. Mulliken RA, Casner MJ. Oral manifestations of systemic disease. Emerg Med Clin N Am. 2000;18:565–75.
64. Durso SC. Oral manifestations of disease. New York: McGraw Hill; 2008.
65. Sebrell WH, Butler RE. Riboflavin deficiency in man: preliminary note. Public Health Rep. 1938;53:2282.
66. Vinodkumar M, Rajagopalan S. Efficacy of fortification of school meals with ferrous glycine phosphate and riboflavin against anemia and angular stomatitis in schoolchildren. Food Nutr Bull. 2009;30:260–4.
67. Sun A, Wu KM, Wang YP, Lin HP, Chen HM, Chiang CP. Burning mouth syndrome: a review and update. J Oral Pathol Med. 2013;42:649–55.
68. Zaridze DG, Trapeznikov NN. Risk factors for cancer of the oral cavity and esophagus in a high incidence region. Vopr Onkol. 1986;32:31–6.
69. Podlodowska J, Szumilo J, Podlodowski W, Staroslawska E, Burdan F. Epidemiology and risk

factors of the oral carcinoma. Pol Merkur Lekarski. 2012;32:135–7.
70. Petridou E, Zavras AI, Lefatzis D, Dessypris N, Laskaris G, Dokianakis G, et al. The role of diet and specific micronutrients in the etiology of oral carcinoma. Cancer. 2002;94:2981–8.
71. Joosten E, Van Den Berg A, Riezler R, Naurath HJ, Lindenbaum J, Stabler SP, et al. Metabolic evidence that deficiencies of vitamin B-12 (cobalamin), folate, and vitamin B-6 occur commonly in elderly people. Am J Clin Nutr. 1993;58:468–76.
72. Kjeldby IK, Fosnes GS, Ligaarden SC, Farup PG. Vitamin B6 deficiency and diseases in elderly people – a study in nursing homes. BMC Geriatr. 2013;13:13.
73. Gonzalez-Gross M, Sola R, Albers U, Barrios L, Alder M, Castillo MJ, et al. B-vitamins and homocysteine in Spanish institutionalized elderly. International journal for vitamin and nutrition research. Internationale Zeitschrift fur Vitamin- und Ernahrungsforschung. J Int Vita Nutr. 2007;77:22–33.
74. McCormick DB. Vitamin B6. In: Bowman BA, Russell RM, editors. Present knowledge in nutrition. 9th ed. Washington, DC: International Life Sciences Institute; 2006.
75. Ulvik A, Midttun O, Pedersen ER, Eussen SJ, Nygard O, Ueland PM. Evidence for increased catabolism of vitamin B-6 during systemic inflammation. Am J Clin Nutr. 2014;100:250–5.
76. Rall LC, Meydani SN. Vitamin B6 and immune competence. Nutr Rev. 1993;51:217–25.
77. Moriwaki K, Kanno Y, Nakamoto H, Okada H, Suzuki H. Vitamin B6 deficiency in elderly patients on chronic peritoneal dialysis. Adv Perit Dial. Conference on Peritoneal Dialysis. 2000;16:308–12.
78. Masse PG, Boudreau J, Tranchant CC, Ouellette R, Ericson KL. Type 1 diabetes impairs vitamin B(6) metabolism at an early stage of women's adulthood. Appl Physiol Nutr Metab. 2012;37:167–75.
79. Corken M, Porter J. Is vitamin B(6) deficiency an under-recognized risk in patients receiving haemodialysis? A systematic review: 2000–2010. Nephrology. 2011;16:619–25.
80. Wilson SM, Bivins BN, Russell KA, Bailey LB. Oral contraceptive use: impact on folate, vitamin B(6), and vitamin B(1)(2) status. Nutr Rev. 2011;69:572–83.
81. Zhou Y, Jiao Y, Wei YH, Zhang GR, Zhang JP, Ren JX, et al. Effects of pyridoxine on the intestinal absorption and pharmacokinetics of isoniazid in rats. Eur J Drug Metab Pharmacokinet. 2013; 38:5–13.
82. Snider DE Jr. Pyridoxine supplementation during isoniazid therapy. Tubercle. 1980;61:191–6.
83. Stone OJ. Pyridoxine deficiency and antagonism produce increased ground substance viscosity with resulting seborrheic dermatitis and increased tumor resistance. Med Hypotheses. 1989;30: 277–80.
84. Clayton PT. B6-responsive disorders: a model of vitamin dependency. J Inherit Metab Dis. 2006;29:317–26.
85. Radler DR, Lister T. Nutrient deficiencies associated with nutrition-focused physical findings of the oral cavity. Nutr Clin Pract. 2013;28:710–21.
86. Foca FJ. Motor and sensory neuropathy secondary to excessive pyridoxine ingestion. Arch Phys Med Rehabil. 1985;66:634–6.
87. Schaumburg H, Kaplan J, Windebank A, Vick N, Rasmus S, Pleasure D, et al. Sensory neuropathy from pyridoxine abuse. A new megavitamin syndrome. N Engl J Med. 1983;309:445–8.
88. Gupta AK, Damji A, Uppaluri A. Vitamin B12 deficiency. Prevalence among South Asians at a Toronto clinic. Can Fam Physician. 2004;50:743–7.
89. Gudgeon P, Cavalcanti R. Folate testing in hospital inpatients. Am J Med. 2015;128(1):56–9.
90. Allen LH. How common is vitamin B-12 deficiency? Am J Clin Nutr. 2009;89:693S–6S.
91. Hunt A, Harrington D, Robinson S. Vitamin B12 deficiency. BMJ. 2014;349:g5226.
92. Cuffe K, Stauffer W, Painter J, Shetty S, Montour J, Zhou W. Update: vitamin B12 deficiency among Bhutanese refugees resettling in the United States, 2012. MMWR. 2014;63:607.
93. Snow CF. Laboratory diagnosis of vitamin B12 and folate deficiency: a guide for the primary care physician. Arch Intern Med. 1999;159:1289–98.
94. Wickramasinghe SN. Diagnosis of megaloblastic anaemias. Blood Rev. 2006;20:299–318.
95. Pontes HA, Neto NC, Ferreira KB, Fonseca FP, Vallinoto GM, Pontes FS, et al. Oral manifestations of vitamin B12 deficiency: a case report. J Can Dent Assoc. 2009;75(7):533–7.
96. Field EA, Speechley JA, Rugman FR, Varga E, Tyldesley WR. Oral signs and symptoms in patients with undiagnosed vitamin B12 deficiency. J Oral Pathol Med. 1995;24:468–70.
97. Graells J, Ojeda RM, Muniesa C, Gonzalez J, Saavedra J. Glossitis with linear lesions: an early sign of vitamin B12 deficiency. J Am Acad Dermatol. 2009;60:498–500.
98. Scully C, Gorsky M, Lozada-Nur F. The diagnosis and management of recurrent aphthous stomatitis: a consensus approach. J Am Dent Assoc. 2003;134:200–7.
99. Stoopler ET, Kuperstein AS. Glossitis secondary to vitamin B12 deficiency anemia. Can Med Assoc J. 2013;185:E582.
100. Itoh I, Ikui A, Ikeda M, Tomita H, Souhei E. Taste disorder involving Hunter's glossitis following total gastrectomy. Acta Otolaryngol Suppl. 2002:159–63.
101. Kuzminski AM, Del Giacco EJ, Allen RH, Stabler SP. Oral cobalamin therapy in patients who absorb it normally. Blood. 1998;92:4879–80.
102. Kuzminski AM, Del Giacco EJ, Allen RH, Stabler SP, Lindenbaum J. Effective treatment of cobalamin deficiency with oral cobalamin. Blood. 1998;92:1191–8.

103. Hess SY, Zimmermann MB, Brogli S, Hurrell RF. A national survey of iron and folate status in pregnant women in Switzerland. Int J Vitam Nutr Res Int J Vitam Nutr Res. 2001;71(5):268–73.
104. Serdula MK, Nichols EK, Aburto NJ, Masa'd H, Obaid B, Wirth J, et al. Micronutrient status in Jordan: 2002 and 2010. Eur J Clin Nutr. 2014;68(10):1124–8.
105. Ma AG, Chen XC, Wang Y, Xu RX, Zheng MC, Li JS. The multiple vitamin status of Chinese pregnant women with anemia and nonanemia in the last trimester. J Nutr Sci Vitaminol. 2004;50:87–92.
106. Hillman RS, Mcguffin R, Campbell C. Alcohol interference with the folate enterohepatic cycle. Trans Assoc Am Phys. 1977;90:145–56.
107. Smith AD. Folic acid fortification: the good, the bad, and the puzzle of vitamin B-12. Am J Clin Nutr. 2007;85:3–5.
108. Okey R, Pencharz R, Lepkovsky S, Vernon ER, Jerome D, Marquette M. Dietary constituents which may influence the use of food cholesterol. I. Eggs: biotin and avidin. J Nutr. 1951;44:83–99.
109. White HB 3rd, Whitehead CC. Role of avidin and other biotin-binding proteins in the deposition and distribution of biotin in chicken eggs. Discovery of a new biotin-binding protein. Biochem J. 1987;241:677–84.
110. Mock DM, Dyken ME. Biotin catabolism is accelerated in adults receiving long-term therapy with anticonvulsants. Neurology. 1997;49:1444–7.
111. Mock DM, Mock NI, Nelson RP, Lombard KA. Disturbances in biotin metabolism in children undergoing long-term anticonvulsant therapy. J Pediatr Gastroenterol Nutr. 1998;26:245–50.
112. Fujimoto W, Inaoki M, Fukui T, Inoue Y, Kuhara T. Biotin deficiency in an infant fed with amino acid formula. J Dermatol. 2005;32:256–61.
113. Tammachote R, Janklat S, Tongkobpetch S, Suphapeetiporn K, Shotelersuk V. Holocarboxylase synthetase deficiency: novel clinical and molecular findings. Clin Genet. 2010;78:88–93.
114. Zempleni J, Hassan YI, Wijeratne SS. Biotin and biotinidase deficiency. Expert Rev Endocrinol Metab. 2008;3:715–24.
115. Moslinger D, Stockler-Ipsiroglu S, Scheibenreiter S, Tiefenthaler M, Muhl A, Seidl R, et al. Clinical and neuropsychological outcome in 33 patients with biotinidase deficiency ascertained by nationwide newborn screening and family studies in Austria. Eur J Pediatr. 2001;160:277–82.
116. Mock DM. Biotin. Washington, DC: ILSI Nutrition Foundation; 1996.
117. Fiume MZ. Final report on the safety assessment of biotin. Int J Toxicol. 2001;20(Suppl 4):1–12.
118. Ravindran RD, Vashist P, Gupta SK, Young IS, Maraini G, Camparini M, et al. Prevalence and risk factors for vitamin C deficiency in north and south India: a two centre population based study in people aged 60 years and over. PLoS One. 2011;6:e28588.
119. Hampl JS, Taylor CA, Johnston CS. Vitamin C deficiency and depletion in the United States: the Third National Health and Nutrition Examination Survey, 1988 to 1994. Am J Public Health. 2004;94:870–5.
120. Schleicher RL, Carroll MD, Ford ES, Lacher DA. Serum vitamin C and the prevalence of vitamin C deficiency in the United States: 2003–2004 National Health and Nutrition Examination Survey (NHANES). Am J Clin Nutr. 2009;90:1252–63.
121. Wrieden WL, Hannah MK, Bolton-Smith C, Tavendale R, Morrison C, Tunstall-Pedoe H. Plasma vitamin C and food choice in the third Glasgow MONICA population survey. J Epidemiol Community Health. 2000;54:355–60.
122. Mosdol A, Erens B, Brunner EJ. Estimated prevalence and predictors of vitamin C deficiency within UK's low-income population. J Public Health (Oxf). 2008;30:456–60.
123. Cahill LE, El-Sohemy A. Vitamin C transporter gene polymorphisms, dietary vitamin C and serum ascorbic acid. J Nutrigenet Nutrigenomics. 2009;2:292–301.
124. Villalpando S, Garcia-Guerra A, Ramirez-Silva CI, Mejia-Rodriguez F, Matute G, Shamah-Levy T, et al. Iron, zinc and iodide status in Mexican children under 12 years and women 12–49 years of age. A probabilistic national survey. Salud Publica Mex. 2003;45(Suppl 4):S520–9.
125. Chiplonkar SA, Agte VV, Mengale SS, Tarwadi KV. Are lifestyle factors good predictors of retinol and vitamin C deficiency in apparently healthy adults? Eur J Clin Nutr. 2002;56:96–104.
126. Raynaud-Simon A, Cohen-Bittan J, Gouronnec A, Pautas E, Senet P, Verny M, et al. Scurvy in hospitalized elderly patients. J Nutr Health Aging. 2010;14:407–10.
127. Netto BD, Moreira EA, Patino JS, Beninca JP, Jordao AA, Frode TS. Influence of Roux-en-Y gastric bypass surgery on vitamin C, myeloperoxidase, and oral clinical manifestations: a 2-year follow-up study. Nutr Clin Pract. 2012;27:114–21.
128. Weinstein M, Babyn P, Zlotkin S. An orange a day keeps the doctor away: scurvy in the year 2000. Pediatrics. 2001;108:E55.
129. Firth N, Marvan E. Oral lesions in scurvy. Aust Dent J. 2001;46:298–300.
130. Yudkin J. Evolution, history, and nutrition: their bearing on oral disease and other diseases of civilization. Dent Pract Dent Rec. 1965;16:60–4.
131. Bacci C, Sivolella S, Pellegrini J, Favero L, Berengo M. A rare case of scurvy in an otherwise healthy child: diagnosis through oral signs. Pediatr Dent. 2010;32:536–8.
132. Gokhale NH, Acharya AB, Patil VS, Trivedi DJ, Thakur SL. A short-term evaluation of the relationship between plasma ascorbic acid levels and periodontal disease in systemically healthy and type 2 diabetes mellitus subjects. J Diet Suppl. 2013;10:93–104.

133. Levine M. New concepts in the biology and biochemistry of ascorbic acid. N Engl J Med. 1986;314:892–902.
134. Amaliya, Timmerman MF, Abbas F, Loos BG, Van Der Weijden GA, Van Winkelhoff AJ, Winkel EG, et al. Java project on periodontal diseases: the relationship between vitamin C and the severity of periodontitis. J Clin Periodontol. 2007;34:299–304.
135. Kroser LS. A four year clinical evaluation of Vitron-C. A new hematinic containing ferrous fumarate and ascorbic acid. West Med. 1965;6:314–5.
136. De Cassia Ribeiro-Silva R, Nunes IL, Assis AM. Prevalence and factors associated with vitamin A deficiency in children and adolescents. J Pediatr. 2014;90:486–92.
137. Mora JO, Gueri M, Mora OL. Vitamin A deficiency in Latin America and the Caribbean: an overview. Rev Panam Salud Publica. 1998;4:178–86.
138. Ahmed F. Vitamin A deficiency in Bangladesh: a review and recommendations for improvement. Public Health Nutr. 1999;2:1–14.
139. Gorstein J, Shreshtra RK, Pandey S, Adhikari RK, Pradhan A. Current status of vitamin A deficiency and the national vitamin A control program in Nepal: results of the 1998 national micronutrient status survey. Asia Pac J Clin Nutr. 2003;12:96–103.
140. Demissie T, Ali A, Mekonen Y, Haider J, Umeta M. Magnitude and distribution of vitamin A deficiency in Ethiopia. Food Nutr Bull. 2010;31: 234–41.
141. Luo M, Estivariz CF, Schleicher RL, Bazargan N, Leader LM, Galloway JR, et al. Prospective analysis of serum carotenoids, vitamin A, and tocopherols in adults with short bowel syndrome undergoing intestinal rehabilitation. Nutrition. 2009;25:400–7.
142. Rana M, Wong-See D, Katz T, Gaskin K, Whitehead B, Jaffe A, et al. Fat-soluble vitamin deficiency in children and adolescents with cystic fibrosis. J Clin Pathol. 2014;67:605–8.
143. Goskowicz M, Eichenfield LF. Cutaneous findings of nutritional deficiencies in children. Curr Opin Pediatr. 1993;5:441–5.
144. Miller SJ. Nutritional deficiency and the skin. J Am Acad Dermatol. 1989;21:1–30.
145. Jolly M. Vitamin A deficiency: a review. II. J Oral Ther Pharmacol. 1967;3:439–51.
146. Sherwin JC, Reacher MH, Dean WH, Ngondi J. Epidemiology of vitamin A deficiency and xerophthalmia in at-risk populations. Trans R Soc Trop Med Hyg. 2012;106:205–14.
147. Hillman JD. Principles of microbial ecology and their application to xerostomia-associated opportunistic infections of the oral cavity. Adv Dent Res. 1996;10:66–8.
148. Silverman S Jr, Eisenberg E, Renstrup G. A study of the effects of high doses of vitamin a on oral leukoplakia (hyperkeratosis), including toxicity, liver function and skeletal metabolism. J Oral Ther Pharmacol. 1965;2:9–23.
149. Rhodus NL, Brown J. The association of xerostomia and inadequate intake in older adults. J Am Diet Assoc. 1990;90:1688–92.
150. Wilson HO, Datta DB. Complications from micronutrient deficiency following bariatric surgery. Ann Clin Biochem. 2014;51(Pt 6):705–9.
151. Yetley EA. Assessing the vitamin D status of the US population. Am J Clin Nutr. 2008;88:558S–64S.
152. Taksler GB, Cutler DM, Giovannucci E, Keating NL. Vitamin D deficiency in minority populations. Public Health Nutr. 2014:1–13.
153. Cashman KD, Muldowney S, Mcnulty B, Nugent A, Fitzgerald AP, Kiely M, et al. Vitamin D status of Irish adults: findings from the National Adult Nutrition Survey. Br J Nutr. 2013;109:1248–56.
154. Brito A, Cori H, Olivares M, Fernanda Mujica M, Cediel G, Lopez De Romana D. Less than adequate vitamin D status and intake in Latin America and the Caribbean: a problem of unknown magnitude. Food Nutr Bull. 2013;34:52–64.
155. Guessous I, Mcclellan W, Kleinbaum D, Vaccarino V, Zoller O, Theler J, et al. Comparisons of serum vitamin d levels, status, and determinants in populations with and without chronic kidney disease not requiring renal dialysis: a 24-hour urine collection population-based study. J Ren Nutr. 2014;24:303–12.
156. Martini LA, Verly E Jr, Marchioni DM, Fisberg RM. Prevalence and correlates of calcium and vitamin D status adequacy in adolescents, adults, and elderly from the Health Survey-Sao Paulo. Nutrition. 2013;29:845–50.
157. Holick MF. McCollum award lecture, 1994: vitamin D – new horizons for the 21st century. Am J Clin Nutr. 1994;60:619–30.
158. Signorello LB, Williams SM, Zheng W, Smith JR, Long J, Cai Q, et al. Blood vitamin d levels in relation to genetic estimation of African ancestry. Cancer Epidemiol Biomark Prev. 2010;19: 2325–31.
159. Goodman JR, Gelbier MJ, Bennett JH, Winter GB. Dental problems associated with hypophosphataemic vitamin D resistant rickets. Int J Paediatr Dent. 1998;8:19–28.
160. Rathore R, Nalawade TM, Pateel D, Mallikarjuna R. Oral manifestations of vitamin D resistant rickets in orthopantomogram. BMJ Case Rep. 2013;12:2013.
161. Souza AP, Kobayashi TY, Lourenco Neto N, Silva SM, Machado MA, Oliveira TM. Dental manifestations of patient with vitamin D-resistant rickets. J Appl Oral Sci. 2013;21(6):601–6.
162. Su JM, Li Y, Ye XW, Wu ZF. Oral findings of hypophosphatemic vitamin D-resistant rickets: report of two cases. Chin Med J. 2007;120:1468–70.
163. Glorieux FH, Pettifor JM. Vitamin D/dietary calcium deficiency rickets and pseudo-vitamin D deficiency rickets. Bonekey Rep. 2014;3:524.
164. Balion C, Griffith LE, Strifler L, Henderson M, Patterson C, Heckman G, et al. Vitamin D,

cognition, and dementia: a systematic review and meta-analysis. Neurology. 2012;79:1397–405.
165. Zambrano M, Nikitakis NG, Sanchez-Quevedo MC, Sauk JJ, Sedano H, Rivera H. Oral and dental manifestations of vitamin D-dependent rickets type I: report of a pediatric case. Oral Surg Oral Med Oral Pathol Oral Radiol Endod. 2003;95:705–9.
166. Dietrich T, Joshipura KJ, Dawson-Hughes B, Bischoff-Ferrari HA. Association between serum concentrations of 25-hydroxyvitamin D3 and periodontal disease in the US population. Am J Clin Nutr. 2004;80:108–13.
167. Krall EA, Wehler C, Garcia RI, Harris SS, Dawson-Hughes B. Calcium and vitamin D supplements reduce tooth loss in the elderly. Am J Med. 2001;111:452–6.
168. Jou PC, Tomecki KJ. Sunscreens in the United States: current status and future outlook. Adv Exp Med Biol. 2014;810:464–84.
169. Zeeb H, Greinert R. The role of vitamin D in cancer prevention: does UV protection conflict with the need to raise low levels of vitamin D? Deutsches Arzteblatt Int. 2010;107:638–43.
170. Bilinski K, Talbot P. Vitamin d supplementation in Australia: implications for the development of supplementation guidelines. J Nutr Metab. 2014;2014:374208.
171. Schoon EJ, Muller MC, Vermeer C, Schurgers LJ, Brummer RJ, Stockbrugger RW. Low serum and bone vitamin K status in patients with longstanding Crohn's disease: another pathogenetic factor of osteoporosis in Crohn's disease? Gut. 2001;48:473–7.
172. Shea MK, Booth SL, Miller ME, Burke GL, Chen H, Cushman M, et al. Association between circulating vitamin K1 and coronary calcium progression in community-dwelling adults: the Multi-Ethnic Study of Atherosclerosis. Am J Clin Nutr. 2013;98:197–208.
173. Urano A, Hotta M, Ohwada R, Araki M. Vitamin K deficiency evaluated by serum levels of undercarboxylated osteocalcin in patients with anorexia nervosa with bone loss. Clin Nutr. 2015;34(3):443–8.
174. Vermeer C. Vitamin K: the effect on health beyond coagulation – an overview. Food Nutr Res. 2012;56.
175. Nowak JK, Grzybowska-Chlebowczyk U, Landowski P, Szaflarska-Poplawska A, Klincewicz B, Adamczak D, et al. Prevalence and correlates of vitamin K deficiency in children with inflammatory bowel disease. Sci Rep. 2014;4:4768.
176. Sikkens EC, Cahen DL, Koch AD, Braat H, Poley JW, Kuipers EJ, et al. The prevalence of fat-soluble vitamin deficiencies and a decreased bone mass in patients with chronic pancreatitis. Pancreatology. 2013;13:238–42.
177. Corbo MD, Lam J. Zinc deficiency and its management in the pediatric population: a literature review and proposed etiologic classification. J Am Acad Dermatol. 2013;69:616–624 e1.
178. Tuerk MJ, Fazel N. Zinc deficiency. Curr Opin Gastroenterol. 2009;25:136–43.
179. Wuehler SE, Peerson JM, Brown KH. Use of national food balance data to estimate the adequacy of zinc in national food supplies: methodology and regional estimates. Public Health Nutr. 2005;8:812–9.
180. Siyame EW, Hurst R, Wawer AA, Young SD, Broadley MR, Chilimba AD, et al. A high prevalence of zinc- but not iron-deficiency among women in rural Malawi: a cross-sectional study. Int J Vitam Nutr Res Int Z Vitam Ernahrungsforschung J Int Vitaminologie Nutr. 2013;83:176–87.
181. Hambidge M. Human zinc deficiency. J Nutr. 2000;130:1344S–9S.
182. Miletta MC, Bieri A, Kernland K, Schoni MH, Petkovic V, Fluck, et al. Transient neonatal zinc deficiency caused by a heterozygous G87R mutation in the zinc transporter ZnT-2 (SLC30A2) gene in the mother highlighting the importance of Zn (2+) for normal growth and development. Int J Endocrinol. 2013;259189.
183. Qian L, Wang B, Tang N, Zhang W, Cai W. Polymorphisms of SLC30A2 and selected perinatal factors associated with low milk zinc in Chinese breastfeeding women. Early Hum Dev. 2012;88:663–8.
184. Changela A, Javaiya H, Changela K, Davanos E, Rickenbach K. Acrodermatitis enteropathica during adequate enteral nutrition. JPEN. 2012;36:235–7.
185. Mayo-Wilson E, Imdad A, Junior J, Dean S, Bhutta ZA. Preventive zinc supplementation for children, and the effect of additional iron: a systematic review and meta-analysis. BMJ Open. 2014;4:e004647.
186. Mayo-Wilson E, Junior JA, Imdad A, Dean S, Chan XH, Chan ES, et al. Zinc supplementation for preventing mortality, morbidity, and growth failure in children aged 6 months to 12 years of age. Cochrane Database Syst Rev. 2014;5:CD009384.
187. Gehrig KA, Dinulos JGH. Acrodermatitis due to nutritional deficiency. Curr Opin Pediatr. 2010;22:107–12.
188. Lott JP, Reeve J, Ko C, Girardi M. Periorificial dermatitis and erosive inguinal plaques in a 57-year-old woman. Acquired zinc deficiency acrodermatitis enteropathica (ADE). JAMA Dermatol. 2013;149:357–63.
189. Heath ML, Sidbury R. Cutaneous manifestations of nutritional deficiency. Curr Opin Pediatr. 2006;18:417–22.
190. Touger-Decker R. Oral manifestations of nutrient deficiencies. Mt Sinai J Med New York. 1998;65:355–61.
191. Dubas LE, Waymire DM, Adams BB. Resident rounds: part II study aid: nutritional deficiencies. J Drugs Dermatol. 2013;12:816–7.
192. Spies TD, Cooper C. The diagnosis of pellagra. Intern Clin. 1937:4.
193. Oldham MA, Ivkovic A. Pellagrous encephalopathy presenting as alcohol withdrawal delirium: a case

series and literature review. Addict Sci Clin Pract. 2012;7:12.
194. Paulionis L, Kane SL, Meckling KA. Vitamin status and cognitive function in a long-term care population. BMC Geriatr. 2005;5:16.
195. Jacobson EL. Niacin deficiency and cancer in women. J Am Coll Nutr. 1993;12:412–6.
196. Ishii N, Nishihara Y. Pellagra among chronic alcoholics: clinical and pathological study of 20 necropsy cases. J Neurol Neurosurg Psychiatry. 1981;44:209–15.
197. Castiello RJ, Lynch PJ. Pellagra and the carcinoid syndrome. Arch Dermatol. 1972;105:574–7.
198. Shah GM, Shah RG, Veillette H, Kirkland JB, Pasieka JL, Warner RR. Biochemical assessment of niacin deficiency among carcinoid cancer patients. Am J Gastroenterol. 2005;100:2307–14.
199. Isaac S. The "gauntlet" of pellagra. Int J Dermatol. 1998;37:599.
200. Lin HP, Wang YP, Chen HM, Kuo YS, Lang MJ, Sun A. Significant association of hematinic deficiencies and high blood homocysteine levels with burning mouth syndrome. J Formosan Med Assoc. 2013;112:319–25.
201. Kohorst JJ, Bruce AJ, Torgerson RR, Schenck LA, Davis MD. A population-based study of the incidence of burning mouth syndrome. Mayo Clin Proc. 2014;89(11):1545–52.
202. Sun A, Lin HP, Wang YP, Chen HM, Cheng SJ, Chiang CP. Significant reduction of serum homocysteine level and oral symptoms after different vitamin-supplement treatments in patients with burning mouth syndrome. J Oral Pathol Med. 2013;42:474–9.
203. Lamey PJ, Hammond A, Allam BF, Mcintosh WB. Vitamin status of patients with burning mouth syndrome and the response to replacement therapy. Br Dent J. 1986;160:81–4.
204. Cho GS, Han MW, Lee B, Roh JL, Choi SH, Cho KJ, et al. Zinc deficiency may be a cause of burning mouth syndrome as zinc replacement therapy has therapeutic effects. J Oral Pathol Med. 2010;39:722–7.
205. Murray EL. Burning mouth syndrome response to high-dose vitamin C. Headache. 2014;54:169.
206. Hugoson A, Thorstensson B. Vitamin B status and response to replacement therapy in patients with burning mouth syndrome. Acta Odontol Scand. 1991;49:367–75.
207. Vucicevic-Boras V, Topic B, Cekic-Arambasin A, Zadro R, Stavljenic-Rukavina A. Lack of association between burning mouth syndrome and hematinic deficiencies. Eur J Med Res. 2001;6:409–12.
208. Aravindhan R, Vidyalakshmi S, Kumar MS, Satheesh C, Balasubramanium AM, Prasad VS. Burning mouth syndrome: a review on its diagnostic and therapeutic approach. J Pharm Bioallied Sci. 2014;6:S21–5.
209. Samaranayake LP, Lamb AB, Lamey PJ, MacFarlane TW. Oral carriage of Candida species and coliforms in patients with burning mouth syndrome. J Oral Pathol Med. 1989;18:233–5.

6 Oral Signs of Connective Tissue Disease

Kenisha R. Heath and Nasim Fazel

In this chapter, we aim to discuss the epidemiology, pathogenesis, differential diagnosis, and treatment of oral manifestations encountered in the autoimmune diseases of Sjögren's syndrome (SS), systemic lupus erythematosus (SLE), systemic sclerosis (SSc), mixed connective tissue disease (MCTD), and dermatomyositis (DM). Systemic autoimmune conditions are estimated to affect 5%–8% of Americans [1]. Oral manifestations are encountered with high frequency and are often the first clinical signs or symptoms of the disease.

Sjögren's Syndrome

Epidemiology

Sjögren's syndrome (SS) is an autoimmune disorder characterized by chronic lymphocytic infiltration of the secretory glands, particularly the salivary and lacrimal glands with reduction of gland function causing dryness of the mucosal surfaces [2]. Sjögren's syndrome may occur alone as primary SS or in association with another autoimmune disease such as rheumatoid arthritis (RA), systemic lupus erythematosus, and systemic sclerosis in which case it is referred to as secondary SS. Although the presence of sicca symptoms is the hallmark of SS, any organ or mucosal surface may be involved. Thus, SS may present with a wide spectrum of clinical manifestations and complications [3].

Until recently there were a number of diagnostic guidelines for primary SS including the Copenhagen, Japanese, Greek, Californian-Fox (CF), and European Community (EC) [4]. The CF and EC criteria were the most commonly used yet they differed so much that almost ten times the number of cases would be diagnosed by the European criteria than by the American [5]. This discrepancy in diagnostic criteria led to great difficulty in determining information regarding prevalence. The American-European Consensus Group classification criteria, aka American-European criteria, were therefore developed to obtain a more uniform classification system and have been used since 2002 as the "gold standard" for the diagnosis of SS [6]. The American-European criteria are based on the presence of at least four out six diagnostic symptoms in which one of the four must include either the presence of anti-60 kD Ro antibodies or supportive histopathology (Table 6.1) [7].

Information regarding the prevalence of SS has been largely difficult to obtain, yet we know that primary SS represents one of the three most common autoimmune disorders with an estimated annual incidence of approximately 7 per 100,000

K. R. Heath
Air Force Institute of Technology, Wright-Patterson AFB, OH, USA

N. Fazel (✉)
Department of Dermatology, University of California, Davis, Sacramento, CA, USA
e-mail: nfazel@ucdavis.edu

N. Fazel (ed.), *Oral Signs of Systemic Disease*, https://doi.org/10.1007/978-3-030-10863-2_6

Table 6.1 Sjögren's syndrome diagnostic criteria[a] based on combined European-American consensus

I. Ocular symptoms – at least one of the following: troublesome dry eyes persisting for more than 3 months, recurrent sensation of sand or gravel in eyes, tear substitute use >3 times/day
II. Oral symptoms – at least one of the following: dry mouth every day >3 months, recurrent swollen salivary glands as an adult, need fluids to aid in swallowing foods
III. Objective evidence of dry eyes – at least one of the following: Schirmer test (<5 mm in 5 min), rose bengal score (>4, according to the van Bijsterveld scoring system)
IV. Objective evidence of salivary gland involvement – salivary gland scintigraphy (delayed uptake, etc.), parotid sialography (at least 1 present), unstimulated salivary flow <1.5 mL in 15 min
V. Histopathological features – lacrimal gland biopsy samples with focus score >1, minor salivary glands, focus score >1 (greater than 50 lymphocytes/4 mm^2 of glandular tissue)
VI. Laboratory abnormality – anti-60-kDa Ro (SS-A)

[a]Four of the six must be present for classification as Sjögren's syndrome, but one of the four must be either V or VI (A)

and a prevalence of 43 per 100,000 [8, 9]. Women are affected more often than men at a ratio of 9:1, and there appears to be two peaks with regard to age, the first occurring during the 20s–30s and the second after menopause [10].

Etiopathogenesis

Despite extensive clinical research, the underlying cause of SS and its pathogenesis remains largely unknown; however, it is believed to be multifactorial. The prevailing hypothesis is that environmental factors, such as a viral infection, trigger inflammation in individuals with a genetic predisposition [11]. In a study published in 2000, Fox and colleagues theorized the pathogenesis as an initial glandular insult leading to cellular necrosis or abnormal apoptosis; Sjögren's SS-A protein is then expressed on the glandular-cell surface; autoimmune T-cells are not effectively destroyed; and the injured gland then produces cytokines that upregulate chemokines. Homing of autoimmune lymphocytes and dendritic cells within the glands then follows. Additionally, major histocompatibility antigens and adhesive molecules are upregulated on epithelial cells in the lacrimal and salivary glands leading to activation of B lymphocytes within the glandular microenvironment. The B lymphocytes, under the influence of T-helper lymphocytes, produce antibodies to SS-A antigens. This triggers the formation of immune complexes, which contain anti-SS-A and ribonucleoproteins that bind to HLA-DR positive dendritic cells. The lymphocytes and epithelial cells secrete pro-inflammatory cytokines that influence the inflammatory response. Meanwhile, defects in post-signal transduction in T-cells leads to apoptosis. It is believed that these immunologic effects in genetically predisposed individuals (i.e., positive for HLA DR3) leads to an immune response to the SS-A antigen. Ultimately, this gives rise to immune complexes that stimulate Toll receptors to yield the characteristic interferon type 1 signature [11].

Clinical Manifestations

Although keratoconjunctivitis sicca symptoms of dry mouth and dry eyes are the hallmarks of the syndrome, any organ or mucosal surface may be involved [12]. Systemic manifestations can be categorized into non-visceral (skin, arthralgia, myalgia) and visceral (lung, heart, kidney, gastrointestinal, endocrine, central and peripheral nervous system).

Non-visceral Manifestations

About 70% of patients with primary SS complain of fatigue noted as the most debilitating symptom and the most common reason for work absences [6]. Myalgias and arthralgias are also very common with approximately 20% of patients experiencing true inflammatory arthritis, which may resemble rheumatoid arthritis (RA) with its symmetrical distribution. Arthritis in SS differs from RA with a higher tendency for relapsing and remitting disease activity and less stiffness.

Cutaneous manifestations of SS often include dry skin, seen in up to 50% of patients, and symptoms of vasculitis such as hypergammaglobulinemic purpura of Waldenstrom, leukocytoclastic vasculitis, and urticarial vasculitis. Cutaneous vasculitis often appears as purpura, urticarial and/or maculopapular lesions. Additionally, vitiligo, alopecia, and Raynaud's phenomenon have been reported in primary SS with Raynaud's occurring in approximately 30% of patients [13].

Cutaneous B- and T-cell lymphomas have been associated with a 40 times greater risk in primary SS patients as compared to the general population. It is reported that 5% of patients with SS develop lymphoma at some point with cutaneous lymphomas appearing far less frequently than the more common B-cell mucosa-associated lymphoid tissue (MALT) lymphomas of the salivary glands or of other extra-nodal sites [14–17].

Visceral Manifestations

Sjögren's syndrome is also associated with visceral manifestations, which can affect multiple organ systems including the gastrointestinal, central and peripheral nervous, pulmonary, renal, and endocrine systems. Gastrointestinal symptoms include esophageal dysmotility and symptoms of gastroesophageal reflux disease (GERD), irritable bowel syndrome, and dysphagia [18]. Neurologic involvement may manifest as a sensory polyneuropathy with burning pain in approximately 20% of patients with SS. Subacute or chronic onset of sensory polyneuropathy occurs over days to months and occurs most commonly in the upper and lower extremities [19, 20]. Headaches also have a high prevalence reported as over 78% in one study. Among the diagnoses, migraine was the most common type at 54% followed by tension-type headaches with a reported prevalence of 24.1% [21].

Renal manifestations can include interstitial nephritis and renal calculi, whereas hypothyroidism represents a common endocrine abnormality [10]. Pulmonary complications in patients with SS are mostly secondary to lymphocytic interstitial pneumonia or bronchiolitis. Most lung lesions are caused by an interstitial infiltrate of lymphocytes diffusely surrounding the bronchioles [3].

Oral Signs and Symptoms

The parotid, submandibular, and sublingual salivary glands are responsible for 90% of oral secretions, with the average adult producing 0.4 mL of saliva per minute or 1.5 L per day. Xerostomia occurs when the rate of salivary flow is reduced to less than 50% and is a hallmark of SS [11, 22]. Dry cracked lips, oral mucosal sores, and denudation of the lingual papillae are the characteristic signs [23] (Figs. 6.1 and 6.2). When xero-

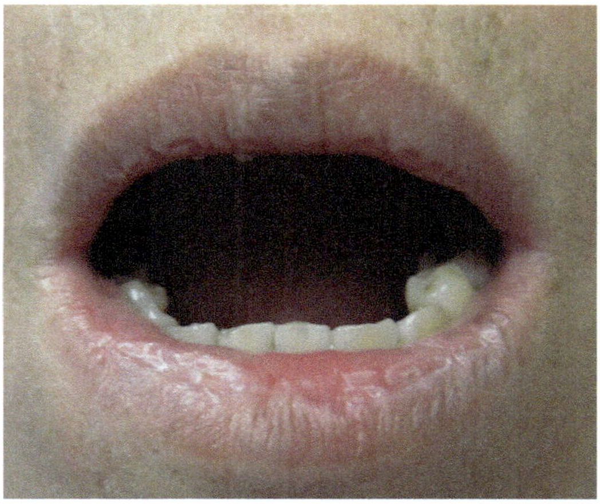

Fig. 6.1 Dry chapped lips as a result of chronic xerostomia secondary to Sjögren's syndrome

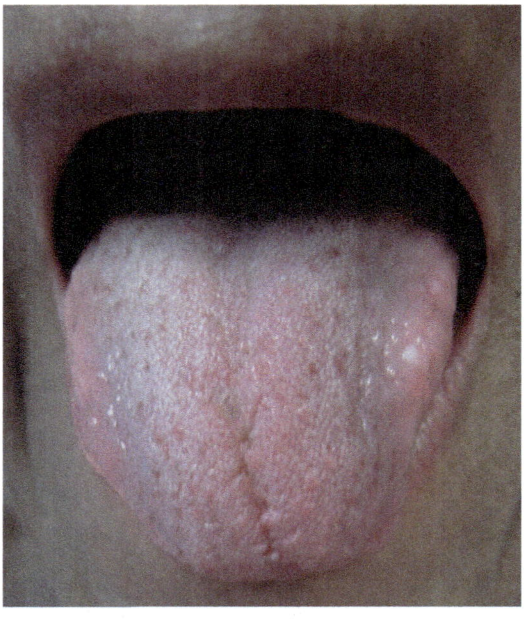

Fig. 6.2 Dry appearance of the tongue with evidence of fissuring

stomia occurs, the protein content of the saliva is also altered, and production of secretory IgA is decreased, which leads to a weakening of the antibacterial defense system against dental caries and oral opportunistic infections [22]. Specifically, chronic erythematous candidiasis is reported in 70%–75% of patients with SS. Candida colonization causes a dry, cracked, and erythematous appearance at the corners of the mouth, erythematous mucosal lesions, denture-associated stomatitis, and glossodynia. Additionally, patients with SS display a much lower parotid salivary pH and buffer capacity when compared to healthy individuals, which can increase the risk of dental caries and erosion [24]. Often dental caries occur at tooth-restoration interfaces and at locations that are not usually prone to caries such as the necks of the teeth. Progressive dental erosion may subsequently lead to tooth loss. As such, SS patients have often been reported to have a higher rate of premature loss of teeth or a higher Decayed, Missing, Filled Teeth (DMFT) index compared with the general population [11, 25].

Other oral symptoms associated with SS include difficulty with chewing, speaking, and swallowing secondary to intraoral dryness as well as sensitivity to flavorful foods, altered or diminished taste, oral pain, and coughing or choking episodes [26]. Finally, swelling of the salivary glands have been commonly reported in the SS patient population with parotid gland swelling, in particular, reported in 30%–40% of patients [27]. When sudden swelling of a single gland occurs, it is suggestive of infection, while chronic asymptomatic involvement of multiple glands with lymphadenopathy is more suggestive of lymphoma [28].

Differential Diagnosis

With respect to the most common SS symptom of xerostomia, it has been proven that a number of medications can also lead to dry mouth. Whereas cholinergic innervation maintains saliva production, use of anticholinergic drugs thereby decreases such production. Diuretics, antidepressants, alpha-adrenergic agents, and antihypertensive agents (beta-blockers, calcium channel blockers, and angiotensin-converting enzyme inhibitors) can also decrease salivary flow [29].

Outside of medications, the differential diagnosis of SS involves consideration for diseases that cause sicca symptoms and/or salivary or lacrimal gland enlargement. The list of possible conditions is quite extensive, but a few discussed in this chapter include age-related sicca syndrome, benign lymphoepithelial sialadenitis and dacryoadenitis, sarcoidosis, human immunodeficiency virus (HIV), graft-versus-host disease (GVHD), and systemic vasculitis.

Age-related sicca syndrome occurs when tear and unstimulated saliva production decline with age. This is most likely a result of age-related histologic alterations in the lacrimal and salivary glands. It can be differentiated from SS because the usual immune-mediated histologic changes seen in SS, and SS-related antibodies (anti-Ro/SSA and anti-La/SSB) are usually absent in these patients [30, 31]. Patients with benign lymphoepithelial sialadenitis and dacryoadenitis show lymphocytic infiltration of the lacrimal and/or major salivary glands with acinar atrophy leading to symptoms similar to those seen in SS and should be considered appropriately. Similarly, sarcoidosis may be considered in the differential diagnosis of patients with parotid and lacrimal gland enlargement. Biopsy may be necessary, if the distinction cannot be readily made based upon the clinical findings [32]. Patients with HIV infection may display diffuse CD8 lymphocytosis syndrome, which may mimic SS, though the incidence has significantly declined with antiretroviral therapy. Those affected may develop parotid gland enlargement, sicca symptoms, and lymphocytic interstitial pneumonitis. Salivary gland biopsies show a CD8-predominant lymphocytic infiltrate, which is helpful in differentiating the virus from SS [33]. Symptoms seen in those with GVHD after allogeneic hematopoietic stem cell transplantation may include dry eyes and dry mouth and should be considered in patients with these presenting symptoms. Additionally, IgG4 plasmacytic infiltration underlies several related forms of lacrimal and salivary gland disease, including orbital inflammatory pseudotumor, chronic sclerosing sialadenitis (Küttner tumor), and Mikulicz disease. These IgG4-related diseases (IgG4-RD) can be distinguished from SS by their associated clinical and laboratory features, and the distinct histopathologic findings seen in IgG4-RD [34].

Systemic vasculitis should also be considered as bilateral parotid and submandibular gland enlargement may occur in Wegener's granulomatosis. It can be differentiated from SS by clinical, laboratory, and histologic differences. Finally, lymphoma and other hematologic malignancies should be considered as malignant infiltration of the parotid glands may also present as bilateral salivary and lacrimal gland enlargement [35, 36].

Treatment

Currently, there is no cure for SS, nor is there any treatment that will restore the irreversible damage to the glands. Alleviating symptoms through medical therapy is the primary goal in the treatment of SS. With that, the treatment of salivary or lacrimal impairment is often approached by one or more of four methods: general measures, replacement, stimulation, and disease-modifying drugs [3].

General measures taken to minimize the loss of water from secretions by evaporation include the use of humidifiers and emollients such as petroleum jelly on the lips to prevent cracking and dryness. Meticulous oral hygiene and regular dental exams are also important [37]. Replacement incorporates the use of saliva substitutes in the form of sprays, lozenges, or gels to relieve oral discomfort and to keep the mouth moist. Compliance with regular use of saliva substitutes can be limited by complaints of an unpleasant taste and can be expensive. Other products used to alleviate dryness include mucin lozenges, oral rinses, and toothpastes containing salivary proteins, which have not been shown to significantly improve saliva production [38].

Increasing evidence suggests that secretory failure of the salivary and lacrimal glands is due to the inhibitory effects of inflammation rather than destruction of exocrine tissue. Thus, salivary stimulants are a reasonable treatment option. However, trials of low-dose steroids or immunosuppressive drugs, such as methotrexate, cyclosporine, and azathioprine, have shown no improvement in lacrimal or salivary function [10]. Hydroxychloroquine, which is effective for many of the extraglandular features of the disease, appears to have no effect on salivary or lacrimal flow [39].

Pilocarpine and cevimeline hydrochloride are cholinergic agents with muscarinic agonist activity used in the treatment of xerostomia. They are effective in increasing salivary flow and improving symptoms of dry mouth. Symptomatic improvement from the use of pilocarpine may take up to 6 weeks with the most prevailing side effects being flushing, sweating, diarrhea, and urinary frequency. Pilocarpine may be started at 5 mg once daily increasing to twice daily after 1 week up to 5 mg four times daily. Cevimeline, believed to be more selective than pilocarpine, predominantly affects the M1 and M3 receptors, which are particularly prevalent in exocrine glands. Two controlled clinical trials showed significant improvement in subjective and objective symptoms of dry eyes and mouth in patients taking cevimeline 30 mg three times daily. A higher dose of 60 mg three times daily was poorly tolerated due to increased side effects of headaches, increased sweating, abdominal pain, and nausea. Due to the side effect profile, pilocarpine should be used first, with preference given to relatively young patients with a good reserve of salivary and lacrimal function [40, 41].

Biologics have also been used to stimulate salivary gland function although studies show conflicting evidence of efficacy with TFN-alpha inhibitors including infliximab and etanercept [42–44]. Because B-cells play a vital role in the pathogenesis of many autoimmune diseases, antibodies that are antagonistic to B-cells have been utilized to manage these diseases. Epratuzumab, the first antagonistic antibody to the B-cell marker CD22, appears to function by immune modulation of B-cells [45]. It functions as a humanized IgG1 monoclonal antibody against the CD22 antigen and downregulates the B-cell receptor [46]. Epratuzumab was originally developed for the treatment of non-Hodgkin's lymphoma and has now been found to be effective in primary SS as well as SLE. Rituximab, known for its tolerance and short-term efficacy, is an anti-CD20 antibody, which is effective in various autoimmune diseases. Rituximab targets B-cells, suggesting that B-cells may play a role in the etiopathogenesis of SS [45, 47].

Additionally, electrical stimulation of the tongue and hard palate has been shown to be useful in stimulating salivary flow in patients with SS and can be considered [48]. Secondary effects of oral candidiasis can be treated with topical and/or systemic antifungal agents [11].

Conclusion

Sjögren's syndrome causes a spectrum of oral problems, including xerostomia, dental caries, candidiasis, and inflammation of the oral mucosa. Swollen sublingual and parotid glands, as well as lymphocytic infiltrates, are a hallmark of SS. Though the exact etiology of SS is unknown, a variety of immunologic factors are thought to be responsible. Oral symptoms secondary to SS can be challenging to treat. Optimal hydration, saliva substitutes, meticulous oral hygiene, and candida prophylaxis are important general measures. Secretory sialagogues have been proven to be the main medical therapy with beneficial effects, if contraindications do not exist as well as biologics.

Systemic Lupus Erythematosus

Epidemiology

Systemic lupus erythematosus (SLE) is a chronic autoimmune disorder characterized by the production of autoantibodies directed against nuclear and cytoplasmic antigens. SLE may affect multiple organ systems causing a multitude of physical and immunologic abnormalities with a relapsing and remitting clinical course [49]. It is the most common autoimmune connective tissue disease in the USA affecting more than 1.5 million people with an estimated prevalence of 20–150 per 100,000 and a female-to-male ratio of 9:1 [50]. It is two to three times more likely to affect African-American females and can occur at any age in both sexes but in women is often diagnosed during the childbearing years [51].

Etiopathogenesis

As in many autoimmune diseases, the underlying pathophysiologic mechanism that triggers the autoimmune response in SLE remains largely unknown. However, genetics, ethnicity, hormonal and immune dysregulation, and environmental factors such as infectious agents, stress, and diet, have all been identified as contributing factors [52].

The characteristic disease findings in SLE include inflammation, abnormalities in the blood vessels, and immune-complex deposition. A hallmark immunologic presentation is generalized autoantibody production directed to self-antigens of the nucleus, cytoplasm, cell surface, soluble IgG, and coagulation factors. Antinuclear antibodies (ANA), in particular, are found in 95% of SLE patients [52]. Antibodies to double-strand (ds) DNA (anti-ds DNA) and Smith antigen (anti-Sm) target small nuclear ribonucleoproteins and are unique to SLE and found in the sera of 40% and 30% of patients, respectively [53]. The production of autoantibodies is believed to initiate an immune-complex-mediated inflammatory response causing tissue injury [54].

Clinical Manifestations

The presenting symptoms of SLE are often nonspecific constitutional signs such as fever, fatigue, and weight loss. Fatigue is seen in approximately 80% of patients, whereas fever can be found in more than 50% of SLE patients [55]. Fever may either be a manifestation of the disorder itself, a symptom related to an infection induced by the disorder, or an adverse drug reaction [56]. Additionally, SLE involves a variety of organs and can lead to musculoskeletal, mucocutaneous, renal, neurologic/psychiatric, cardiovascular, and hematologic manifestations all of which have the tendency to exhibit flares followed by periods of remission [57].

Musculoskeletal symptoms usually include arthralgias, arthritis, avascular necrosis of bone (osteonecrosis), and myopathy. The arthritis and arthralgias of SLE tend to be migratory and symmetrically affecting the small joints, yet any joint may be affected [58]. Periarticular structures may also be become inflamed, leading to tendonitis, tenosynovitis, and tendon rupture. Avascular necrosis is mostly seen in larger joints such as the hip and knee with resultant degrees of disability. Mobility is further impaired by myalgias and muscle weakness, which commonly affects the neck, pelvis, thighs, shoulders, and upper arms [59].

Lupus nephritis, one of the most concerning manifestations of SLE, causes substantial morbidity and mortality. A wide variety of other renal disorders may present as well, such as renal amyloidosis, focal segmental glomerulosclerosis, IgA and IgM nephropathy, and necrotizing glomerulitis [60].

Gastrointestinal signs and symptoms occur frequently in SLE patients with two of the most common being mesenteric vasculitis and thrombosis. These are significant in that both can lead to life-threatening ischemia, perforation, and infarction [61].

The most common pulmonary manifestation is pleuritis; however, even parenchymal disease, such as pneumonitis, acute respiratory distress, diffuse alveolar hemorrhage, chronic interstitial pneumonitis, and shrinking lung syndrome can be seen [62]. Vascular involvement, acute reversible hypoxemia, pulmonary embolism, pulmonary arterial hypertension, and obstructive lung disease and upper airway disease are also seen in patients with SLE [63].

Cardiovascular disease (CVD) seen in SLE include valvular heart disease associated with Libman-Sacks disease lesions, sterile vegetations, serositis associated with pericardial disease, and venous and arterial thrombosis associated with antiphospholipid antibodies. Research suggests that such association between SLE and CVD strictly depends on a combination of risk factors for CVD, which should be thoroughly assessed in all SLE patients [64].

The central nervous system is often affected in SLE patients, which can lead to neurologic and psychiatric symptoms. The two most common neurologic manifestations in SLE patients are seizures and cerebrovascular disease, such as stroke, transient ischemic attack, and venous sinus thrombosis. Common psychiatric manifestations are depression and cognitive dysfunction, yet additional symptoms such as headaches, mood disorders, acute confusional states, and anxiety may also occur [65, 66].

Blood disorders are common in SLE patients and can present with significant clinical manifestations. The main hematological findings are cytopenia (including anemia, thrombocytopenia, neutropenia, and leukopenia) and thrombophilia [67].

Approximately 30% of SLE patients suffer from ocular involvement. Keratoconjunctivitis sicca, in which one or both eyes display persistent dryness, is the most common manifestation. Optic neuritis and ischemic optic neuropathy cause the most devastating symptoms as a result of damage to the optic nerve. Additionally, retinal vaso-occlusion similar to diabetic and hypertensive retinopathy may seriously threaten visual acuity [68].

With as much as 85% involvement, the skin is one of the most frequently affected organs in SLE patients and, in some cases, may be the only organ involved [69]. Cutaneous manifestations include the malar rash and discoid lesions. These lesions spread centrifugally and may be painful and pruritic [57]. Areas most frequently affected are the face, scalp, ears, and neck [70].

Oral Signs and Symptoms

Variations exist in reported rates of oral manifestations in lupus ranging from a low prevalence to more than 50%. This wide range is likely secondary to the fact that routine oral examinations are not always included in physical examinations. Nevertheless, as one of the criteria for establishing a diagnosis of SLE, oropharyngeal manifestations of the disease are important [49]. Oral ulcerations affecting the gingiva, buccal mucosa, hard and soft palate, as well as the tongue and lips may occur [71, 72] (Figs. 6.3 and 6.4). The classic oral lupus lesion is a whitish plaque with erythema in the center and keratotic striae at the periphery with or without telangiectasias. However, the pattern of the oral lesions may differ among different types of lupus [73]. Most lesions are round, but they may also be linear, fissured, or ulcerated lesions, which most commonly affect the hard palate. In the bullous form of SLE, multiple blisters may be seen, which may affect the entire oropharyngeal cavity. Other oropharyngeal signs and symptoms include oral candidiasis with a prevalence ranging from 4% to 75%; dysphagia, with a prevalence ranging from 11% to 75%; and xerostomia, with a prevalence of 1%–100% [57].

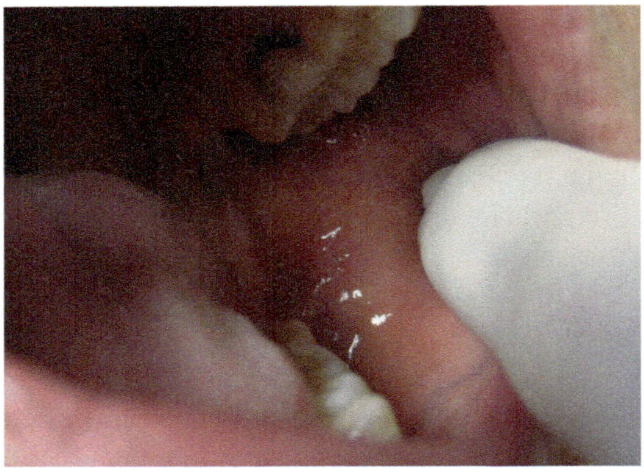

Fig. 6.3 Mucosal ulcerations involving the left buccal mucosa, inferiorly

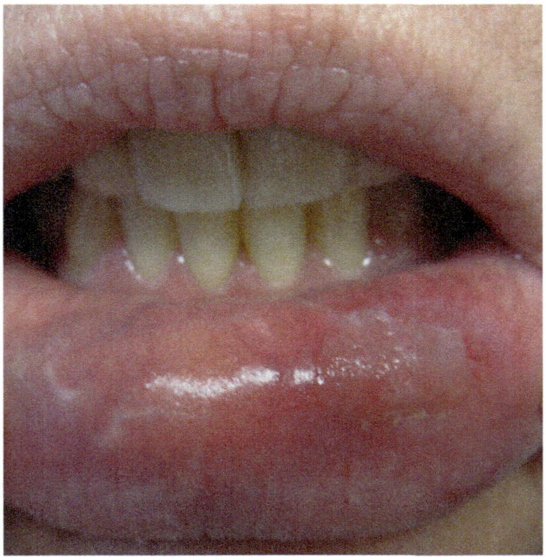

Fig. 6.4 Ulceration of the lower labial mucosa

Skin or intraoral biopsy is generally required for diagnosis where histologic characteristics include lichenoid mucositis with acanthosis and deep perivascular infiltrate, hyperkeratosis with keratotic plugs, liquefaction necrosis, thickening of the basement membrane, atrophy of the rete ridges, edema in the lamina propria, a subepithelial mononuclear infiltrate, and periodic acid-Schiff-positive deposits. Direct immunofluorescence is often positive and shows linear deposits of IgG or IgM and/or C3 in the basement membrane zone. The base of the ulcer often reveals CD4+ T lymphocytes [74, 75].

Differential Diagnosis

Due to multisystem involvement and its various manifestations, the diagnosis of SLE may be difficult with a fairly broad differential diagnosis. SLE should be considered in any patient who has features affecting two or more organ systems [72]. While a comprehensive list of all possible alternative diagnoses is too broad to review, a few are listed in this discussion.

Although rare, a few drugs are associated with causing a lupus-like syndrome or exacerbating preexisting disease. These include sulfonamides, penicillin, minocycline, and NSAIDs [72].

Early rheumatoid arthritis (RA) may be difficult to distinguish from the arthritis of SLE since both conditions may cause joint tenderness and swelling. Additionally, symptoms more frequently seen in later stages of RA such as swan neck deformities, ulnar deviation, and soft tissue laxity can also be seen in patients with SLE. Plain radiographs may help distinguish the two, whereas joint erosions are infrequent in SLE but characteristic of rheumatoid arthritis.

Mixed connective tissue disease (MCTD), characterized by overlapping features of SLE, systemic sclerosis (SSc), polymyositis (PM), and the presence of high titers of antibodies against U1 ribonucleoprotein (RNP), is often difficult to diagnose since many of its characteristic features occur sequentially and often over a period of years. Furthermore, some patients with MCTD may evolve into another connective tissue disease, including SLE [76]. Therefore, it is important to consider MCTD in the differential diagnosis of SLE.

Patients with undifferentiated connective tissue disease (UCTD) have signs and symptoms suggestive of a systemic autoimmune disease but do not satisfy the classification criteria for a defined connective tissue disease. These patients may have symptoms such as arthritis and arthralgias, Raynaud's phenomenon, and serological findings that are difficult to distinguish from early phases of SLE [77].

Patients with systemic sclerosis (SSc) and SLE share similar symptoms. The coexistence of Raynaud's phenomenon and gastroesophageal reflux is typically observed in SSc, but these findings may also be seen in patients with SLE. Histology may help differentiate the two as well as laboratory investigations including ANA, which is frequently positive in both SLE and SSc, while other serologies such as anti-double-stranded DNA (dsDNA) and anti-Smith (Sm) antibodies are more commonly present in SLE [78].

Constitutional symptoms, skin lesions, neuropathy, and renal dysfunction commonly seen in SLE can also be seen in the setting of medium and small vessel vasculitides such as polyarteritis nodosa, granulomatosis with polyangiitis, or microscopic polyangiitis.

Dermatomyositis (DM) and polymyositis (PM) should also be considered in the differential diagnosis of SLE especially for those presenting with myositis or proximal muscle weakness. A positive ANA is observed in approximately 30% of patients with DM and PM, compared to a much larger proportion in SLE. The characteristic skin findings of DM including Gottron's papules, heliotrope rash, photodistributed poikiloderma, and the absence of SLE findings such as oral ulcers, arthritis, nephritis, and hematologic abnormalities can differentiate the two [78].

Other conditions to consider in the differential diagnosis include Adult Still's disease (ASD), serum sickness, fibromyalgia, multiple sclerosis, malignancies, and infections such as cytomegalovirus, Epstein-Barr virus, human parvovirus B19, human immunodeficiency virus, and the hepatitis B and C viruses [78].

Treatment

The treatment course for SLE varies from patient to patient given that it is a multiorgan system disease. Therapy usually involves nonsteroidal anti-inflammatory drugs (NSAIDs), corticosteroids, antimalarial agents, and immunosuppressive drugs. These drugs may be used alone or in combination depending upon the severity of symptoms.

Arthritis and serositis are often controlled with NSAIDs or aspirin. Use of these agents requires vigilance on part of the physician because they can detrimentally affect renal function or cause drug-induced hepatitis. Treatment with chloroquine and hydroxychloroquine is a consideration, if arthritis symptoms are not controlled with NSAIDs. Similarly, NSAIDS are used initially in the treatment of pleurisy and pericarditis. Corticosteroids should be considered, if symptom relief is not found with NSAIDs and infection and thromboembolic phenomena have been ruled out. Cutaneous manifestations have traditionally been responsive to topical corticosteroids or antimalarial agents. Severe discoid lupus and cutaneous vasculitis, however, usually necessitate the use of systemic corticosteroids. Steroid therapy is also initiated to treat patients with thrombocytopenia and hemolytic anemia. Immunosuppressive agents should be considered, if no response is seen with steroid therapy. Cyclophosphamide and glucocorticoids have shown efficacy in treating lupus nephritis and angiopathy [72].

There are limited controlled studies on the management of SLE-associated oral lesions. Potent topical corticosteroids are often administered initially; however, intralesional corticosteroids may also be considered. Thalidomide, clofazimine, and methotrexate have also been used for treatment [79, 80].

Conclusion

The mucocutaneous lesions of LE and the multisystem manifestations of SLE significantly impact the dental health of affected individuals. SLE-associated oral lesions are often challenging to treat and require a range of different medications from topical steroids to potent systemic immunosuppressive therapy. Oral lesions occur in approximately 20%–30% of patients. However, the impact of renal, neuropsychiatric, cardiovascular, and hematologic disease often influences the management of oral disease.

Systemic Sclerosis

Epidemiology

Systemic sclerosis (SSc) is a chronic, immune-mediated condition within the scleroderma spectrum of disorders characterized by inflammation and fibrotic changes, which can compromise the function of multiple organ systems [81]. Systemic sclerosis is relatively rare with an estimated prevalence of 1–2/10,000. There appears to be two peaks of onset; in the early 1930s and mid-1950s with a female predominance of 5:1, though environmentally induced disease is generally more common in men [82, 83]. The disease often occurs in conjunction with other autoimmune diseases such as SLE [84].

Etiopathogenesis

Like many other autoimmune disorders, the pathogenesis of SSc and scleroderma itself is poorly understood though immune activation, vascular damage, and increased deposition of collagen are known to be important factors in the development of the disease [85]. Generally, it is believed that an early immunologic event leads to vascular changes that results in activation of fibroblasts.

Approximately 95% of patients with SSc have circulating autoantibodies directed at one or more antigens including topoisomerase I (formerly called Scl-70), centromere antigens, fibrillarin, ribonucleic acid (RNA) polymerase, PM-Scl, and fibrillin-1 [86–88]. The inciting event causing the production of these autoantibodies, unfortunately, is unknown though several theories exist.

The hallmark of SSc is the development of fibroblasts capable of producing and depositing excess matrix. This may be the result of a net excess of positive activating signals, a reduction in inhibitory signals, or both. Interactions with extracellular matrix components like collagen fibers and fibronectin influence inhibition of collagen synthesis by normal dermal fibroblasts while modulating cell morphology, proliferative capacity, and cytokine responsiveness.

Clinical Manifestations

Raynaud's phenomenon is commonly seen in patients with SSc characterized by an initial white color change to the skin due to exposure to cold temperatures. As a consequence, the reduced blood supply to the fingers, toes, nose, or earlobes may lead to cyanosis. Other manifestations include smooth, taut, stretched, and mask-like facies due to subcutaneous collagen deposition (Fig. 6.5). More serious sequelae

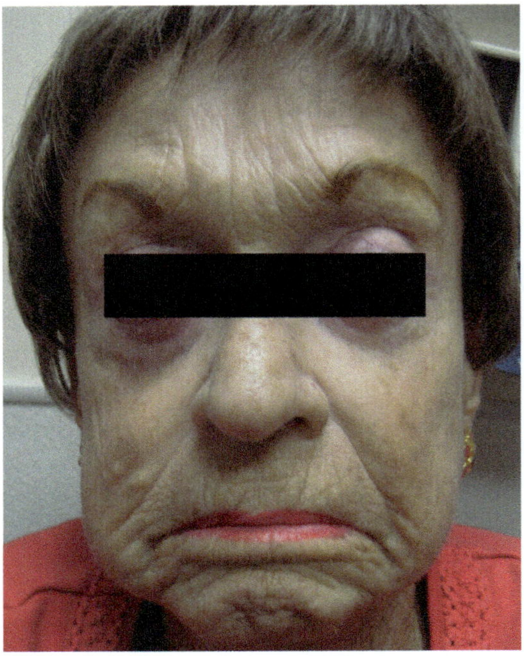

Fig. 6.5 Characteristic mask-like facies and thinned lips

of SSc include fibrosis of the lungs, heart, kidneys, and gastrointestinal tract, which may lead to organ failure. Additionally, gastrointestinal symptoms such as dysphagia and heartburn are not uncommon [89].

The most widely used classification of SSc is based on the extent of skin sclerosis and recognizes two major subsets, limited cutaneous systemic sclerosis (LCSS) and diffuse cutaneous systemic sclerosis (DCSS). LCSS typically presents with a long history of antecedent Raynaud's phenomenon that is often severe and associated with recurrent digital ulceration. Skin involvement is limited to areas distal to the knees and elbows and often affects the wrists and ankles. Changes in the face and neck are also usually present. Other hallmark features include cutaneous telangiectasias, which are often seen on the palms and periorally, and subcutaneous calcinosis. Esophageal dysmotility and gastroesophageal reflux disease can also be seen. Diffuse cutaneous systemic sclerosis is present when sclerosis occurs proximal to the elbows or knees or affects the trunk. Affected skin is often intensely pruritic and loss of specialized skin structures occurs leading to changes in the pattern of perspiration and loss of hair growth. Pain and swelling of the extremities is common and may be mistaken for inflammatory arthropathy [83].

Oral Signs and Symptoms

Oral manifestations of SSc are variable, but approximately 70% of patients develop microstomia, difficulty opening the mouth, as well as a pursed lip appearance due to constriction of the mouth from perioral collagen deposition [90] (Fig. 6.6). Also, fibrosis of the tongue and esophagus results in limited mobility and dysphagia. Gingival recession is also common, and salivary gland fibrosis can lead to severe xerostomia and dental caries. Radiographic changes include an increased width of the periodontal ligament spaces in all quadrants and mandibular resorption that tends to be more pronounced in the posterior regions [84]. Diffuse widening of the periodontal ligament space is noted in the entire dentition. The mandible exhibits resorption of the ramus along with the coronoid processes, mental tubercle, and condyles on panoramic radiography [91].

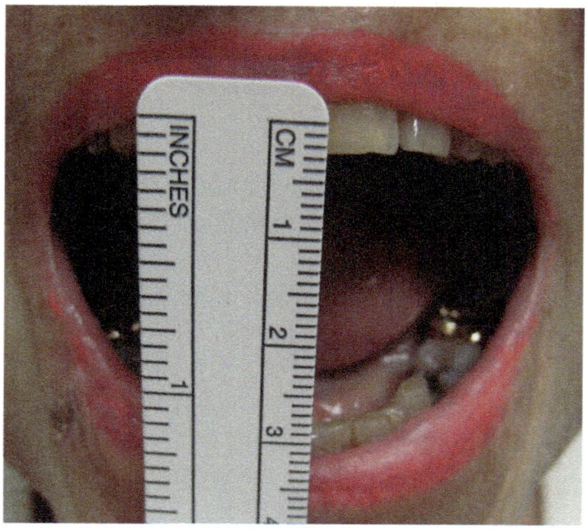

Fig. 6.6 Limited oral aperture due to sclerosis of the perioral tissues

Differential Diagnosis

The differential diagnosis of SSc is broad and determined by the salient clinical features of the particular patient. The coexistence of Raynaud's phenomenon and gastroesophageal reflux disease is strongly suggestive of SSc. These disorders occur frequently in otherwise healthy persons or in association with various diseases, drugs, and environmental exposures; thus, their presence may be of limited diagnostic value. The combination of pitting scars at the fingertips and evidence of interstitial lung disease prominent at the lung bases is strongly suggestive of SSc [92].

Exposure to drugs, toxins, or harmful environmental factors must be considered when evaluating patients with indurated skin. Additionally, some endocrine disorders (e.g., diabetes mellitus and hypothyroidism), renal disease, and infiltrative disorders can also cause scleroderma-like skin changes [92].

Other conditions to consider in the differential diagnosis of SSc are scleromyxedema, diabetes mellitus, myxedema due to hypothyroidism, nephrogenic systemic fibrosis, amyloidosis, eosinophilic fasciitis, chronic GVHD, drug-induced scleroderma, and environmental exposure to organic solvents [92].

Treatment

Organ-based treatment has frequently been the approach to therapy because of the vast array of symptoms caused by SSc. Treatment of localized sclerotic skin includes ultraviolet A1 (UVA-1) light therapy, highly potent topical glucocorticoids, calcipotriol (a vitamin D analog), and methotrexate [92]. Combinations of high-dose systemic glucocorticoids and methotrexate have also been utilized with careful screening for scleroderma renal crisis. Furthermore, antihistamines have been useful for pruritus along with topical corticosteroids. Calcium channel blockers have been helpful in patients with SSc-related calcinosis and Raynaud's phenomenon. In treatment-resistant cases, surgical intervention with a sympathectomy has been tried.

Meticulous dental hygiene is imperative in SSc patients, due to predisposition to caries and periodontal disease and potential limitations with dental care resulting from microstomia and flexion contractures.

Conclusion

Systemic sclerosis is a multifaceted disease with a complex and poorly understood pathogenesis due to immunologically triggered fibrosis. Our limited understanding of the pathogenesis of the disease has hampered the development of effective therapies. Therefore, life-threatening complications should be managed aggressively.

Mixed Connective Tissue Disease

Epidemiology

Mixed connective tissue disease (MCTD) is a systemic autoimmune disease first described in 1972 as a condition displaying mixed features of SLE, SSc, polymyositis/dermatomyositis (PM/DM), and rheumatoid arthritis in connection with the presence of high titers of anti-U1 ribonucleoprotein (anti-U1 RNP) antibodies [93]. The prevalence and incidence of MCTD is unclear; however, it is known that the condition is much more common in women than in men.

Etiopathogenesis

Like other autoantibody-mediated diseases, the development of MCTD appears to be the result of a complex interaction between genetic and environmental factors. Furthermore, autoimmunity is often driven by components of subcellular particles such as spliceosomes, which are complex nuclear particles involved in the processing of pre-messenger RNA into mature "spliced RNA." Certain components of the spliceosome are common targets of autoimmunity in the diffuse connective tissue diseases such as small nuclear ribonucleoprotein particles (snRNPs) and heterogeneous nuclear RNP particles (hnRNPs) [94]. Also, like in many other autoimmune diseases, autoantibodies are widely recognized as the hallmark of the disease. Specifically, the presence of anti-RNP antibodies is required for the diagnosis of MCTD. Patients with MCTD display a very vigorous antibody response characterized by hypergammaglobulinemia [95]. Additionally, anti-U1 RNP antibodies have demonstrated Ig class switching from IgM to IgG as evidenced by variable region mutations, a feature typical of T-cell dependent B-cell maturation [96]. In fact, T-cells play a central role in the pathogenesis of many murine models of autoimmunity. Additional evidence of T-cell involvement in the pathogenesis of MCTD includes the dense T-cell lymphocytic infiltrate found at sites of tissue injury and experimental findings that human RNP-reactive T-cells can provide B-cell help in anti-RNP autoantibody production [97, 98].

Clinical Manifestations

Early clinical manifestations of MCTD often include fever, malaise, arthralgias and myalgias. Although almost any organ system can be affected by MCTD, there are four clinical features that point toward MCTD rather than other connective tissue disorders: Raynaud's phenomenon, the absence of severe renal and central nervous system disease, the presence of severe arthritis and the insidious onset of pulmonary hypertension, and anti-U1 RNP antibodies [99–101]. Raynaud's phenomenon (RP) is one of the most consistent features of MCTD, which appears in approximately 75%–90% of patients and may precede other clinical manifestations by months or years [102]. Also, almost 70% of patients develop swollen hands and sausage-like digits [99]. Superficial vasculitis of the digits, acrosclerosis, calcinosis cutis, discoid plaques, and a malar rash can also occur [100].

Joint involvement varies from minimal arthralgias, arthritis, erosions typical of rheumatoid arthritis to arthritis mutilans. In general, polyarthralgia is an early and common symptom in MCTD, occurring in approximately 60% of patients, and may be accompanied by joint deformities with radiographic changes. Rheumatoid factor can be positive in up to 70% of patients with MCTD [99, 103, 104]. Between 80% and 90% of patients develop muscle involvement. Proximal muscles are more frequently affected with elevation of creatinine kinase; however, it does not present a specific pattern that differentiates it from other connective tissue diseases with muscle involvement. Electromyography is typical of inflammatory myopathy, although, focal myositis may also occur [99].

Pulmonary abnormalities are found in about 85% of MCTD patients though most have an asymptomatic course. Fibrosis, interstitial lung disease, pulmonary arterial hypertension, dyspnea, and pleuritic chest pain can arise. Radiographic findings include interstitial changes, pleural effusions, pneumonic infiltrates, and pleural thickening [105].

Approximately 30% of MCTD patients have symptomatic heart disease. The most frequent manifestation is pericarditis (10%–29%), which is usually mild. Myocarditis, conduction disturbances, and abnormal left ventricular diastolic filling (26%) have also been detected by echocardiography. Furthermore, vasculopathy in MCTD is usually similar to SSc and is characterized by intimal proliferation and hypertrophy of the media that affects small and medium-sized vessels [106, 107].

Gastrointestinal involvement is common (66–74%) and often represents a major feature of overlap with SSc. Esophageal dysfunction is the most prevalent gastrointestinal manifestation, which is initially subclinical but often presents as dysphagia when symptomatic. Esophageal dysmotility and gastroesophageal reflux disease occur more frequently in patients who have clinical manifestations mostly related to SSc rather than SLE. Other gastrointestinal manifestations described include mesenteric vasculitis, colonic perforation, protein-losing enteropathy, acute pancreatitis, hemoperitoneum, diarrhea, and chronic active hepatitis [108].

Renal involvement is one of the major complications of MCTD though often asymptomatic. In some studies, it has been observed in approximately 25% of patients [109]. Severe renal disease is rare, and the presence of anti-U1 RNP antibodies may be protective against the development of diffuse proliferative glomerulonephritis (GNF). Membranous and mesangial GNF are the most common presentation although focal or diffuse proliferative GNF can also be present. In addition, immune-complex-mediated nephritis has been reported [110].

Leukopenia, anemia of chronic disease, broad-based hypergammaglobulinemia, and positive Coombs test without hemolysis are the most frequently reported hematological features. Interestingly, although they are not specific for MCTD, anemia and leukopenia tend to correlate with disease activity and usually improve with treatment. Other less common features include thrombocytopenia, thrombotic thrombocytopenic purpura (TTP), and red cell aplasia [102].

Trigeminal neuralgia is the most common manifestation of the peripheral nervous system in MCTD. Headaches and peripheral neuropathies have also been reported. Some patients can develop aseptic meningitis with increased concentrations of interferon gamma (IFN-γ), interleukin-6 (IL-6), and higher titers of anti-

U1-RNP antibodies in cerebrospinal fluid (CSF) than in serum. In fact, titers of anti-U1 RNP antibodies in CSF correlate well with disease activity [111, 112].

Oral Signs and Symptoms

There is very little described regarding oral symptoms of MCTD likely because the oral manifestations are less characteristic in MCTD than in other more common autoimmune disorders. Oral symptoms associated with other autoimmune conditions such as xerostomia and limited mouth opening, however, can arise in MCTD [113].

Differential Diagnosis

Mixed connective tissue disease should be suspected in patients with Raynaud's phenomenon and non-deforming, nonerosive arthritis or arthralgia. Such cases are sometimes misdiagnosed as rheumatoid arthritis because these patients frequently have high titers of rheumatoid factor. It appears that moderate to severe erosive arthritis is uncommon in anti-RNP positive patients even in the presence of prolonged elevations of RF. The combination of subacute or chronic cutaneous lupus erythematosus, Raynaud's phenomenon, and arthralgia is frequently observed by dermatologists and appears to have a high association with anti-RNP antibodies [114, 115].

Distinguishing MCTD from SLE, SSc, and RA can be challenging in some cases, particularly because many patients who have anti-U1 RNP antibodies satisfy the criteria for SLE or SSc. Additionally, patients may experience an evolution of symptoms from MCTD to SLE. It has also been a challenge to distinguish MCTD from PM/DM; however, its association with HLA class II alleles can be helpful in making this distinction. In MCTD, HLA-DR1, HLA -DR2, and HLA -DR4 are the main HLA-associated alleles [115]. SLE is mainly associated with HLA-DR2 and HLA-DR3, SSc with HLA-DR3 or HLA-DR5, and PM/DM with HLA-DR3 [102, 116].

Treatment

Patients diagnosed with MCTD were initially described as having a good prognosis and being extremely responsive to corticosteroid therapy. However, subsequent long-term studies have revealed that not all patients have a benign clinical course and that not all clinical manifestations are responsive to steroids [93]. Some patients may have mild self-limited disease, whereas others may develop severe major organ involvement with life-threatening manifestations. Unfortunately, there are no controlled clinical trials for the treatment of MCTD; thus, treatment must largely rely upon the conventional therapies that are used to treat similar clinical manifestations in other rheumatic diseases such as SLE, SSc, and PM [117]. In any case, therapy should be individualized for each patient based on the specific organs involved and the severity of underlying disease activity. Inflammatory manifestations such as fever, serositis, myositis, arthritis, and skin rash usually respond to steroid treatment, whereas clinical sclerodermatous manifestations such as sclerodactyly, moderate esophageal disease, sclerodermatous bowel disease, and pulmonary interstitial disease more often require cytotoxic immunosuppressive treatment. In general, corticosteroids (prednisone and methylprednisolone) and cytotoxic agents (most often cyclophosphamide) are the most frequently used immunosuppressants. Antimalarials such as hydroxychloroquine, methotrexate, and different types of vasodilators have also been used with varying degrees of success [118]. Fever, fatigue, nonspecific arthralgias, or myalgias usually respond to NSAIDs, hydroxychloroquine, or low-dose prednisone depending on the severity [99]. Gastrointestinal disease in MCTD can be treated with conventional treatment such as proton pump inhibitors, H2-receptor antagonists, and lifestyle modifications, together with esophageal pH monitoring in patients with persistent reflux symptoms [108].

Conclusion

MCTD has a wide spectrum of clinical manifestations with long-term studies revealing that some patients experience mild self-limited disease, whereas others develop severe major organ involvement. The worst prognosis and highest mortality are associated with the presence of pulmonary arterial hypertension. Treatment of MCTD is individualized depending upon the specific clinical manifestations and potential need for aggressive treatment for life-threatening manifestations. Further prospective clinical trials are needed to evaluate its clinical course, long-term prognosis, and response to therapy.

Dermatomyositis

Epidemiology

The idiopathic inflammatory myopathies (IIM) comprise a heterogeneous group of autoimmune muscle disorders characterized by progressive muscle weakness. Although they are uncommon conditions, their importance has increasingly been recognized because of the associated morbidity and mortality. Dermatomyositis (DM) is a subtype of IIM with characteristic cutaneous manifestations. In 1975, Bohan and Peter wrote a classic article that suggested a set of criteria to aid in the diagnosis and classification of dermatomyositis and polymyositis (PM). These included progressive, proximal, and symmetric weakness, increased concentration of muscle enzymes, abnormal electromyogram, abnormal muscle biopsy sample, and compatible cutaneous disease [119]. Dermatomyositis has many signs and symptoms that involve the orofacial regions and is therefore relevant to oral health care providers.

Information about the incidence and prevalence of DM is limited because of the rarity of the disease. Yet a population-based study confirmed an incidence of 9.63 cases per million persons and a bimodal age distribution of children under 18 years and adults in their late 40s to early 60s [120]. Several studies have found a preponderance of female over male patients, commonly 1.5–2.0:1 with an equal sex ratio in older patients with malignancy. The average age at diagnosis is approximately 40 years, whereas that associated with malignancy is 55 years. DM/PM associated with a connective tissue disease occurs more often in younger women with a higher prevalence in African-Americans [121, 122].

Etiopathogenesis

The etiology of DM is unknown; however, there appears to be immunogenetic markers correlated with the disease. Like other autoimmune disorders, it is possible that DM is due to an interaction between environmental factors and an immunogenetic predisposition to the disease [123]. Studies of histocompatibility antigen prevalence have demonstrated that HLA-B8, -B14, -DR3, -DRw52, and -DQA1 are associated with dermatomyositis [124]. Both juvenile and adult forms have been associated with infectious agents such as influenza A or B1 and hepatitis B, although little scientific evidence has demonstrated a virus as the causative factor. Additionally, a small study hypothesized that a host response to Coxsackie B virus could be related to the pathophysiology of juvenile DM. Picornaviruses have also been thought to be a possible cause of the disease. Finally, one study found that 29 of 58 patients with DM had positive serologic titers for the protozoa Toxoplasma gondii [122].

Clinical Manifestations

A characteristic feature of DM is skin rash, particularly on the face, which precedes, accompanies, or follows progressive proximal muscle weakness. The skin lesions can be transient, atypical, or completely absent. When the rash does occur, it typically presents as a violaceous to dusky erythema of the eyelids and periorbital area with or without edema. This is known as the heliotrope rash, which is characteristic of DM and rarely seen in SLE or scleroderma. Additionally, raised violaceous papules affecting the metatarsophalangeal and interphalangeal joints are considered a pathognomonic sign of DM, known as Gottron's papules. Telangiectasia within the lesions is common [125]. These lesions may be clinically confused with lesions of lupus erythematosus or with papulosquamous disorders, such as psoriasis or lichen planus. Poikiloderma, the combination of atrophy, dyspigmentation, and telangiectasias in a photosensitive distribution, is also common in DM. Although poikiloderma may occur in any sun-exposed site, the classic areas of involvement are the upper back (described as shawl sign), and the V of the neck and chest (known as the V-sign) [126]. Histopathological assessment will aid in differentiation from psoriasis and lichen planus but cannot distinguish the cutaneous lesions of dermatomyositis from those of lupus erythematosus [123]. Several other cutaneous features are characteristic of the disease, which include malar erythema and periungual and cuticular telangiectasia [126].

Muscular involvement in DM is characterized by symmetric weakness that develops over weeks to months in the proximal muscles, as evidenced by difficulty walking upstairs, getting up from a chair, or combing one's hair. Fatigue, myalgias, and muscle tenderness are common symptoms as well. Typically, deep tendon reflexes are unchanged, and muscle atrophy occurs late in the course of the disease. Lumbar lordosis or Trendelenburg gait can also be seen [127]. Arthralgias and/or arthritis may be present in up to one fourth of patients with inflammatory myopathy. The usual picture is one of generalized arthralgias accompanied by morning stiffness. The small joints of the hands, wrists, and ankles may be involved with symmetrical non-deforming arthritis that is nonerosive [123]. Muscle weakness may not be present until late in the course of the disease or may be completely absent as seen in amyopathic DM. Symptoms of DM usually begin gradually with onset of low-grade fever and/or weight loss or fatigue [125].

Pulmonary disease occurs in DM in about 15%–30% of patients, often presenting as interstitial pneumonitis, which is more frequent in patients with esophageal involvement. Lung disease may be a direct complication of muscle disease, such as hypoventilation or aspiration in patients with dysphagia, or might be a result of treatment, as with opportunistic infections or drug-induced hypersensitivity pneumonitis. Pulmonary involvement is associated with a poor prognosis [128]. Cardiac manifestations may occur in up to 50% of patients, but only a small proportion of these patients have symptoms. Various abnormalities have been described, including conduction defects and arrhythmias. Cardiac conditions such as congestive heart failure, pericarditis, and valvular disease may also occur but are much less frequent [129]. Gastrointestinal manifestations include esophageal reflux, delayed gastric emptying, esophageal dysmotility, decreased intestinal motility, and rectal incontinence [122]. A wide variety of malignancies have been reported in patients with DM to include non-Hodgkin's lymphoma, ovarian, nasopharyngeal, lung, pancreatic, stomach, and colorectal cancer. Malignancy is more common in older patients and is rarely seen in children [130].

Oral Signs and Symptoms

Esophageal disease, manifested by dysphagia, is estimated to be present in 15–50% of patients with inflammatory myopathy. The dysphagia can be proximal or distal. Proximal dysphagia is caused by involvement of striated muscles of the pharynx or proximal esophagus, which correlates with the severity of muscle disease and is responsive to steroids. Distal esophageal involvement is more common in patients who have an overlap with scleroderma or another collagen vascular disease. Dysphagia is associated with a poor prognosis and correlates with the presence of pulmonary involvement [126].

Mucous membrane involvement is reported in 10%–20% of cases with mucosal edema and intraoral telangiectasias being the most common oral signs. Marginal gingivitis is believed to be a special sign of the capillary changes in DM [131]. Calcification can also affect the skin and mucosa in DM. Obliteration of the pulp chamber of the teeth may also occur. Patients also have a significantly higher prevalence of dental caries, dental plaque accumulation, and gingival inflammation and therefore are at higher risk for premature loss of the teeth. These symptoms are attributable to decreased salivary flow as can be seen in other autoimmune diseases [132].

Though the risk of oral malignancy in those with DM is unclear, several cases of oral cancer associated with DM have been reported. Squamous cell carcinoma of the tongue, for example, occurred following transient ulcers in the same area in a 19-year-old male patient, 1 year after the onset of DM. Another study reported squamous cell carcinoma of the tongue arising after steroid therapy in an elderly DM patient [125].

Differential Diagnosis

The diagnosis of DM has been largely based on the combination of classic skin manifestations, proximal muscle weakness, and elevated serum creatine kinase (CK), which is the most sensitive diagnostic enzyme test. Levels of this enzyme can increase by a factor of 50 in active DM but can be normal as well [127]. Muscle biopsy characteristically reveals perifascicular muscle fiber atrophy of two to ten layers, which is considered diagnostic even in the absence of inflammation [133]. The inflammatory infiltration of B-cells and CD4 T-cells, when present, is mainly perivascular and peripheral to the fascicles. Serum autoantibodies are common in DM patients, and ANA is frequently positive. Myositis-specific antibodies have been identified in DM such as the anti-Jo-1 antibody, often associated with interstitial lung disease and partially responsive to therapy, and anti-Mi-2 antibodies, which are considered DM specific and associated with treatment responsiveness [125]. Although studies have shown that these serum markers correlate with disease activity, response to therapy, and prognosis, the findings have not been consistent. Therefore, their clinical applications are limited. Muscle biopsies and electromyography can be used as confirmatory tests, while noninvasive diagnostic procedures such as MRI and ultrasound are also helpful [125, 134]. The characteristic skin findings in combination with muscle weakness and appropriate laboratory data can provide straightforward evidence for the diagnosis of DM. Unfortunately, many cases do not present in this manner.

Differential diagnoses of early skin manifestations of dermatomyositis include polymorphic light eruption, SLE, contact dermatitis, lichen planus, seborrheic dermatitis, psoriasis, and atopic dermatitis. The facial erythema seen in DM should be differentiated from lupus erythematosus, rosacea, seborrheic dermatitis, and atopic dermatitis. Clinical distinction may be difficult in some cases, but histopathological assessment is helpful [126].

Other conditions to consider in the differential diagnosis of DM include trichinosis which can cause periorbital swelling and edema similar to that seen in DM, HIV infection, and drugs such as penicillamine, NSAIDs, practolol, hydroxyurea, and pravastatin [122].

Treatment

The goal of treatment is to manage symptoms and prevent further disability, which most often requires a multidisciplinary approach in the medical management of these patients. Corticosteroid treatment represents the mainstay of therapy for DM. Traditionally, prednisone 0.5–1.0 mg/kg is given and continued for at least 6 weeks after myositis symptoms are clinically controlled and enzymes normalize. The dose is then slowly tapered over a period lasting 1.5–2 times as long as the period of active treatment. Approximately 25% of patients will not respond to systemic corticosteroids. Early intervention with steroid-sparing agents, therefore, may be an effective alternative. These include immunosuppressive agents such as methotrexate, azathioprine, cyclophosphamide, mycophenolate mofetil, chlorambucil, or cyclosporin. Some studies report that 50%–75% of patients treated with these agents will respond with a decrease in enzyme concentrations or a decrease in required corticosteroid dose. In a recent report, Ramanan et al. demonstrated that the early addition of methotrexate allowed a more aggressive taper of corticosteroid therapy and resulted in equal control with less steroid-related toxicity [123]. Additionally, hydroxychloroquine in doses of 200–400 mg per day is effective in about 80% of patients when used as a steroid-sparing agent [135]. Patients who do not respond to hydroxychloroquine can be switched to chloroquine phosphate (250–500 mg/day), or combination therapy with quinacrine hydrochloric acid 100 mg twice daily can be considered [136]. Patients who fail to respond to immunosuppressive agents may respond to combination therapy with etanercept, infliximab, or rituximab. Furthermore, a double-blind, placebo-controlled study demonstrated the benefits of high-dose intravenous immune globulin for recalcitrant DM.

Conclusion

Dermatomyositis, a condition primarily of the skin and muscles, frequently involves other organ systems. Though the pathogenesis is not completely understood, common clinical symptoms and treatment recommendations have been acknowledged. Corticosteroids, immunosuppressive agents, biologic agents, and/or intravenous immune globulin are effective therapies for the myopathy of DM. Skin disease is best managed with sun protection, topical corticosteroids, antimalarials, methotrexate, and/or intravenous immune globulin [122].

References

1. Autoimmune Diseases Coordinating Committee. Department of Health and Human Services, National Institutes of Health, National Institute of Allergy and Infectious Disease; 2002. NIH Publication No. 03-5140.
2. Jonsson R, Bowman SJ, Gordon TP. Sjögren's syndrome. In: Koopman WJ, Moreland LW, editors. Arthritis and allied disorders (a textbook of rheumatology). 15th ed. Philadelphia: Lippincott Williams & Wilkins; 2005. p. 1681–706.
3. Venables PJ. Management of patients presenting with Sjogren's syndrome. Best Pract Res Clin Rheumatol. 2006;20(4):791–807.
4. Skopouli FN, Drosos AA, Papaioannou T, Moutsopoulos HM. Preliminary diagnostic criteria for Sjögren's syndrome. Scand J Rheumatol. 1986;61(Suppl):22–5.
5. Manoussakis MN, Georgopoulou C, Zintzaras E, Spyropoulou M, Stavropoulou A, Skopouli FN, et al. Sjögren's syndrome associated with systemic lupus erythematosus: clinical and laboratory profiles and comparison with primary Sjögren's syndrome. Arthritis Rheumatol. 2004;50:882–91.
6. Vitali C, Bombardieri S, Moutsopoulos HM. Classification criteria for Sjogren's syndrome: a revised version of the European criteria proposed by the American European consensus group. Ann Rheum Dis. 2002;61:554–8.
7. Langegger C, Wenger M, Duftner C, Dejaco C, Baldissera I, Moncayo R, et al. Use of the European preliminary criteria, the Breiman classification tree and the American-European criteria for diagnosis of primary Sjögren's syndrome in daily practice: a retrospective analysis. Rheumatol Int. 2007;27:699–702.
8. Uhlig T, Kvien TK, Jensen JL, Ax T II. Sicca symptoms, saliva and tear production, and disease variables in 636 patients with rheumatoid arthritis. Ann Rheum Dis. 1999;58:415–22.
9. Qin B, Wang J, Yang Z, Yang M, Ma N, Huang F, Zhong R. Epidemiology of primary Sjögren's syndrome: a systematic review and meta-analysis. Ann Rheum Dis. 2015;74(11):1983–9.
10. Fox R. Sjögren's syndrome. Lancet. 2005;366:321–31.
11. Matthews SA, Kurien BT, Scofield RH. Oral manifestations of Sjögren's syndrome. J Dent Res. 2008;87:308.
12. Roguedas AM, Misery L, Sassolas B, Le Masson G, Pennec YL, Youinou P. Cutaneous manifestations of primary Sjögren's syndrome are underestimated. Clin Exp Rheumatol. 2004;22:632–6.
13. Alexander EL, Provost TT. Cutaneous manifestations of primary Sjögren's syndrome: a reflection of vasculitis and association with anti-Ro (SSA) antibodies. J Investig Dermatol. 1983;80:386–91.
14. Jubert C, Cosnes A, Clerici T, Gaulard P, Andre P, Revuz J, et al. Sjogren's syndrome and cutaneous B cell lymphoma revealed by anetoderma. Arthritis Rheumatol. 1993;36:133.
15. Stroehmann A, Dorner T, Lukowsky A, Feist E, Hiepe F, Burmester GR. Cutaneous T cell lymphoma in a patient with primary biliary cirrhosis and secondary Sjogren's syndrome. J Rheumatol. 2002;29:1326.
16. Selva-O'Callaghan A, Perez-Lopez J, Solans-Laque R, Lopez-Peig C, Angel-Bosch GJ, Vilardell-Tarres M. Primary cutaneous large B-cell lymphoma of the legs in a patient with primary Sjogren's syndrome. Clin Exp Rheumatol. 2003;21:672.
17. Sarzi-Puttini P, Doria A, Girolomoni G, Kuhn A. The skin in systemic autoimmune diseases. In: Bombardieri S, Baldini C, editors. Handbook of systemic autoimmune diseases, Ch 12 Mucocutaneous manifestations of Sjogren's syndrome: Elsevier B.V.; 2006. https://doi.org/10.1016/S1571-5078(05)05012-9.
18. Mandl T, Ekberg O, Wollmer P, Manthorpe R, Jacobsson L. Dysphagia and dysmotility of the pharynx and oesophagus in patients with primary Sjögren's syndrome. Scand J Rheumatol. 2007;36:394–401.
19. Delande S, de Seze J, Fauchais AL, Hachulla E, Stojkovic T, Ferriby D, et al. Neurologic manifestations in primary Sjögren syndrome: a study of 82 patients. Medicine. 2004;83:280–91.
20. Barendregt PJ, Van den Bent MJ, Van Raaijvan den Aarssen VJ, Van den Meiracker AH, Vecht CJ,

Markusse HM. Involvement of the peripheral nervous system in primary Sjögren's syndrome. Ann Rheum Dis. 2001;60:876–81.
21. Napeñas JJ, Rouleau TS. Oral complications of Sjögren's syndrome. Oral Maxillofac Surg Clin N Am. 2014;26:55–62.
22. Astor FC, Hanft KL, Ciocon JO. Xerostomia: a prevalent condition in the elderly. Ear Nose Throat J. 1999;78:476–9.
23. Mavragani CP, Moutsopoulos NM, Moutsopoulos HM. The management of Sjögren's syndrome. Nat Clin Pract Rheumatol. 2006;2:252–61.
24. Perdson AM, Reibel J, Nordgarden H, Bergrem HO, Jensen JL, Nauntofte B. Primary Sjögren's syndrome: salivary gland function and clinical oral findings. Oral Dis. 1999;5:128–38.
25. Gonzalez S, Sung H, Sepulveda D, Gonzalez MJ, Molina C. Oral manifestations and their treatment in Sjögren's syndrome. Oral Dis. 2014;20(2):153–61.
26. Soto-Rojas AE, Kraus A. The oral side of Sjögren syndrome. Diagnosis and treatment. A review. Arch Med Res. 2002;33:96–106.
27. Pertovaara M, Korpela M, Uusitalo H, Pukander J, Miettinen A, Helin H, et al. Clinical follow up study of 87 patients with sicca symptoms (dryness of eyes or mouth, or both). Ann Rheum Dis. 1999;58:423–7.
28. Harris NL. Lymphoid proliferations of the salivary glands. Am J Clin Pathol. 1999;111:S94–103.
29. Russell SL, Reisine S. Investigation of xerostomia in patients with rheumatoid arthritis. J Am Dent Assoc. 1998;129:733–9.
30. Percival RS, Challacombe SJ, Marsh PD. Flow rates of resting whole and stimulated parotid saliva in relation to age and gender. J Dent Res. 1994;73(8):1416–20.
31. Scott J. Qualitative and quantitative observations on the histology of human labial salivary glands obtained post mortem. J Biol Buccale. 1980;8(3):187–200.
32. Greenburg G, Anderson R, Sharpstone P, James DG. Enlargement of parotid gland due to sarcoidosis. Br Med J. 1964;2(5413):861–2.
33. Kazi S, Cohen PR, Williams F, Schempp R, Reveille JD. The diffuse infiltrative lymphocytosis syndrome. Clinical and immunogenetic features in 35 patients. AIDS. 1996;10(4):385.
34. Cheuk W, Chan JK. IgG4-related sclerosing disease: a critical appraisal of an evolving clinicopathologic entity. Adv Anat Pathol. 2010;17(5):303.
35. Liu SY, Vlantis AC, Lee WC. Bilateral parotid and submandibular gland enlargement: rare features of Wegener's granulomatosis. J Laryngol Otol. 2003;117(2):148–50.
36. Feinstein AJ, Ciarleglio MM, Cong X, Otremba MD, Judson BL. Parotid gland lymphoma: prognostic analysis of 2140 patients. Laryngoscope. 2013;123(5):1199.
37. Amarasena R, Bowman S. Sjögren's syndrome. Clin Med. 2007;7:53–6.
38. Van der Reijden WA, Vissink A, Veerman E, Nieuw-Amerongen AV. Treatment of oral dryness related complaints (xerostomia) in Sjögren's syndrome. Ann Rheum Dis. 1999;58:465–73.
39. Kruize AA, Hene RJ, Kallenberg CG, van Bijsterveld OP, van der Heide A, Kater L, et al. Hydroxychloroquine treatment for primary Sjogren's syndrome; a two year, double blind cross over trial. Ann Rheum Dis. 1993;52:60–4.
40. Petrone D, Condemi JJ, Fife R, Gluck O, Cohen S, Dalgin P. A double-blind, randomized, placebo-controlled study of cevimeline in Sjogren's syndrome patients with xerostomia and keratoconjunctivitis sicca. Arthritis Rheum. 2002;46:748–54.
41. Fife RS, Chase WF, Dore RK, Wiesenhutter CW, Lockhart PB, Tindal E, et al. Cevimeline for the treatment of xerostomia in patients with Sjögren syndrome: a randomized trial. Arch Intern Med. 2002;162:1293–300.
42. Thanou-Stavraki A, James JA. Primary Sjögren's syndrome: current and prospective therapies. Semin Arthritis Rheum. 2008;37(5):273–92.
43. Steinfeld SD, Demols P, Salmon I, Kiss R, Appelboom T. Infliximab in patients with primary Sjögren's syndrome: a pilot study. Arthritis Rheumatol. 2001;44:2371–5.
44. Sankar V, Brennan MT, Kok MR, Leakan RA, Smith JA, Manny J, et al. Etanercept in Sjögren's syndrome: a twelve-week randomized, double-blind, placebo-controlled pilot clinical trial. Arthritis Rheumatol. 2004;50:2240–5.
45. Goldenberg DM. Epratuzumab in the therapy of oncological and immunological diseases. Expert Rev Anticancer Ther. 2006;6:1341–53.
46. Steinfeld SD, Tant L, Burmester GR, Teoh NK, Wegener WA, Goldenberg DM, et al. Epratuzumab (humanized anti-CD22 antibody) in primary Sjögren's syndrome: an open-label phase I/II study. Arthritis Res Ther. 2006;8:129.
47. Ramos-Casals M, Brito-Zerón P. Emerging biological therapies in primary Sjögren's syndrome. Rheumatology. 2007;46:1389–96.
48. Steller M, Chou L, Daniels TE. Electrical stimulation of salivary flow in patients with Sjögren's syndrome. J Dent Res. 1988;67:1334–7.
49. Fortuna G, Brennan M. Systemic lupus erythematosus epidemiology, pathophysiology, manifestations, and management. Dent Clin N Am. 2013;57:631–55.
50. Schur PH, Hahn BH. Epidemiology and pathogenesis of systemic lupus erythematosus. In: Basow DS, editor. UpToDate. Netherlands: Wolters Kluwer; 2013. Retrieved 17 Sept 2014.
51. Pons-Estel GJ, Alacron GS, Scofield L, Reinlib L, Cooper GS. Understanding the epidemiology and progression of systemic lupus erythematous. Semin Arthritis Rheum. 2010;39:257–68.
52. Pisetsky DS. Systemic lupus erythematosus. A. Epidemiology, pathology, and pathogenesis. In: Klippel JH, Crofford LJ, Stone JH, Weyand CM, editors. Primer on the rheumatic diseases. Atlanta: The Arthritis Foundation; 2001. p. 329–52.
53. Tan EM, Cohen AS, Fries JF, Masi AT, McShane DJ, Rothfield NF, et al. The 1982 revised criteria for

the classification of systemic lupus erythematosus. Arthritis Rheumatol. 1982;25(11):1271–7.
54. Boumpas DT, Fessler BJ, Austin HA, Balow JE, Klippel JH, Lockshin MD. Systemic lupus erythematosus: emerging concepts. Part 2: dermatologic and joint disease, the antiphospholipid antibody syndrome, pregnancy and hormonal therapy, morbidity and mortality, and pathogenesis. Ann Intern Med. 1995;123(1):42–53.
55. Tench CM, McCurdie I, White PD, D'Cruz DP. The prevalence and associations of fatigue in systemic lupus erythematosus. Rheumatology. 2000;39:1249–54.
56. Stahl NI, Klippel JH, Decker JL. Fever in systemic lupus erythematosus. Am J Med. 1979;67:935–40.
57. Brennan M, Valerin M, Napenas J, Lockhart PB. Oral manifestations of patients with lupus erythematosus. Dent Clin N Am. 2005;49:127–41.
58. Grossman JM. Lupus arthritis. Best Pract Res Clin Rheumatol. 2009;23:495–506.
59. Cronin ME. Musculoskeletal manifestations of systemic lupus erythematosus. Rheum Dis Clin N Am. 1988;14:99–116.
60. Borchers AT, Leibushor N, Naguwa SM, Cheema GS, Shoenfeld Y, Gershwin ME. Lupus nephritis: a critical review. Autoimmun Rev. 2012;12:174–94.
61. Tian XP, Zhang X. Gastrointestinal involvement in systemic lupus erythematosus: insight into pathogenesis, diagnosis and treatment. World J Gastroenterol. 2010;16:2971–7.
62. Quadrelli SA, Alvarez C, Arce SC, Paz L, Sarano J, Sobrino EM, et al. Pulmonary involvement of systemic lupus erythematosus: analysis of 90 necropsies. Lupus. 2009;18:1053–60.
63. Kamen DL, Strange C. Pulmonary manifestations of systemic lupus erythematosus. Clin Chest Med. 2010;31:479–88.
64. Frostegard J. SLE, atherosclerosis and cardiovascular disease. J Intern Med. 2005;257:485–95.
65. Hanly JG, Fisk JD, McCurdy G, Fougere L, Douglas J. Neuropsychiatric syndromes in patients with systemic lupus erythematosus and rheumatoid arthritis. J Rheumatol. 2005;32:1459–66.
66. Mok CC, Lau CS, Wong RW. Neuropsychiatric manifestations and their clinical associations in southern Chinese patients with systemic lupus erythematosus. J Rheumatol. 2001;28:766–71.
67. Hepburn AL, Narat S, Mason JC. The management of peripheral blood cytopenias in systemic lupus erythematosus. Rheumatology (Oxford). 2010;49:2243–54.
68. Palejwala NV, Walia HS, Yeh S. Ocular manifestations of systemic lupus erythematosus: a review of the literature. Autoimmune Dis. 2012;2012:290898. https://doi.org/10.1155/2012/290898.
69. Uva L, Miguel D, Pinheiro C, Freitas JP, Gomes MM, Filipe P. Cutaneous manifestations of systemic lupus erythematosus. Autoimmune Dis. 2012;2012:834291.
70. Tebbe B, Orfanos CE. Epidemiology and socioeconomic impact of skin disease in lupus erythematosus. Lupus. 1997;6(2):96–104.
71. Ghosh A. Cutaneous manifestations of systemic lupus erythematosus. Indian J Rheumatol. 2007;2(4):156–64.
72. Louis PJ, Fernandes R. Review of systemic lupus erythematosus. Oral Surg Oral Med Oral Pathol. 2001;91:512–6.
73. Menta M, Nico S, Apparecida M, Vilela C, Ararigoia E, Rivitti SV. Oral lesions in lupus erythematosus: correlation with cutaneous lesions. Eur J Dermatol. 2008;18(4):376–81.
74. Lourenco SV, De Carvalho FR, Boggio P, Sotto M, Vilela MA, Rivitti E, et al. Lupus erythematosus: clinical and histopathological study of oral manifestations and immunohistochemical profile of the inflammatory infiltrate. J Cutan Pathol. 2007;34(7):558–64.
75. Lopez-Labady J, Villarroel-Dorrego M, Gonzalez N, Perez R, Mata de Henning M. Oral manifestations of systemic and cutaneous lupus erythematosus in a Venezuelan population. J Oral Pathol Med. 2007;36(9):524–7.
76. Cappelli S, Bellando Randone S, Martinović D, Tamas MM, Pasalić K, Allanore Y, et al. To be or not to be, ten years after: evidence for mixed connective tissue disease as a distinct entity. Semin Arthritis Rheum. 2012;41(4):589–98.
77. Mosca M, Tani C, Neri C, Baldini C, Bombardieri S. Undifferentiated connective tissue diseases (UCTD). Autoimmun Rev. 2006;6(1):1.
78. Schur PH, Wallace DJ. Diagnosis and differential diagnosis of systemic lupus erythematosus in adults. In: UpToDate; 2014. Retrieved 12 Sept 2014 from http://www.uptodate.com/contents/diagnosis-and-differential-diagnosis-of-systemic-lupus-erythematosus-in-adults?source=search_result&search=Differential+diagnosis+of+systemic+lupus+erythematosus&selectedTitle=1%7E150.
79. Brown RS, Flaitz CM, Hays GL, Trejo PM. The diagnosis and treatment of discoid lupus erythematosus with oral manifestations only: a case report. Compendium. 1994;15(6):724–32.
80. Boehm IB, Boehm GA, Bauer R. Management of cutaneous lupus erythematosus with low dose methotrexate: indication for modulation of inflammatory mechanisms. Rheumatol Int. 1998;18(2):59–62.
81. Ferri C, Valentini G, Cozzi F, Sebastiani M, Michelassi C, La Montagna G, et al. Systemic sclerosis: demographic, clinical, and serologic features and survival in 1,012 Italian patients. Medicine. 2002;81(2):139–53.
82. Chung L, Lin J, Furst DE, Fiorentino D. Systemic and localized scleroderma. Clin Dermatol. 2006;24(5):374–92.
83. Denton CP. Systemic sclerosis. Medicine. 2002:36–40.
84. Cleveland DB, Rinaggio J. Oral and maxillofacial manifestations of systemic and generalized disease. Endod Top. 2003;4:69–90.
85. Black CM. The aetiopathogenesis of systemic sclerosis: thick skin – thin hypotheses. In: The Parkes Weber Lecture 1994. J R Coll Phys Edinb. 1995;29(2):119.

86. Reveille JD, Solomon DH. Evidence-based guidelines for the use of immunologic tests: anticentromere, Scl-70, and nucleolar antibodies. American College of Rheumatology Ad Hoc Committee of Immunologic Testing Guidelines. Arthritis Rheumatol. 2003;49(3):399.
87. Tan FK, Arnett FC, Antohi S, Saito S, Mirarchi A, Spiera H, et al. Autoantibodies to the extracellular matrix microfibrillar protein, fibrillin-1, in patients with scleroderma and other connective tissue diseases. J Immunol. 1999;163(2):1066.
88. Bunn CC, Black CM. Systemic sclerosis: an autoantibody mosaic. Clin Exp Immunol. 1999;117(2):207.
89. Islam NM, Bhattacharyya I, Cohen DM. Common oral manifestations of systemic disease. Otolaryngol Clin N Am. 2011;44:161–82.
90. Chan LS, Ahmed AR, Anhalt GJ, Bernauer W, Cooper KD, Elder MJ, et al. The first international consensus on mucous membrane pemphigoid. Arch Dermatol. 2002;138:370–9.
91. Rout PG, Hamburger J, Potts AJ. Orofacial radiological manifestations of systemic sclerosis. Dentomaxillofac Radiol. 1996;25:193–6.
92. Varga J. Diagnosis and differential diagnosis of systemic sclerosis (scleroderma) in adults. In: UpToDate; 2014. Retrieved 09 Oct 2014 from http://www.uptodate.com/contents/diagnosis-and-differential-diagnosis-of-systemic-sclerosis-scleroderma-inadults?source=search_result&search=systemic+sclerosis&selectedTitle=4%7E150.
93. Minkin W, Rabhan N. Mixed connective tissue disease. Arch Dermatol. 1976;112:1535–8.
94. Bennett RM. Anti-U1 RNP antibodies in mixed connective tissue disease. In: UpToDate; 2014. Retrieved 12 Oct 2014 from http://www.uptodate.com/contents/anti-u1-rnp-antibodies-in-mixed-connective-tissue-disease?source=search_result&search=mixed+connective+tissue+disease&selectedTitle=4%7E73.
95. Sharp GC. Diagnostic criteria for classification of MCTD. In: Kasukawa R, Sharp GC, editors. Mixed connective tissue. Diseases and anti-nuclear antibodies. Amsterdam: Elsevier; 1987. p. 23–32.
96. Greidinger EL, Hoffman RW. Autoantibodies in the pathogenesis of mixed connective tissue disease. Rheum Dis Clin N Am. 2005;31:437–50.
97. Datta SK, Zhang L, Xu L. T-helper cell intrinsic defect in lupus that break peripheral tolerance to nuclear autoantigens. J Mol Med. 2005;83:267–78.
98. Hoffman RW. T cells in the pathogenesis of systemic lupus erythematosus. Clin Immunol. 2004;113:4–13.
99. Bennett RM, O'Connell DJ. The arthritis of mixed connective tissue disease. Ann Rheum Dis. 1987;37(5):397–403.
100. Pope JE. Other manifestations of mixed connective tissue disease. Rheum Dis Clin N Am. 2005;31(3):519.
101. Hassoun PM. Pulmonary arterial hypertension complicating connective tissue diseases. Sem Respir Crit Care Med. 2009;30(4):429.
102. Ortega-Hernandez OD, Shoenfeld Y. Mixed connective tissue disease: an overview of clinical manifestations, diagnosis and treatment. Best Pract Res Clin Rheumatol. 2012;26:61–72.
103. Ramos-Niembro F, Alarcon-Segovia D, Hernandez-Ortiz J. Articular manifestations of mixed connective tissue disease. Arthritis Rheum. 1979;22:43–51.
104. Mimura Y, Ihn H, Jinnin M, Asano Y, Yamane K, Tamaki K. Rheumatoid factor isotypes in mixed connective tissue disease. Clin Rheumatol. 2006;25(4):572.
105. Sullivan WD, Hurst DJ, Harmon CE, Esther JH, Agia GA, Maltby JD, et al. A prospective evaluation emphasizing pulmonary involvement in patients with mixed connective tissue disease. Medicine. 1984;63(2):92.
106. Alpert MA, Goldberg SH, Singsen BH, Durham JB, Sharp GC, Ahmad M, et al. Cardiovascular manifestations of mixed connective tissue disease in adults. Circulation. 1983;68:1182–93.
107. Ungprasert P, Wannarong T, Panichsillapakit T, Cheungpasitporn W, Thongprayoon C, Ahmed S, et al. Cardiac involvement in mixed connective tissue disease: a systematic review. Intern J Cardiol. 2014;171(3):326–30.. Epub 2013 Dec 29
108. Marshall JB, Kretschmar JM, Gerhardt DC, Winship DH, Winn D, Treadwell EL, et al. Gastrointestinal manifestations of mixed connective tissue disease. Gastroenterology. 1990;98:1232–8.
109. Kitridou RC, Akmal M, Turkel SB, Ehresmann GR, Quismorio FP Jr, Massry SG. Renal involvement in mixed connective tissue disease: a longitudinal clinicopathologic study. Semin Arthritis Rheum. 1986;16:135–45.
110. Bennett RM, Spargo BH. Immune complex nephropathy in mixed connective tissue disease. Am J Med. 1977;63:534–41.
111. Klasser GD, Balasubramaniam R, Epstein J. Topical review-connective tissue diseases: orofacial manifestations including pain. J Orofac Pain. 2007;21:171–84.
112. Fujita Y, Fujii T, Nakashima R, Tanaka M, Mimori T. Aseptic meningitis in mixed connective tissue disease: cytokine and anti-U1RNP antibodies in cerebrospinal fluids from two different cases. Mod Rheumatol. 2008;18:184–8.
113. Gonzales TS, Coleman GC. Periodontal manifestations of collagen vascular disorders. Periodontology. 2000;1999(21):94–105.
114. Prystowsky SD. Mixed connective tissue disease. West J Med. 1980;132:288–93.
115. Hoffman RW, Sharp GC, Deutscher SL. Analysis of anti-U1 RNA antibodies in patients with connective tissue disease. Association with HLA and clinical manifestations of disease. Arthritis Rheum. 1995;38:1837–44.
116. Ha Hassan AB, Nikitina-Zake L, Padyukov L, Karlsson G, Gupta M, Lundberg IE, et al. MICA4/HLA-DRB1*04/TNF1 haplotype is associated with

mixed connective tissue disease in Swedish patients. Hum Immunol. 2003;64:290–6.

117. Kim P, Grossman JM. Treatment of mixed connective tissue disease. Rheum Dis Clin N Am. 2005;31:549–65.
118. Lundberg I. The prognosis of mixed connective tissue disease. Rheum Dis Clin N Am. 2005;31:535–47.
119. Bohan A, Peter JB. Polymyositis and dermatomyositis (first of two parts). N Engl J Med. 1975;292:344–7.
120. Na SJ, Kim SM, Sunwoo IN, Choi YC. Clinical characteristics and outcomes of juvenile and adult dermatomyositis. J Kor Med Sci. 2009;24:715–21.
121. Medsger TA, Dawson WN, Masi AT. The epidemiology of polymyositis. Am J Med. 1970;48:715–23.
122. Kovacs SO, Kovacs SC. Dermatomyositis. J Am Acad Dermatol. 1998;39(6):899–920.
123. Callen JP, Wortmann RL. Dermatomyositis. Clin Dermatol. 2006;24:363–73.
124. Appleyard ST, Dunn MJ, Dubowitz V, et al. Increased expression of HLA ABC class I antigens by muscle fibers in Duchenne muscular dystrophy, inflammatory myopathy, and other neuromuscular disorders. Lancet. 1985;1:361–3.
125. Tanaka TI, Geist SM. Dermatomyositis: a contemporary review for oral health care providers. Med Manag Pharmacol Updat. 2012;114(5):e1–8.
126. Callen JP. Dermatomyositis. Lancet. 2000;355:53–7.
127. Dalakas MC. Polymyositis, dermatomyositis, and inclusion-body myositis. N Engl J Med. 1991;325:1487–98.
128. Marie I, Hatron P-Y, Hachulla E, Wallaert B, Michon-Pasturel U, Devulder B. Pulmonary involvement in polymyositis and in dermatomyositis. J Rheumatol. 1998;25:1336–43.
129. Gonzalez-Lopez L, Gamez-Nava JI, Sanchez L, Rosas S, Suarez-Almazor M, Cardona-Munoz C, et al. Cardiac manifestations in dermato-polymyositis. Clin Exp Rheumatol. 1996;14:373–9.
130. Hill CL, Zhang Y, Sigurgeirsson B, Pukkala E, Mellemkajaer L, Airio A, et al. Frequency of specific cancer types in dermatomyositis and polymyositis: a population-based study. Lancet. 2001;357:96–100.
131. Keil H. The manifestations in the skin and mucous membranes in dermatomyositis, with special reference to the differential diagnosis from systemic lupus erythematosus. Ann Intern Med. 1942;16:828–31.
132. Sanger RG, Kirby JW. The oral and facial manifestations of dermatomyositis with calcinosis. Oral Surg Oral Med Oral Pathol Oral Radiol. 1973;35:476–88.
133. Mammen AL. Dermatomyositis and polymyositis: clinical presentation, autoantibodies, and pathogenesis. Ann N Y Acad Sci. 2010;1184:134–53.
134. Curiel RV, Jones R, Brindle K. Magnetic resonance imaging of the idiopathic inflammatory myopathies: structural and clinical aspects. Ann N Y Acad Sci. 2009;1154:101–14.
135. Woo TY, Callen JP, Voorhees JJ, Bickers DR, Hanno R, Hawkins C. Cutaneous lesions of dermatomyositis are improved by hydroxychloroquine. J Am Acad Dermatol. 1984;10:590–600.
136. Zieglschmid-Adams ME, Pandya AG, Cohen SB, Sontheimer RD. Treatment of dermatomyositis with methotrexate. J Am Acad Dermatol. 1995;32:754–7.

7 Oral Signs of Vesiculobullous and Autoimmune Disease

Michael Z. Wang, Julia S. Lehman, and Roy Steele Rogers III

Oral Pemphigus Vulgaris

Epidemiology

Oral pemphigus vulgaris is a rare disease in Northern Europe and the USA, with an incidence of 1–5 per 1,000,000 per year [1], while Mediterranean and Jewish populations have reported a higher prevalence and incidence [2]. The female to male ratio is reported between 1: 1 and 2.25: 1, with a higher rate in pregnant women. The age of onset is commonly in the fourth to sixth decade, with an earlier onset observed in Asian, Middle Eastern, and African patients [2]. The majority of patients, approximately 66–92%, present with oral lesions only [2].

M. Z. Wang
Department of Dermatology, Mayo Clinic, Rochester, MN, USA

J. S. Lehman (✉)
Departments of Dermatology and Laboratory Medicine and Pathology, Mayo Clinic, Rochester, MN, USA
e-mail: lehman.julia@mayo.edu

R. S. Rogers III
Department of Dermatology, Mayo Clinic Arizona, Scottsdale, AZ, USA

Etiopathogenesis

The erosion, ulceration, and vesiculation of oral pemphigus vulgaris is caused by loss of intercellular adhesion through an autoimmune response affecting the desmosomes. IgG polyclonal antibodies, predominantly IgG4, react against the extracellular domain of desmoglein (dsg) 3, a cadherin-type epithelial cell adhesion protein. In isolated oral disease, dsg 1 autoantibodies are usually absent.

Pemphigus has a strong genetic linkage to HLA class II subtypes, including DR4, DRw14, DQB1*0503, and B15, all of which may play an important role in T lymphocyte recognition of dsg 3 peptides. Medications are also known etiological factors, including thio-medications represented by penicillamine and captopril and nonthiol-medications such as rifampin, diclofenac, and phenol drugs. The relationship between herpesvirus infections and pemphigus vulgaris has been suggested by the epitope spreading pathogenesis theory [3–5]. Additional observations reported in the literature include higher incidences with pesticide exposure, pregnancy, and a lower incidence in smokers.

Clinical Manifestations

Patients with pemphigus vulgaris develop painful erosions of the oral mucosa, typically prior to development of cutaneous erosions.

N. Fazel (ed.), *Oral Signs of Systemic Disease*, https://doi.org/10.1007/978-3-030-10863-2_7

Signs and Symptoms

The diagnosis of oral pemphigus vulgaris is based on clinical, histopathological, and direct immunofluorescence (DIF) studies along with serum tests. Oral pemphigus vulgaris may involve any oral mucosal surface. Lesions most commonly affect buccal, palatal, and lip locations, areas that are frequently subjected to frictional trauma. Extra-oral mucosal involvement includes conjunctival, nasal, tracheal, upper esophageal, and anogenital surfaces. Erythematous and edematous mucosal lesions are seen, with prominent erythema of the gingiva (Fig. 7.1). Fragile, fluid-filled vesicles and bullae are rarely observed as they rupture soon after their formation, leaving behind painful erosions and ulcerations of varying sizes with ragged, ill-defined borders. A collar of detached epithelium may be observed. Some lesions have a whitish fibromembranous exudate covering the ulcer base. The lesions are slow-healing, and the surrounding mucosa is fragile resulting in a positive Nikolsky sign. Lesions can rapidly progress and become confluent.

The characteristic histopathological picture is one of suprabasilar clefting from acantholysis, with associated lymphocytic or mixed inflammation and the likely presence of eosinophils. In the early stages, eosinophilic spongiosis may be seen with little or no acantholysis. Intercellular IgG and C3 deposition within the epidermis is seen on DIF. The same pattern is seen in indirect immunofluorescence testing (IIF) performed on monkey esophagus epithelium. The sensitivity of DIF testing is 92%, and the predictive value of a positive test is 87% [6].

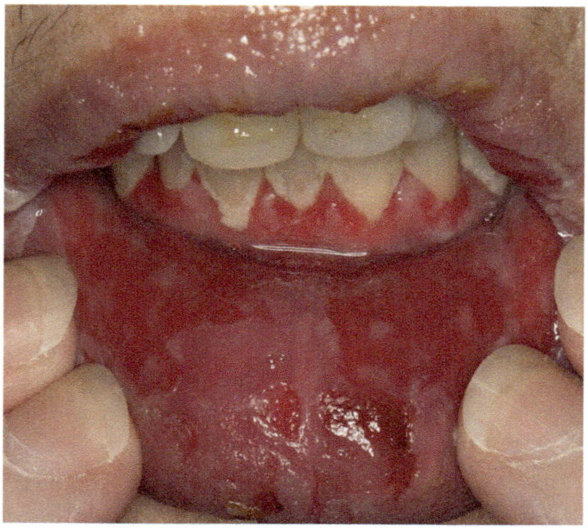

Fig. 7.1 Pemphigus vulgaris. Mucosal lip erosions with erosive gingivitis

Differential Diagnosis

Many oral mucosal diseases, including acute herpetic gingivostomatitis, aphthous stomatitis, paraneoplastic pemphigus, mucous membrane pemphigoid, dermatitis herpetiformis (DH), lichen planus, systemic lupus erythematosus, erythema multiforme (EM), and Stevens-Johnson syndrome, may present as raw, erythematous, and eroded oral mucosal erosions and ulcerations. Thus, with clinical appearance alone, the diagnosis of pemphigus vulgaris is difficult. Hence, lesional biopsy of nonulcerated mucosa for histopathology and perilesional DIF examination is crucial. Other potentially valuable investigations include IIF, dsg 3 antibody serology, bullous pemphigoid 180 and 230 antibody serology, herpes simplex virus and varicella zoster virus polymerase chain reaction tests, culture for candida, antinuclear antibody screening, and endoscopy, if tracheal or esophageal involvement is suspected.

Treatment Recommendations

Prior to the 1950s, pemphigus vulgaris was nearly uniformly fatal within years, and it continues to be potentially fatal due to interference with oral intake and skin denudation. Since then, great strides have been made with effective treatment options. Early diagnosis permits early aggressive therapy with a favorable likelihood of sustained remission off of therapy. Therefore, the initial goal is to induce disease remission, followed by a maintenance period using the minimum medication required to achieve disease control, and then ultimately treatment withdrawal. Occasional blisters are acceptable. These indicate that the patient is not being over-treated. A serological marker for following disease activity is dsg 3, given its higher value is associated with a higher chance of having more severe disease [7].

The mainstay of treatment for pemphigus vulgaris is systemic immunosuppression, usually achieved with corticosteroids. Rituximab is emerging as a first-line therapy for severe pemphigus vulgaris. Adjuvant options that have a corticosteroid-sparing effect include azathioprine, mycophenolate mofetil, IVIG, cyclophosphamide, topical epidermal growth factor [8], and extracorporeal photopheresis. Treatments that require further investigation include methotrexate, cyclosporine, tetracyclines, dapsone, chlorambucil, and plasma exchange [9, 10]. When systemic corticosteroids are contraindicated, combination therapy with rituximab and IVIG is suggested [5]. For limited, mild disease and suppression of disease activity in the setting of a low dsg 3 titer, topical antibiotics, class 1 topical corticosteroids, and tacrolimus can be considered. Intralesional corticosteroids can be used for resistant localized lesions, while intralesional rituximab has been proposed.

Minimization of oral irritation, gentle oral hygiene, pain control, and adequate nutrition are also essential parts of disease management. In addition, superimposed oral candidiasis or herpetic stomatitis should also be treated [1–23].

Paraneoplastic Pemphigus/Paraneoplastic Autoimmune Multiorgan Syndrome

Epidemiology

The epidemiology for paraneoplastic pemphigus (PNP)/paraneoplastic autoimmune multiorgan syndrome (PAMS) is unknown, given that it is extraordinarily rare. From reported cases in the literature, there is no gender predilection. Cases have been reported in all age groups, though it does occur more often in older individuals.

Etiopathogenesis

PNP is an autoimmune blistering disease first described by Anhalt et al. in 1990 [24], and more recently the name of paraneoplastic autoimmune multiorgan syndrome (PAMS) was suggested to reflect its frequent multiorgan involvement [25]. PNP can be the presenting symptom of an underlying disease or arise years after the underlying disease has been treated. The disease is associated with non-Hodgkin lymphoma (38.6%), chronic lymphocytic leukemia (18.4%), Castleman disease (18.4%), malignant and benign thymoma (5.5%), a variety of carcinomas (8.6%), and sarcomas (6.2%). Rare associations with Waldenstrom's macroglobulinemia, Hodgkin lymphoma, and malignant melanoma have been reported. Its most frequent associations are hematologic neoplasms or disorders of lymphoid origin, of which Castleman disease is the most likely association in children.

The pathogenesis of PNP is a combination of humoral immunity and cell-mediated cytotoxicity [25]. The exact mechanism of epidermal damage is unknown. Current hypotheses include:

1. Tumor-produced antibodies target epidermal antigens.
2. Autoimmunity due to cross-reaction of tumor antigens and epidermal antigens.
3. Elevated IL-6 associated with Castleman disease promotes B cell differentiation and drives immunoglobulin production.
4. Epitope spreading from malignancy induced lichenoid interface dermatitis.
5. Epidermal damage by cytotoxic T lymphocyte-mediated cellular immunity. The cytotoxic mechanism could offer an explanation to the severe and refractory clinical course of PNP.

Circulating autoantibodies found in PNP include desmoglein (dsg) 1 and 3, plectin, desmoplakin I and II, bullous pemphigoid antigen 1, envoplakin, periplakin, and alpha 2 macroglobulin-like 1 protein [26, 27]. Interestingly, multiple members of the plakin and desmoglein family may be targeted, indicating that alterations in these protein families may contribute to the pathogenesis of the disease. The multitude of autoantibodies detected in this disease may also explain its highly varied clinical presentations. In addition, genetic associations are found for HLA-DRB1*03 in Caucasians and HLA-Cw14 in the Chinese.

Clinical Manifestations

A polymorphic cutaneous skin eruption is seen with an extensive, painful, and persistent stomatitis. The onset may follow or precede the discovery of an underlying malignancy. Rare cases without an associated neoplasm have been reported. The clinical course is distinguished by resistance to treatment.

Oral Signs and Symptoms

PNP/PAMS commonly presents as diffuse and severe stomatitis and conjunctivitis with polymorphic cutaneous findings (Figs. 7.2 and 7.3). Hemorrhagic stomatitis is frequently the presenting symptom and characteristically involves the vermilion border of the lips. Any location within the oral cavity may be affected, with the lateral tongue being the most frequent site. Extra-oral mucosal involvement can arise including the esophageal, gastric, duodenal, colonic, respiratory, and urogenital mucosa.

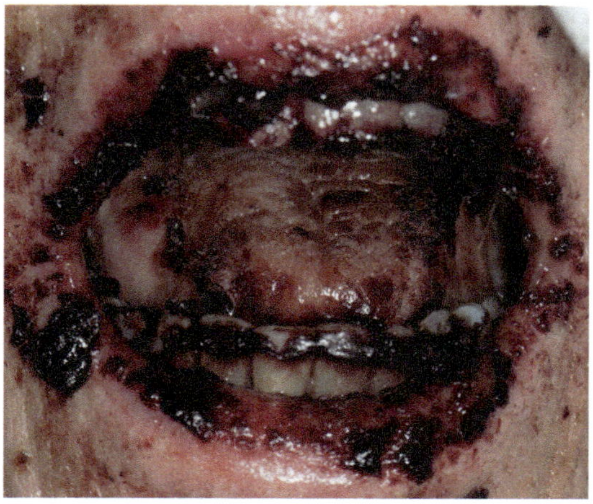

Fig. 7.2 Paraneoplastic autoimmune multiorgan syndrome (paraneoplastic pemphigus). Erosive stomatitis with hemorrhagic crust that extends onto the vermilion lip with tongue involvement

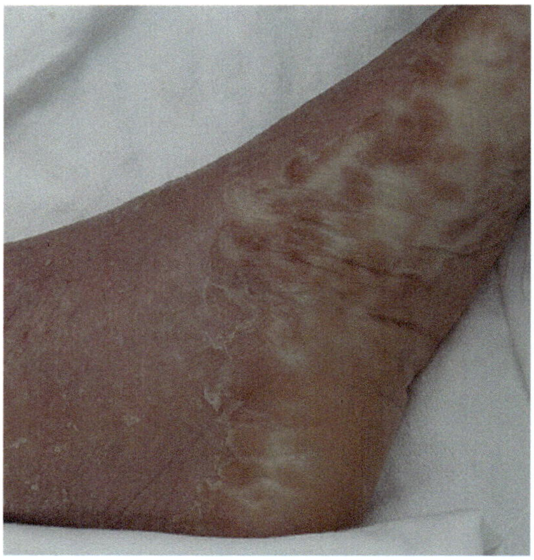

Fig. 7.3 Paraneoplastic autoimmune multiorgan syndrome (paraneoplastic pemphigus) with cutaneous involvement. Atypical targetoid lesions on the plantar foot

The cutaneous findings may mimic bullous pemphigoid, pemphigus vulgaris, pemphigus vegetans, erythema multiforme, graft-versus-host disease, lichen planus, and psoriasis. The presence of acral vesicles or erythema multiforme-like lesions in the setting of stomatitis should heighten the suspicion for PNP/PAMS. Frequently, Nikolsky sign is also positive.

Multiple organ involvement is seen in PNP/PAMS, with bronchiolitis obliterans being the most prominent. It can be assessed by pulmonary function testing but frequently is not detected on chest radiographs. Examples of other organ involvement include cardiomyopathy, glomerulonephritis, and myasthenia gravis. Patients with erythema multiforme-like skin lesions, histologic evidence of keratinocyte necrosis, and extensive lesions at presentation are at increased risk for severe PNP/PAMS.

In oral lesions, suprabasal acantholysis is a commonly observed histopathological feature. An additional distinctive feature is dyskeratotic keratinocytes that can be present at all levels of the epidermis and more prevalent in acantholytic areas. Both lichenoid and vacuolar interface changes may be observed with or without acantholysis. A combination of the above histopathological features may be observed in PNP. Eosinophils are rare.

Characteristically, in PNP/PAMS, DIF testing shows IgG and C3 deposition on epithelial cell surfaces and variably along the basement membrane zone (BMZ). The combination of epithelial cell surface and BMZ DIF staining has low sensitivity (27–41%) and high specificity (97–98%) for PNP, while BMZ fluorescence is frequently missing [28, 29]. IIF testing has good sensitivity (75–86%) and specificity (83–98%) for PNP [29, 30]. IIF is tested with rat bladder, showing cell surface and BMZ staining.

The recent proposal for diagnostic criteria [31] includes major criteria of:

- Polymorphous mucocutaneous eruption
- Painful and persistent stomatitis
- Respiratory involvement
- Concurrent internal neoplasia
- Immuno-precipitation of 190, 210 (doublet), 230, and 250 kDa bands

And minor criteria of:

- Acantholysis and/or subepidermal split
- DIF showing both intercellular and linear BMZ staining of the epidermis
- IIF of rodent bladder epithelium showing cell surface and BMZ staining
- Lack of correlation of dsg 3 and dsg 1 lab values

Differential Diagnosis

The differential diagnosis of PNP includes major aphthous stomatitis, chemotherapy-induced stomatitis, bullous pemphigoid, pemphigus vulgaris, mucous membrane pemphigoid, erythema multiforme, Stevens-Johnson syndrome, toxic epidermal necrolysis, graft-versus-host disease, lichen planus, persistent herpes simplex virus infection, and *Mycoplasma* pneumoniae-associated mucositis.

Treatment Recommendations

Treatment of PNP/PAMS requires a multidisciplinary approach, including dermatology, oncology, or hematology specialists, as clinically indicated, as well as pulmonologists, if the patient develops bronchiolitis obliterans. Though PNP/PAMS may respond to aggressive immunosuppression with high-dose corticosteroids and often concurrent immunosuppressants including azathioprine, cyclosporine, and mycophenolate mofetil, the risk of immunosuppression in the context of underlying malignancy should be considered carefully. Newer promising treatment options include rituximab, alemtuzumab, and daclizumab. The efficacy of plasmapheresis and IVIG are disputed in the literature. High-dose cyclophosphamide therapy has also been reported. Supportive management including pain control, moisturization, body temperature management, hydration, and nutrition is essential. Reduction of cutaneous colonization by methods such as dilute acetic acid wet dressings and systemic treatment of early infections are also crucial.

Despite treatment, survival is commonly less than 1 year, with 75–90% mortality. Infection is the leading cause of death in patients with PNP/PAMS. Oral erosions are more persistent compared to cutaneous lesions. Manifestations of PNP/PAMS may not respond to treatment of the underlying malignancy. Excision of benign tumors is reported with success, in which autoantibodies were drastically reduced postoperatively. However, the subsequent resolution of PNP/PAMS required 6–18 months [24–54].

Bullous Pemphigoid

Epidemiology

Bullous pemphigoid (BP) is the most common autoimmune blistering disorder, with an annual incidence of 6–21 cases per million. In persons over 80 years old, the incidence substantially rises to 150–330 per million per year [55, 56]. Oral involvement in BP is seen in 10–30% of patients.

Etiopathogenesis

Blister and erosion formation in BP originate from autoantibodies targeting bullous pemphigoid antigen 1 (BPAG 1) and bullous pemphigoid antigen 2 (BPAG 2), with the NCA 16 region of the BPAG 2 as the main autoantibody target in the BMZ of the skin and mucous membranes. Circulating polyclonal IgG antibodies are present in the majority of BP patients, predominantly IgG3.

Triggers include trauma, burns, radiotherapy, infections, and vaccination. Medications associated with BP include penicillamine, furosemide, phenacetin, ACE inhibitors, ibuprofen, penicillin, and spironolactone. Potential infectious causes include cytomegalovirus, Epstein-Barr virus, human herpesvirus 6, hepatitis viruses, *Helicobacter pylori*, and *Toxoplasma gondii*. A genetic link in BP is HLA-DQβ1*0301.

Clinical Manifestations

When the oral mucosa is affected in BP, severely painful desquamative gingivitis (DG) with discrete vesicles and erosions is the most common presentation. The oral presentation is usually accompanied by cutaneous blisters.

Oral Signs and Symptoms

A minority of patients with BP present with oral lesions. Oral mucosal disease is associated with a slower response to treatment. Oral lesions of BP may be painful. Oral bullae and vesicles are smaller and more fragile compared to their cutaneous counterparts; hence, discrete erosions with areas of sparing are more commonly the clinical presentation. When the oral mucosa is involved, scarring is a possibility. Severe DG may be an oral presentation of BP, a feature shared with MMP. Gingival involvement commonly affects a large area with an overlying thin white membrane. Nikolsky's sign is negative. Extra-oral mucosal sites including ocular, nasal, pharyngeal, perianal, vulvar, and urethral surfaces can be affected. BP tends to be a chronic condition, with exacerbations and remissions over months to years.

The cutaneous histopathological findings of BP are characterized by a subepithelial split with the presence of eosinophils. Varied lymphocytic, neutrophilic, and histiocytic infiltrates are present in the upper dermis. The histopathology of the non-bullous phase of BP shows eosinophilic spongiosis or urticarial changes.

Direct immunofluorescence (DIF) testing of perilesional skin shows IgG and C3 deposition along the basement membrane zone (BMZ), and IIF testing conducted on monkey esophagus shows linear fluorescence at the BMZ. IIF with human salt-split skin substrate shows epidermal deposition. In patients with only cutaneous lesions, DIF of the oral mucosa is positive 80% of the time [57]. Serological study with ELISA for anti-BPAG 1 and anti-BPAG 2 antibodies serves as further confirmation.

Differential Diagnosis

Oral vesicular and bullous lesions may be seen with mucous membrane pemphigoid, bullous lichen planus, dermatitis herpetiformis, and bullous systemic lupus erythematosus. Given the fragility of oral bullae and vesicles, erosive oral diseases are also in the differential diagnosis, including acute herpetic gingivostomatitis, linear IgA bullous dermatosis, paraneoplastic pemphigus/paraneoplastic autoimmune multiorgan syndrome, lichen planus, erythema multiforme, and Stevens-Johnson syndrome. In this setting, cutaneous findings of intact tense bullae would support a clinical diagnosis of BP; however, clinicians should be mindful that the cutaneous presentation of BP is not always bullous. The differential diagnosis for DG includes acute necrotizing ulcerative gingivostomatitis (ANUG) and acute herpetic gingivostomatitis (AHGS) where erythema, edema, and necrosis occur at the interdental papillae. MMP may also present with DG and may also involve the conjunctiva, other extra-oral mucosal sites, and the skin. If a BP patient has a bleeding disorder or is taking anticoagulation medications, hemorrhagic bullae can be observed, mimicking angina bullosa haemorrhagica.

Treatment Recommendations

Though BP can be considered benign, untreated BP could cause significant morbidity and even mortality. While treating BP, clinicians need to be mindful of the patient's comorbidities and the treatment side effects. Topical corticosteroids alone may be successful in localized oral BP. Due to the slower treatment response when oral involvement is present, more aggressive systemic treatment should be considered. Systemic treatment options include monotherapy with tetracycline, niacinamide, or erythromycin, tetracycline with niacinamide, and corticosteroids. Immunomodulators may be used alone or as corticosteroid-sparing agents, including azathioprine, methotrexate, cyclophosphamide, chlorambucil, and dapsone. Rituximab is emerging as an effective treatment for severe bullous pemphigoid. Secondary bacterial and fungal infections should be documented and treated. Patient education for minimization of oral irritation, gentle oral hygiene, and adequate nutrition are also essential [55–64].

Mucous Membrane Pemphigoid

Epidemiology

The prevalence of mucous membrane pemphigoid (MMP) is estimated at 0.8–2 per million, with oral disease occurring in 85% and ocular disease in 65%. Although MMP can be seen in a wide range of age groups, the elderly population is more often targeted. The mean age is in the seventh decade, with a slight female predominance.

Etiopathogenesis

MMP is a heterogeneous group of diseases characterized by subepithelial blistering with potential for scarring, which predominantly involves the mucous membranes. Linear deposition of IgG, IgA, IgM, and C3 can be seen along the epithelial BMZ. Known target antigens in MMP include bullous pemphigoid antigen 1 (BPAG1), C-terminus and ecto-domains of bullous pemphigoid antigen 2 (BPAG2), laminin-332, alpha-3 chain of laminin-311, type VII collagen, integrin alpha-6 and beta-4 subunits, and uncein. An unidentified mucosal 168-kDa antigen is also recognized [65]. Ocular MMP is associated with integrin beta-4, oral MMP is linked to alpha-6 integrin, while MMP with solid cancers are related to laminin-332. Multiple antigen targets can be found concomitantly in individual patients. The precise mechanism of the disease pathogenesis is unclear and is a subject of ongoing research. The fibrotic process in MMP may be related to inflammatory cytokines such as interleukin-4 [66]. Genetically, HLA-DQB1*0301 allele is found to be increased in MMP patients [67, 68].

Clinical Manifestations

Oral manifestations of MMP are desquamative gingivitis (DG) and bullous and erosive lesions of the oral mucosa. This is often accompanied by ocular and other mucous membrane manifestations. MMP may present with mucosal lesions alone. Mucous membrane pemphigoid can be a paraneoplastic phenomenon in some patients, so a diligent search for an underlying neoplasm is warranted.

Oral Signs and Symptoms

MMP is a chronic inflammatory blistering disease with a diverse range of clinical presentations that can affect any or all mucous membranes, with oral involvement being the most frequent. The most commonly affected oral sites are the gingiva and palate; however, all oral sites are potential targets. Extra-oral MMP sites include the eyes, nose, larynx, nasopharynx, esophagus, anogenital mucosa, and skin [69]. Ocular

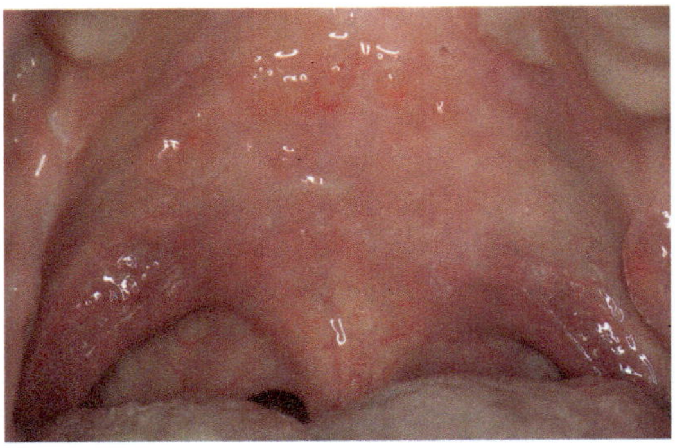

Fig. 7.4 Mucous membrane pemphigoid. Multiple bullae on the hard palate with erosions on the soft palate

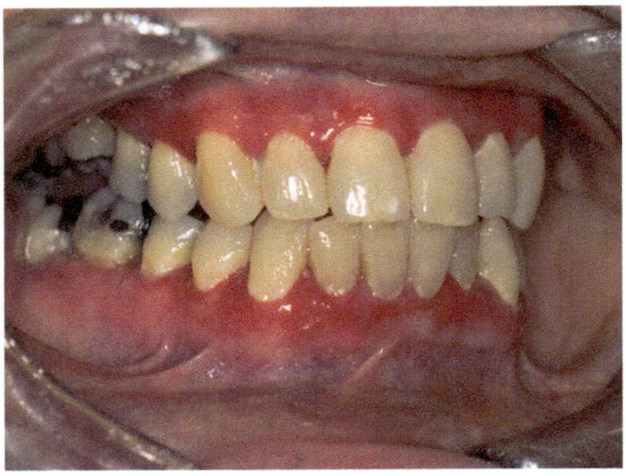

Fig. 7.5 Mucous membrane pemphigoid. Desquamative gingivitis with fibrous tracts at the labial sulcus

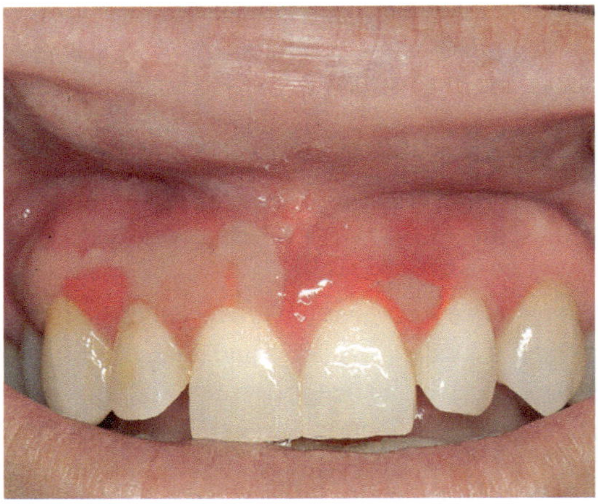

Fig. 7.6 Mucous membrane pemphigoid. Erosive gingivitis

involvement may occur independent of oral symptoms. There is occasional involvement of the skin. Though scarring is not always observed, its presence may lead to functional impairment, such as blindness and airway obstruction. When the oral mucosa is the sole site affected, the risk for scarring is lower [69].

The mucosal manifestations in the oral cavity are commonly irregularly shaped erythematous patches and desquamative erosions, while atrophic changes and vesicles are occasionally present. Nikolsky sign can be positive. The vesicles may remain for 3 days before rupturing (Fig. 7.4), and subsequent erosions can heal in approximately 2–3 weeks [70]. Secondary bacterial infection of the ulcer base by oral flora can produce suppurative inflammation, while patients are also at risk for local and disseminated herpes virus infections when on immunosuppressive therapy [71, 72]. Patchy or diffuse DG is a characteristic finding in MMP. Gingival symptoms range from glazed erythema to chronic soreness and loss of stippling (Fig. 7.5). The gingival desquamation and erythema is slow to heal, which may persist for several years, if left untreated (Fig. 7.6). Clinical findings may be more severe at areas of friction and in the setting of poorly fitting dentures [70].

A perilesional biopsy for direct immunofluorescence studies is essential for the diagnosis of MMP. In MMP, the subepithelial split is present in the absence of acantholysis. Direct immunofluorescence (DIF) findings account for half of the diagnostic criteria for MMP, along with clinical features. Perilesional DIF is required to demonstrate linear deposition of IgG, C3, and/or IgA at the BMZ. However, false negativity can be seen in long-standing lesions or in lesional biopsies [73]. A severe and persistent disease course is associated with involvement of multiple BMZ antigens and dual IgG and IgA deposition along the BMZ [74].

Indirect immunofluorescence testing serves to detect circulating autoantibodies in MMP patients. As a result of MMP's heterogeneous nature, salt-split skin testing can show deposition at the epithelial side, dermal side, or a combination of both sides or no reactivity. Epidermal reactivity on salt-split skin suggests that the target antigens could be beta-4 integrin, BPAG1, and BPAG2, while dermal reactivity suggests target antigens being type VII collagen, laminin-332, and laminin-311. Serologies for autoantibodies are frequently negative, due to low circulating antibody concentrations. An additional adjunctive testing method for detecting IgG and IgA autoantibodies of BPAG2 NC16a subunit can be performed from whole saliva [75].

Differential Diagnosis

Through histopathology and DIF testing, MMP can be distinguished from pemphigus, non-MMP drug-induced cicatrization, oral lichen planus, lupus erythematosus, graft-versus-host disease, erythema multiforme, and SJS/TEN. Due to shared histopathological and DIF features, clinical differentiation must be made between MMP and BP, anti-p200 pemphigoid, anti-p105 pemphigoid, anti-p450 pemphigoid, linear IgA bullous dermatosis (LABD), and epidermolysis bullosa acquisita (EBA). Clinically, MMP is predominantly mucosal, whereas cutaneous disease predominates in BP, LABD, and EBA. When DG is the primary feature, differential diagnosis includes MMP, lichen planus, pemphigus, contact stomatitis, and estrogen imbalance from menopause or hysterectomy.

Treatment Recommendations

The goals of MMP treatment are disease control, symptomatic relief, and prevention of complications. The treatment choice should be guided by sites of involvement, severity, and progression. Ocular, genital, nasopharyngeal, esophageal, and laryngeal mucosal involvement may evolve into long-lasting functional deficit. Hence, careful questioning of symptoms and clinical examination of all mucosal areas is critical. When relevant, consultation with ophthalmology and other specialties should be sought. Minimization of irritation, trauma, secondary infection, and malnutrition is also an integral part of management.

Rapidly evolving and severe MMP can be treated by a combination of systemic corticosteroids and cyclophosphamide. Immunosuppressive medications such as azathioprine may also act as adjunctive therapy to systemic corticosteroids. Rituximab is found to be effective in recalcitrant MMP, and its addition to conventional therapy increases the likelihood of disease control and may also result in faster remission. Multiple courses of Rituximab treatment are frequently needed. When MMP is under control, systemic corticosteroids should be tapered. IVIG is also under investigation for MMP treatment, and disease-modifying potential has been found for beta-4 integrin-related MMP [68]. Plasmapheresis and etanercept have been reported to be effective in isolated cases [76, 77].

When the disease is limited to the oral mucosa, systemic dapsone therapy is very effective with a 50% remission, off treatment outcome [78]. Local treatment with high potency topical corticosteroids or calcineurin inhibitors may be administered initially. Other treatment options include tetracycline, nicotinamide, colchicine, low-dose systemic corticosteroids, and immunosuppressant therapy. Surgical relief of scarred tissue can be considered once the disease is in remission [65–92].

Lichen Planus

Epidemiology

Oral lichen planus (OLP) is observed in up to 4% of the population, with varying prevalence depending on geographic regions. All ethnicities are affected [93], with a higher prevalence in women than men [94]. In contrast, OLP is rare in children and adolescents, and it typically affects adults between the age of 30 and 60 years old [95].

Etiopathogenesis

The pathogenesis of OLP is hypothesized to be a T cell-mediated chronic inflammatory disorder. Investigations toward antigen-specific and nonspecific mechanisms are ongoing. Moreover, studies on the genetic aspects of the disease are also one of the focuses for understanding the disorder, including polymorphism of interferon gamma and tumor necrosis factor-alpha (TNF-α) genes. Studies also demonstrated associations between OLP and human leukocyte antigen (HLA) types, including HLA DRB1*11 and DQB1*03, HLA-B8, B16, DR1, and DRw9. Erosive OLP is associated with HLA-B51, Bw57, DR2, DR3, and DR9 [96]. Hepatitis C virus (HCV)-related LP is associated with HLA-DR6.

Inciting factors include medications, psychological (stress), mechanical (hard toothbrush, poor oral habits, sharp teeth, rough dental implants), chemical (alcohol, smoking, contact allergens, irritating foods), and viral infections (HCV). Medication offenders include nonsteroidal anti-inflammatory agents, ACE inhibitors, and beta-blockers, among many others. Examples of contact allergens are gold and amalgam restorations in which case patch testing can provide direction for dental work modifications. HCV is shown to be correlated with OLP, but this correlation is controversial for the US population. Hence, HCV testing can be considered when there are identified risk factors.

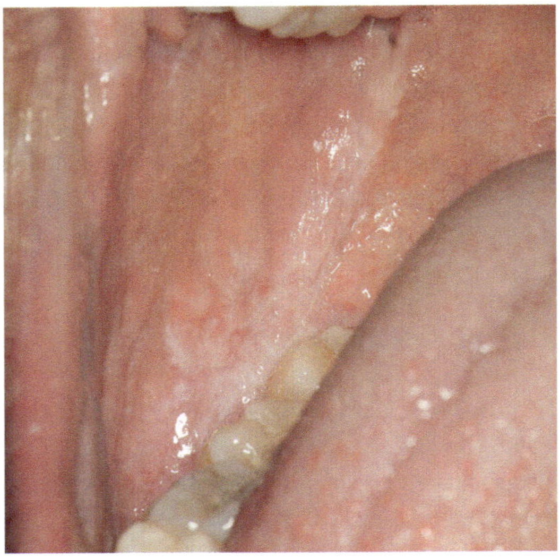

Fig. 7.7 Reticular oral lichen planus. Wickham striae represented by lacy white plaque involving the posterior buccal mucosa

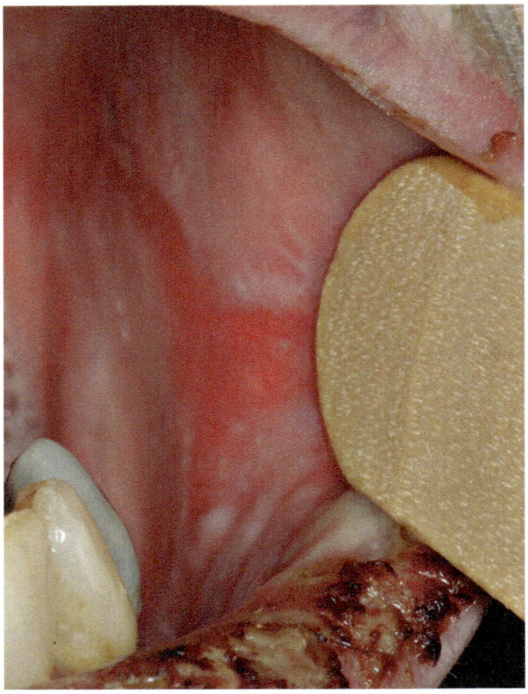

Fig. 7.8 Erosive oral lichen planus. Lacy white striae with central erythroplakia on the buccal mucosa. Yellow crust overlying extensive erosions involving the lip

Clinical Manifestations

OLP can present as white reticular plaques, erythematous and atrophic patches, bullae, erosions, or as a combination of these. OLP is commonly found in the buccal mucosa, but it can also be found in other locations of the oral cavity.

Signs and Symptoms

There are three clinical subtypes of OLP based on the Eisen Classification, which are reticular, erythematous, and erosive presentations. The three clinical subtypes may coexist with one another. Reticular OLP is represented by Wickham's striae (white reticular plaques) on an erythematous background (Fig. 7.7), while erythematous OLP is distinguished by mucosal atrophy (Fig. 7.8). Erosions, ulcers, and occasionally bullae are found in erosive OLP (Fig. 7.9). Symptomatically, OLP can range from being asymptomatic to having debilitating pain. The most common location is the buccal mucosa. Lingual, vestibular, and gingival involvement are also common (Fig. 7.10). It is prudent to be vigilant regarding oral malignancy in the setting of

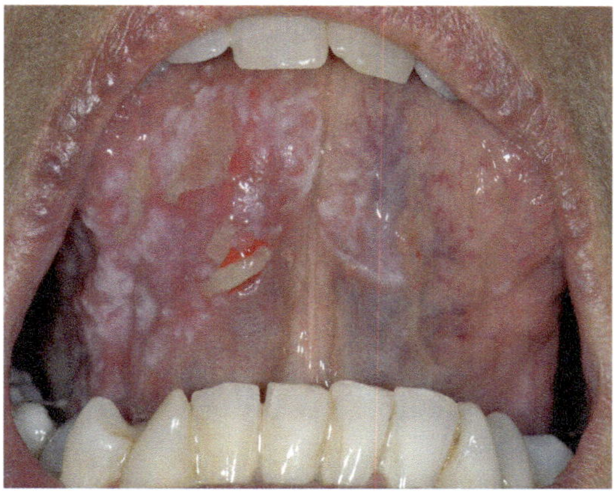

Fig. 7.9 Oral lichen planus. Ulcerations involving the ventral tongue

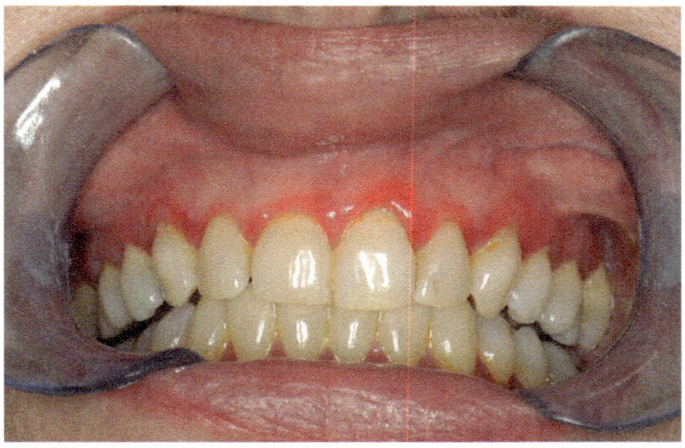

Fig. 7.10 Oral lichen planus. Desquamative gingivitis

OLP, especially when the OLP is atrophic or erosive. However, malignant transformation of OLP is controversial, with reports of 0.4–1.5% incidence [97]. Potential complications also include interference with speech and eating.

Genital lesions are noted in 20% of OLP patients; hence, it is an important component of the physical examination. Other extra-oral sites involved are the conjunctiva, ears, esophagus, and less commonly the bladder, nasal mucous membranes, larynx, and anus. Of note, the majority of OLP cases occur without cutaneous involvement (85%).

Histopathologically, OLP is characterized by a dense infiltrate of lymphocytes, interface dermatitis with Civatte bodies, and "saw-toothing" of the rete ridges. Supporting histopathological features include compact orthokeratotic hyperkeratosis, irregular acanthosis, or epidermal atrophy. Histopathologically, OLP can be indistinguishable from graft-versus-host disease (GVHD), so the distinction requires clinicopathologic correlation. Direct immunofluorescence (DIF) testing of perilesional mucosa can demonstrate cytoid bodies and shaggy fibrinogen deposition at the BMZ.

Differential Diagnosis

The differential diagnosis of OLP includes oral lichenoid drug eruption, leukoplakia, lupus erythematosus, EM, GVHD, herpetic gingivostomatitis, cicatricial pemphigoid, and DH. If there are uncertainties in the clinical diagnosis, biopsy for histopathologic examination, PCR analysis for the herpes simplex virus, antinuclear antibody, DIF and indirect immunofluorescence studies, or colonoscopy can be informative.

Treatment Recommendations

Currently, there is no curative treatment for OLP, and the treatment goal is aimed at symptom alleviation and prevention or early detection of malignant transformation. Essential behavioral guidance should be given to patients regarding gentle yet effective oral hygiene, alcohol and tobacco withdrawal, and trauma prevention. Patients should be steered away from potential sources of oral irritation including mechanical trauma, contact allergens, and irritant foods. Psychological support is often important given the chronic and painful nature of OLP. Regular monitoring for malignancy is advised, and persistent ulceration should trigger heightened suspicion for malignancy.

Treatment should be tailored to each patient's individual needs. For treatment of mild disease and maintenance, lifestyle modifications with topical treatments are most appropriate. With severe flares and uncontrollable diseases, addition of systemic treatment is necessary. Topical medications include corticosteroids, calcineurin inhibitors, cyclosporine, retinoids, and rapamycin. Systemic therapeutic options include corticosteroids, immunomodulators (azathioprine, cyclosporine, methotrexate, and mycophenolate mofetil), antimicrobials (dapsone, doxycycline, and metronidazole), biologics (TNF-α inhibitors, rituximab), hydroxychloroquine, thalidomide, retinoids, mesalamine, and curcuminoids [93–104].

Table 7.1 Malignancies in EM [110]

Hematologic malignancies
Leukemias
Lymphomas
Solid organ cancers
Gastric adenocarcinoma
Renal cell carcinoma
Extrahepatic cholangiocarcinoma

Erythema Multiforme

Epidemiology

The incidence of erythema multiforme (EM) is unknown with oral involvement seen in up to 90% of patients. EM may occur in both genders, at any age, with a slight female predominance when occurring in young adults [105, 106].

Etiopathogenesis

EM is a reactive disorder to a multitude of potential triggers, most commonly associated with herpes simplex virus (HSV) infection. It is believed that autoreactive T lymphocytes mediate keratinocyte apoptosis in EM [107]; however, there is no known unifying mechanism for autoreactive T cell generation, given the large variety of potential triggers. EM minor and major both can be caused by viral infections, whereas EM major is also associated with bacterial infections and medications, differing from Stevens-Johnson syndrome and toxic epidermal necrolysis (SJS/TEN) triggers that are frequently due to medications [108].

Viral causes are not limited to HSV; other viral agents including smallpox, vaccinia virus, varicella zoster virus, Epstein-Barr virus, cytomegalovirus, hepatitis viruses, coxsackievirus, influenza, parvovirus B19, and HIV may also contribute to EM [107]. Parasites as well as fungi such as dermatophytes and deep fungal infections are also known triggers of EM [107, 109].

Bacterial respiratory infections known to trigger EM include *Mycoplasma pneumoniae*, *Mycobacterium* tuberculosis, *Mycobacterium* avium complex, *Chlamydophila* psittaci, *Corynebacterium* diphtheriae, hemolytic *Streptococci*, *Streptococcus* pneumonia, legionellosis, and psittacosis [107]. *Mycoplasma pneumoniae* in particular is known to cause severe mucositis. Gastrointestinal and urinary tract infections related to EM include *Proteus*, *Salmonella*, *Vibrio parahaemolyticus*, and *Yersinia* [107]. Sexually transmitted diseases triggering EM include chlamydia, *Lymphogranuloma venereum*, *Neisseria meningitidis*, and *Treponema pallidum*. Vector-borne or zoonotic diseases can also be the triggers, which include borreliosis, rickettsia, typhoid, cat scratch disease, and tularemia [107]. Common bacterial infections may also cause EM, such as *Staphylococcus*, *Streptococcus*, *Pseudomonas*, and *Mycobacterium* organisms [107].

A wide range of medications can induce EM, such as nonsteroidal anti-inflammatory drugs, sulfonamides, anticonvulsants, other antibiotics, and allopurinol. Systemic conditions triggering EM include pregnancy, GVHD, inflammatory bowel disease, sarcoidosis, lupus erythematosus, polyarteritis nodosa, and Behcet's disease. Underlying malignancy is rare, but hematologic cancers and solid organ cancers have been reported (Table 7.1) [107].

Clinical Manifestations

Extensive lip and oral mucosal erosions appear with acute cutaneous targetoid lesions over several days. Common preceding events include HSV infection, *Mycoplasma*-related pneumonia, and new medications.

Oral Signs and Symptoms

EM is an acute disease sharing the same spectrum with SJS/TEN. Within EM, it is further divided into EM minor and major based on the clinical appearance [111].

The onset of EM can begin 1–2 weeks after a triggering event. The typical duration of EM is 1–4 weeks; however, 10–37% of patients are affected by recurrent EM. EM minor accompanied by mucosal involvement is typically mild and limited to one mucosal site, without systemic symptoms. EM major is described as severe mucosal disease with bullous lesions and systemic symptoms (Fig. 7.11). Oral lesions can be the only presentation in nearly half of EM patients. Extra-oral mucosal involvement includes the eyes, nose, esophagus, and genitalia.

Oral lesions are typically most pronounced anteriorly and more likely to involve non-keratinized mucosa (buccal, labial, and alveolar mucosae, ventral tongue, floor of the mouth, and soft palate). The vermilion border is also frequently affected. Mucosal vesicles and bullae rapidly rupture becoming erosions, accompanied by erythema and swelling, hemorrhagic crusting, and mucosal sloughing. When diffuse, the clinical presentation can be indistinguishable from other erosive oral diseases.

Cutaneous features of EM include typical or palpable atypical targetoid lesions (only two zones or poorly defined border) on the face and extremities, whereas SJS/TEN presents with macular atypical target lesions or purpuric macules that are predominantly truncal or generalized. Nikolsky sign is negative in EM.

The histopathological features of EM are vacuolar degeneration of the BMZ with dyskeratotic keratinocytes through all layers of the epidermis. Severe papillary edema, subepithelial and intraepithelial vesiculation, and a perivascular lymphocytic infiltrate may be observed. These changes are more prominent in early-stage lesions. Nonspecific immune deposits of IgM, C3, and fibrin may be detected on DIF testing, whereas IIF testing is negative. In severe cases, complete blood count, liver and renal function tests, chest X-ray, and cultures (blood, sputum, urine, stool, and wound) should be considered along with HSV and mycoplasma serologies.

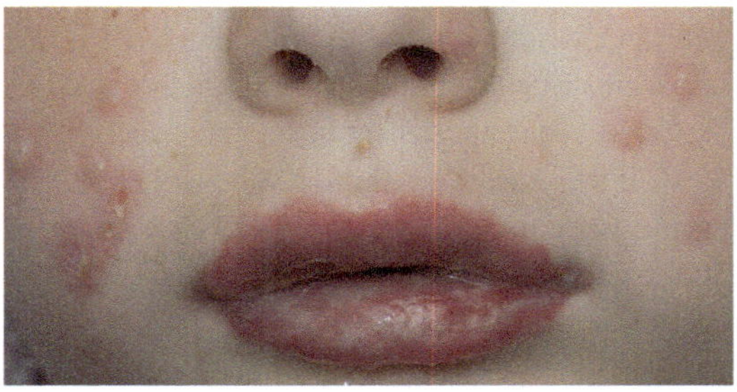

Fig. 7.11 Mucosal involvement in erythema multiforme major. Two zones of color with a polycyclic outline at the margin of the lip with multiple vesicular lesions on the face

Differential Diagnosis

The differential diagnosis of EM includes major aphthous stomatitis, chemotherapy-induced stomatitis, bullous pemphigoid, pemphigus vulgaris, PNP/PAMS, MMP, SJS/TEN, GVHD, lichen planus, persistent HSV infection without EM, and non-EM *Mycoplasma pneumoniae*-induced mucositis. When mucositis is extensive, GVHD, SJS/TEN, pemphigus vulgaris, and PNP/PAMS must be considered due to high morbidity and mortality. Compared to pemphigus vulgaris, EM rarely shows severe gingivitis. When cutaneous involvement is sparse, *Mycoplasma pneumoniae*-induced mucositis is proposed to be an independent entity from EM; however, oral mucosa-limited EM is not uncommonly reported. The differentiation is made with the aid of a detailed history, review of systems, careful oral examination, HSV PCR, biopsy for histopathological examination, DIF, and IIF.

Treatment Recommendations

Precipitating infections should be treated and potential triggers removed. EM minor may only require topical corticosteroids, while EM major requires systemic treatment. The mainstay of therapy is systemic corticosteroids tapered over approximately 3 weeks. Alternative and adjunctive treatment options for recurrent or chronic EM include dapsone, mycophenolate mofetil, azathioprine, cyclophosphamide, cyclosporine, levamisole, thalidomide, IVIG, and interferon-alpha.

Prophylactic antiviral therapy for at least 6 months is recommended in the treatment of HSV-related and idiopathic recurrent EM. Cyclosporine can also provide benefit to control recurrent EM [112]. Supportive care with analgesics and nutrition is essential, and hospital care is recommended when symptoms are severe. Ophthalmological care should be initiated early when ocular involvement is suspected [105–123].

Stevens-Johnson Syndrome and Toxic Epidermal Necrolysis

Epidemiology

The combined annual incidence of SJS/TEN is estimated to be up to seven per million cases [124]. The disease is found in all age groups but more commonly in female and Asian descendants. HIV-infected patients have a thousand-fold increase in the prevalence of SJS/TEN [125]. Mucosal involvement is present in nearly all SJS/TEN patients.

Etiopathogenesis

In SJS/TEN, the ultimate consequence is extensive keratinocyte death leading to the clinical manifestations of full-thickness denudation of the skin. The epidermal apoptosis is mediated by T cells, in particular, $CD8^+$ cytotoxic T cells and natural killer cells. The $CD8^+$ cytotoxic T cells are enhanced by the upregulation of CD137/CD137 ligand system. Other T cells and the innate immune system are also activated in SJS/TEN, with both Th1 and Th2 helper T cells involved. On the other hand, increased CD40/CD40 ligand presence in the epidermis and dermis enhances innate immunity and inflammatory cytokine release. Additionally, other contributors, such as Fas ligand, granulysin, nitric oxide, and tumor necrosis factor-alpha, may also be involved in the disease process.

SJS/TEN is most often caused by antiepileptic medications and allopurinol. Other common causative agents include antibiotics (sulfonamides, tetracyclines, aminopenicillins, cephalosporins, and quinolones), sulfasalazine, and nonsteroidal anti-inflammatory drugs.

A genetic component of SJS/TEN is present in various ethnic groups. In Han Chinese with SJS/TEN, strong associations are found between aromatic anticonvulsants (carbamazepine, phenytoin, oxcarbazepine, lamotrigine) and HLA-B*1502, as well as allopurinol and HLA-B*5801. The same associations between carbamazepine and HLA-B*1502 are also found in Thai, Malaysian, and South Indian populations. For individuals of European descent, an association between carbamazepine and HLA-A*3101, allopurinol and HLA-B*5801, as well as abacavir and HLA-B*5701 have been reported. Similar to Han Chinese patients, an association of allopurinol-induced SJS/TEN with HLA-B*5801 has also been identified in African-Americans patients.

Clinical Manifestations

Widespread mucocutaneous denudation occurs in SJS/TEN, frequently with constitutional symptoms and multi-organ involvement.

Oral Signs and Symptoms

SJS/TEN is a life-threatening disease that is more severe than EM major, with widespread denudation affecting both mucosa and skin. Lesions can affect the eyes, pharynx, larynx, esophagus, and genitalia. Scarring of the conjunctiva in SJS/TEN is a well-known sequela of the disease.

Constitutional symptoms that accompany SJS/TEN include fever, sore throat, headache, arthralgia, and myalgia. Multiple organs may be affected by SJS/TEN, including the lungs, kidneys, liver, heart, and brain.

The disease has a sudden onset, and in some cases oral lesions precede cutaneous involvement. Mucosal involvement frequently affects two or more sites, including oral, conjunctival, nasal, and genital sites. The buccal mucosa, palate, and vermilion border of the lips are the most frequently affected oral sites. Characteristic features of the lesions are painful, diffuse, irregular, and hemorrhagic erosions that can be seen with gray-white pseudomembranes and hemorrhagic crusting. A positive Nikolsky sign and Asboe Hansen sign may also present in this condition. Long-term oral sequelae include xerostomia, periodontal disease, gingival inflammation, synechiae, and dysesthesia.

The differentiation of SJS and TEN is based upon clinical appearance. SJS has less than 10% of the body surface area (BSA) detachment, with erythematous or purpuric macules or flat atypical target lesions. SJS and TEN overlap has BSA detachment between 10% and 30%. TEN may cause more than 30% BSA detachment. Frequently, the extent and severity of epidermal detachment is not correlated with the severity of the oral presentation (Table 7.2).

Histopathological features include full-thickness epidermal necrosis, subepidermal splitting, and endothelial apoptosis. Strong staining of high-mobility group protein B1 (HMGB1) in necrotic keratinocytes is a potential emerging marker for SJS/TEN. In addition, Bcl-2 expression in the dermal infiltrate is also considered as a potential marker.

Table 7.2 The severity of illness is measured by Severity of Illness Score for Toxic Epidermal Necrolysis (SCORTEN). One point is added for each criterion [126]:

HPI factors:
Age >40
Cancer or hematologic malignancy
BSA detachment on day 1 >10%
Vitals and labs:
Heart rate >120 beats per minute
Serum urea level (>10 mmol/l, or 28 mg/dl)
Serum bicarbonate level (<20 mmol/l)
Serum glucose level (>14 mmol/l, or 252 mg/dl)
Total score (mortality rate)
0–1 (3.2%)
2 (12.2%)
3 (35.5%)
4 (58.3%)
≥5 (90.0%)

Differential Diagnosis

Early presentations of SJS/TEN can be difficult to differentiate from EM major. In general, SJS/TEN tend to show increased keratinocyte apoptosis and epidermal necrosis compared to EM, although the microscopic features of these entities do overlap. Generally, the clinical course will help to distinguish these entities.

The clinical presentation of EM includes the presence of classic cutaneous target lesions (three zones with defined border) or palpable raised atypical targetoid lesions (only two zones or poorly defined border), whereas SJS/TEN commonly presents with flat atypical targetoid lesions. In addition, SJS/TEN tends to have epidermal exfoliation and bullae formation.

Other differential diagnoses include acute herpetic gingivostomatitis, aphthous stomatitis, PNP/PAMS, MMP, linear IgA dermatosis, lichen planus, systemic lupus erythematosus, staphylococcal-scalded skin syndrome (SSSS), and GVHD. Of these, SSSS is distinguished by the absence of mucosal involvement. PNP/PAMS may mimic the targetoid lesions in SJS/TEN and EM. However, PNP/PAMS and other autoimmune bullous diseases are identified through patterns noted in DIF testing. Acute GVHD is difficult to distinguish from SJS/TEN, by sharing similarities in presentation of a bullous eruption with erosions, as well as full-thickness epidermal necrosis. In addition, a clinical history of bone marrow and/or allogeneic hematopoietic stem cell transplant within weeks, diarrhea and elevation of liver enzymes may be seen as extracutaneous manifestations of GVHD.

Treatment Recommendations

When BSA involvement is over 30%, hospitalization is required, and the mortality of the disease can be 30–40% despite all possible efforts, with Chinese descendants having the highest mortality. When less than 10% of the BSA is affected with no severe systemic involvement, the mortality rate is less than 5%, and complete recovery can be achieved in 2–6 weeks when managed appropriately. Prevention and timely treatment of sepsis is crucial as it is the most common cause of death. After recovering from the acute phase of TEN, 5-year survival rate is 65% [124, 127, 128].

The initial treatment of SJS/TEN rests on the identification of a suspect causative agent and its removal. Intensive care is crucial. Burn units can be helpful in caring for patients with extensive epidermal damage. Supportive effort is directed at complications of large BSA denudation, including temperature dysregulation, infection, and caloric and fluid loss. An ambient temperature of 30–32 °C may be the optimal range. Though systemic prophylactic antibiotic therapy is not recommended, diluted vinegar wet dressings and other forms of topical decolonization measures, as well as gentle debridement of crusting, are essential. Sustaining adequate nutrition and hydration are vital, and vigilance over electrolyte imbalance is critical. Use of a Foley catheter may prevent urethral stricture but should be balanced against the risk of acquired infection. Collaboration among a team of intensivists and specialists is indispensable to the care of patients with SJS/TEN [129].

Corticosteroids can be a beneficial treatment for SJS/TEN when topical care is optimized, especially when infection control and prevention have been effectively managed. IVIG has been suggested as a treatment for SJS/TEN. However, data on its efficacy have been conflicting. Recent investigative studies suggest that cyclosporine may offer a greater mortality benefit over IVIG. Furthermore, plasmapheresis, TNF-α inhibitors, N-acetylcysteine, and other adjuvant therapies have emerged as promising treatment alternatives that are currently awaiting further substantiating data [129].

Prevention of recurrence is critical in SJS/TEN survivors, with avoidance of causative medications and their cross-reacting agents. In Asian descendants, HLA-B*1502 testing before carbamazepine initiation and HLA-B*5801 testing before allopurinol initiation may be considered. Among those of European heritage, descendant testing for HLA-B*5701 can be considered prior to abacavir administration [114, 124–130].

Dermatitis Herpetiformis

Epidemiology

Dermatitis herpetiformis (DH) is most common in patients of northern European heritage and is rarely seen in Asian and African-American patients. The prevalence of DH is 12–753 per million [131, 132] worldwide, with 112 per million reported in Utah [133]. The incidence of DH is 4–26 per million per year [132]. Oral lesions are rare in DH. The male to female ratio is 1.44–2:1, and the age of onset is broad but commonly in the third and fourth decades. In patients with gluten sensitivity enteropathy (GSE), 16% of men and 9% of women are diagnosed with DH.

Etiopathogenesis

DH is associated with GSE, but, clinically, gastrointestinal symptoms are frequently lacking. The pathogenesis of DH involves both the intestinal tract and the skin. The initial event in DH is theorized to be a loss of tolerance to gluten in the gut through risk factors such as pregnancy, enteric infections, lymphoma, or tumors. Interaction of transglutaminase (TTG) with wheat peptides induces T cell activation and IgA autoantibody production [132]. Subsequently, IgA autoantibodies deposit at the dermoepidermal junction (DEJ) due to events such as dermal pressure, trauma, and sunlight exposure. It is hypothesized that IgA deposition activates complement, which in turn induces cytokine and metalloproteinase production as well as neutrophil chemotaxis. These events cause subepidermal clefting at the lamina lucida and nonspecific connective tissue breakdown at the DEJ, leading to vesicle formation [132].

DH has a strong genetic linkage to HLA class II including HLA-DR3, DQ2, and DQ8 [132, 134]. Furthermore, presence of the MYO9B gene on chromosome 9p13 is strongly associated with GSE, but the association with DH is weak [132]. Autoimmune diseases are frequently associated with DH; in particular, thyroid diseases are the most commonly related disorders. Other associated diseases include type 1 diabetes mellitus, lupus erythematosus, Sjögren syndrome, sarcoidosis, vitiligo, pernicious anemia, and rheumatoid arthritis. Therefore, screening with thyroid stimulating hormone, anti-thyroid peroxidase antibody, glucose, hemoglobin A1C, complete blood count, antinuclear antibody (ANA), and vitamin B 12 are among further investigations to consider in a patient with DH. Splenic atrophy and lymphoma are complications associated with long-standing untreated DH and GSE [135].

Clinical Manifestations

Oral involvement is rare in DH but intraoral vesicles and erosions can be seen. Cutaneous involvement is characteristically pruritic vesicles that are heavily excoriated. The typical anatomic distribution includes the extensor elbows and knees, upper back, scalp, and sacrum.

Oral Signs and Symptoms

Although oral lesions are rare in DH, they can be the initial manifestations as early as 6 months prior to the onset of a cutaneous eruption. The buccal mucosa and the surfaces underneath dentures are the oral locations often affected in DH. Vesicles, pseudo-vesicles, erythematous erosions, and purpura are potential oral findings in DH. Small papules can be found on the maxillary ridge and alveolar mucosa, which may coalesce into plaques extending onto the hard palate. Oral lesions are typically burning or painful. Enamel defects are found in 80% of childhood and 53% of adult DH cases, which most frequently present as horizontal grooves. Cutaneous lesions are commonly extremely pruritic erosions on extensor surfaces and acral purpura.

On histopathology, neutrophilic microabscesses in the dermal papillae with fibrin, leukocytoclastic debris, and edema are observed. These findings are nonspecific. Separation at the BMZ may occur, and occasional apoptotic keratinocytes may be present above the papillary microabscesses. In early lesions, lymphocytic inflammation may be prominent.

DIF of perilesional normal-appearing skin or mucosa is paramount, with the pathognomonic features of granular deposition of IgA along the DEJ and stippling in the dermal papillae. DIF testing on oral biopsy can be positive without clinically active oral disease, and in contrast, DIF testing of the oral mucosa is negative in celiac disease without DH. IIF with IgA on monkey esophagus endomysium (EMA) has sensitivity of 90% and specificity of 96% [136].

Laboratory testing for IgA autoantibodies to TTG has a sensitivity of 89.1% and specificity of 97.6% for the diagnosis of DH [137]. Other testable autoantibodies have targets against gliadin and endomysium. Autoantibody serologies are less sensitive when patients do not exhibit total villus atrophy. These serological tests are especially useful when DIF testing is negative and may serve as an alert for sampling errors. In this situation, appropriate considerations include rebiopsy and gastroenterology work-up. When a patient has selective IgA deficiency, IgG serological testing should be used instead of IgA; however, it has lesser diagnostic sensitivity.

Differential Diagnosis

DH-associated diseases, such as GSE, lupus erythematosus, and Sjögren syndrome, may have oral symptoms independently or in conjunction with DH. Enamel defects found in celiac disease without DH are the same as enamel defects found in DH. Other oral clinical differential diagnoses include viral infections, other immunobullous disorders, and bullous lichen planus.

Treatment Recommendations

In some patients, DH can be treated successfully with a gluten-free diet. Some patients require additional treatment with dapsone, which is the standard agent used for DH treatment. It inhibits neutrophil chemotaxis and adhesion. Dapsone also protects cells from neutrophil-mediated injuries and decreases inflammation by blocking prostaglandin and leukotriene production. Alternative therapeutic agents include sulfamethoxypyridazine, sulfasalazine, and sulfapyridine. With medical treatment, cutaneous lesions are expected to improve in 2 days and clear in a week. However, without a gluten-free diet, relapse of skin symptoms is equally rapid. Dapsone does not treat gastrointestinal involvement, nor does it lower the risk for lymphoma and the development of splenic atrophy. Hence, a gluten-free diet is essential. It is helpful to solicit the guidance of dietitians. With dietary changes, dapsone may be tapered and discontinued in 1–2 years. DIF findings may take years to resolve and therefore are not helpful in disease monitoring. It is advisable to avoid iodides and nonsteroidal anti-inflammatory drugs other than ibuprofen as they may aggravate DH symptoms [138]. In addition, screening of family members is a reasonable consideration [131–147].

Linear IgA Bullous Dermatosis

Epidemiology

Approximately half of linear IgA bullous dermatosis (LABD) patients may present with minor oral lesions [148–150], though in rare patients, oral involvement may be severe. Laryngeal involvement can lead to scarring and airway constriction. Mucous membrane lesions are rare in children. Onset of adult LABD is usually in the sixth decade of life. Within adult onset LABD, females outnumber males 2:1 [151, 152].

Etiopathogenesis

LABD was originally hypothesized to be a variant of BP or DH, but it is now recognized as a separate entity. LABD is defined by linear deposition of IgA along the BMZ, specifically at the lamina lucida and sublamina densa, causing subepidermal separation. Low titers of circulating IgA autoantibodies can be found in one-third of patients. LABD autoantibodies target multiple anchoring filaments, including Ladinin 1 (LAD 1) and bullous pemphigoid antigen 2.

LABD has a wide variety of potential causes, including medications, infections (typhoid, tuberculosis, HSV, VZV, and upper respiratory infection), autoimmune diseases (inflammatory bowel diseases, multiple sclerosis, systemic lupus erythematosus, and rheumatoid arthritis), and malignancies (Hodgkin and non-Hodgkin lymphoma, chronic lymphocytic leukemia, plasmacytoma, multiple myeloma, and esophageal squamous cell carcinoma). Among medications, vancomycin is the number one cause of drug-induced LABD, while other implicated medications include diclofenac, lithium, captopril, cyclosporine, glyburide, iodine contrast, interferon gamma, phenytoin, somatostatin, and sulfamethoxazole/trimethoprim. LABD is also associated with gluten-sensitive enteropathy up to 25–33% of the time, but it is drastically less common compared to DH. In addition, immune complex glomerulonephritis is a potential consequence of LABD.

Clinical Manifestations

Oral presentation of LABD involves painful vesicles, bullae, and erosions that could lead to scarring.

Oral Signs and Symptoms

Ordinarily, oral symptoms of LABD are minor compared to cutaneous symptoms. However, exclusively oral LABD has been reported in the literature. LABD can involve any oral site, as well as extra-oral mucosal sites including the nose, conjunctiva, and genitalia. The principal oral symptoms of LABD are painful vesicles and bullae that progress to ulcerations and erosions with resultant scarring that can be extensive (Figs. 7.12 and 7.13). Generalized DG, gingival hyperplasia, and erosive cheilitis are also clinical features observed in oral LABD. Cutaneous symptoms are valuable in establishing a diagnosis, including extensor surface distribution, clusters of discrete bullae termed as the “jewel

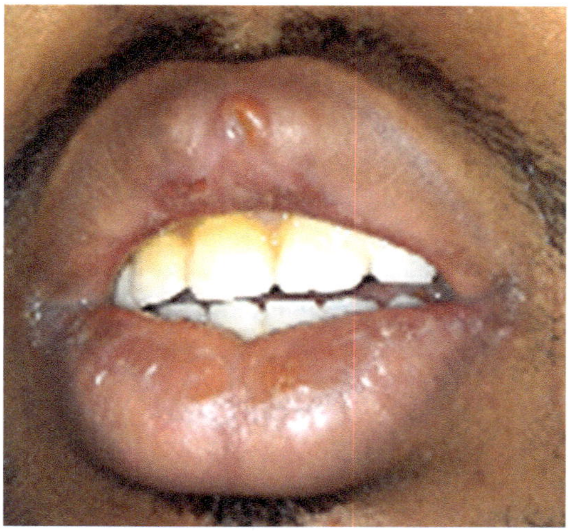

Fig. 7.12 Linear IgA bullous dermatosis. Annular vesiculobulla on the lip

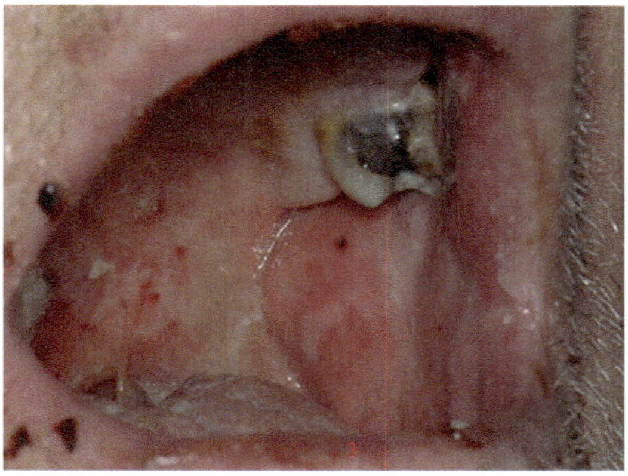

Fig. 7.13 Intraoral linear IgA bullous dermatosis. Irregular superficial erosions and ulcerations extensively involving the buccal mucosa and palate

sign," and vesicles or bullae at the border of annular lesions known as "string of pearls." Unlike the oral mucosa, cutaneous lesions heal without scarring. Depending on the cause, LABD may be chronic, with acute exacerbations and very few cases of spontaneous remission. Removal of an offending medication may lead to complete resolution of LABD.

On histopathology, LABD is characterized by subepidermal separation with neutrophilic papillitis. Micro-abscesses are seen in 50% of specimens, with a variable eosinophil infiltrate. DIF studies showing linear IgA deposition at the BMZ is the diagnostic hallmark of LABD. Occasionally, the co-existence of IgG and C3 linear deposition with IgA is observed. In these cases, IgA is much stronger and more prominent in LABD compared to MMP. Using anti-IgG conjugates, IIF testing is negative in LABD. However, linear deposition along the BMZ can be seen on monkey esophagus using anti-IgA conjugates. Either epidermal, dermal, or mixed patterns may be seen on IIF testing using human salt-split skin substrate.

Differential Diagnosis

Oral clinical findings of LABD could resemble BP, pemphigus vulgaris, MMP, bullous lichen planus, epidermolysis bullous acquisita, DH, EM, and SJS/TEN. MMP and LABD share the characteristic of mucosal scarring, while linear IgA deposition at the BMZ is reported in a minority of patients with MMP, making differentiation of these two diagnoses difficult [153].

Treatment Recommendations

Recognition of drug-induced LABD can lead to withdrawal of the implicated agent and resolution of the disease. In non-drug-induced forms of LABD, oral lesions are frequently refractory to treatment. Topical treatments and dapsone monotherapy are often not effective. There have been reported successes with dapsone combined with low-dose systemic corticosteroids. Other treatments include sulfapyridine, mycophenolate mofetil, tetracycline with nicotinamide, and colchicine. Oral hygiene, trauma prevention, pain control, and treatment of secondary infections are also essential in the management of LABD [143, 148–161].

Epidermolysis Bullosa

Epidemiology

In the USA, it is estimated that there are 50 epidermolysis bullosa (EB) cases per million live births. The incidence is much lower in Japan, with only 7.8 per million live births. It is estimated that there are approximately 400,000 people with EB worldwide. EB is a heterogeneous group of diseases categorized into four phenotypic types: EB simplex (EBS), dystrophic EB (DEB), junctional EB (JEB), and Kindler syndrome. EBS comprises the overwhelming majority, accounting for 92% of the EB cases. DEB and JEB are 5% and 1% of the total EB population, respectively, whereas Kindler syndrome (also known as mixed EB) is the rarest among the four categories. The remaining 2% of EB cases are unclassified.

Oral involvement is frequent in all major forms of EB, 58.6% in generalized EBS, 34.7% in localized EBS, 83.3% in Herlitz subtype of JEB, 91.6% in non-Herlitz JEB, 81.1% in dominant DEB, 100% in generalized recessive DEB, and 92.3% in localized recessive DEB.

Etiopathogenesis

EBS is caused by intraepidermal cleavage at the basal layer, resulting from gene mutations including plakophilin-1, desmoplakin, keratin-5, keratin-14, plectin, and alpha6-beta4 integrin. JEB affects the lamina lucida, due to mutations in laminin 332, type XVII collagen, and alpha6-beta4 integrin. DEB affects the sublamina densa, owing to the mutations in type VII collagen. Kindler syndrome is due to loss-of-function mutations in the FERMT1, a gene encoding the focal adhesion protein, fermitin family homolog-1, primarily found in basal keratinocytes.

The phenotype of each EB subtype is related to the mutated gene and the impact on its protein function (Table 7.3). For example, laminin 332 is broadly expressed in the skin and most other epithelia and participates in the attachment, migration, and organization of cells into tissues during embryonic development. Since it is expressed during tooth development, individuals with alteration in laminin 332 have defects in both tooth enamel and oral mucosal integrity. The junctional epithelium is critical for the function of ameloblasts that produce dental enamel. Type VII collagen plays a critical role in the integrity of the oral mucosa, but it is not involved in the development of teeth.

Clinical Manifestations

The clinical presentation varies widely depending on different types of EB. Generally, oral blisters and erosions can be seen. The presence or absence of dental caries, dental enamel defects, periodontal disease, oral architectural changes, scarring, cutaneous features, and systemic symptoms can aid in the clinical differentiation of EB subtypes.

Oral Signs and Symptoms

EBS, JEB, and DEB all may cause blistering with minor mechanical friction. The resultant erosion and secondary infection can lead to death. The most lethal form of EB is the Herlitz subtype of JEB, with a mortality rate reaching 87% within the 1st year of life. If infancy is survived, patients will continue to suffer a high risk of SCC, scarring, and disfigurement. The scarring can lead to symblepharon and other ocular symptoms, dysphagia when the esophagus is affected, as well as fusion of the fingers and toes. The lining of internal organs can be affected by EB as well. Kindler syndrome presents with sun sensitivity and subsequent acral blistering, erythema, and pruritus. Poikiloderma, atrophy and wrinkling of acral dorsum, and phimosis are also features of Kindler syndrome.

Clinical manifestations and severity vary dramatically between different types of EB. Oral blistering can be seen in all forms of EB. EBS oral lesions are most often localized to areas of trauma and heal without scarring. The Dowling-Meara subtype of EBS can be associated with scarring. Severe oral mucosal diseases are seen in autosomal recessive EBS and EBS with pyloric atresia. Localized areas of gingival hyperkeratosis can also be seen in EBS. Tongue fissuring is a feature found in plakophilin deficiency. Blister formation and oral ulceration can be severe in JEB, in particular the Herlitz type, generalized non-Herlitz type, and LOC syndrome. Despite its severity, JEB heals without scarring. Extreme fragility of oral and perioral mucosa is seen in DEB, especially in recessive DEB, which can

Table 7.3 Overview of EB subtypes and their associated proteins and genes [162, 163]

EB type	Subcategory	EB subtype	Protein	Gene
EBS	Suprabasal	Lethal acantholytic EB	Plakophilin-1	PKP1
		Plakophilin deficiency	Desmoplakin	DSP
		Superficialis	Unknown	
	Basal	Localized (Weber-Cockayne)	Keratin 5, Keratin 14	KRT5, KRT14
		Dowling-Meara	Keratin 5, Keratin 14	KRT5, KRT14
		Other generalized (Koebner)	Keratin 5, Keratin 14	KRT5, KRT14
		Mottled pigmentation	Keratin 5	KRT5
		Migratory circinate	Keratin 5	KRT5
		Autosomal recessive	Keratin 14	KRT14
		Muscular dystrophy	Plectin	PLEC1
		Ogna	Plectin	PLEC1
		Pyloric atresia	a6b4 integrin	ITGA6, ITGB4
JEB	Herlitz	Herlitz	Laminin 332	LAMA3, LAMB3, LAMC2
	Non-Herlitz	Non-Herlitz, generalized	Laminin 332, Collagen XVII	LAMA3, LAMB3, LAMC2, COL17A1
		Non-Herlitz, inversa	Laminin 332	LAMA3, LAMB3, LAMC2
		Non-Herlitz, localized	Collagen XVII	COL17A1
		LOC syndrome	Alpha chain of Laminin 332	LAMA3
		Pyloric atresia	a6b4 integrin	ITGA6, ITGB4
		Late onset	Unknown	
DEB	Dominant	Generalized	Collagen VII	COL7A1
		Acral	Collagen VII	COL7A1
		Pretibial	Collagen VII	COL7A1
		Pruriginosa	Collagen VII	COL7A1
		Nails only	Collagen VII	COL7A1
		Bullous dermolysis of the newborn	Collagen VII	COL7A1
	Recessive	Severe generalized (Hallopeau-Siemens)	Collagen VII	COL7A1
		Generalized other	Collagen VII	COL7A1
		Inversa	Collagen VII	COL7A1
		Pretibial	Collagen VII	COL7A1
		Pruriginosa	Collagen VII	COL7A1
		Centripetalis	Collagen VII	COL7A1
		Bullous dermolysis of the newborn	Collagen VII	COL7A1
Mixed EB	Kindler syndrome	–	Kindlin-1	KIND1

severely hinder the neonate's ability to suckle. Oral blistering in Kindler syndrome can also be severe and prominent in neonates with scarring potential, and the fragility diminishes with age (Table 7.4).

The Herlitz type of JEB is characterized by exuberant perioral granulation tissue leading to microstomia and loss of lip mobility. Oral architecture, salivation, and soft tissue mobility are preserved both in EBS and JEB. Enamel defects are distinctive features of JEB. Patients with JEB are at higher risk of developing dental caries. Enamel developmental defects include hypoplasia, pitting, horizontal bands, and white mottled enamel, which most prominently affects the molars. Despite the absence of enamel defects in DEB, the combination of scarring and limited ability in maintaining oral hygiene frequently leads to dental caries for DEB patients as well. Kindler syndrome can have enamel hypoplasia, as well as marked periodontal disease. This is due to kindlin-1, which affects adhesion of the oral

Table 7.4 Suggestive findings in Kindler syndrome [164]

Mucosal symptoms
Oral
Gingivitis, mucositis, and fragility
Enamel hypoplasia
Periodontitis
Premature loss of teeth
Labial leukokeratosis
Ocular
Conjunctivitis and scarring
Corneal erosion
Ectropion
Cutaneous symptoms
Fragility and trauma-induced blistering
Skin atrophy
Nail atrophy
Poikiloderma
Axillary freckling
Photosensitivity
Hyperkeratosis of palms and soles
Pseudosyndactyly
Extracutaneous involvements
Esophageal stenosis
Colitis, bloody diarrhea
Rectal fissures and stenosis
Urethral stenosis and strictures
Vaginal stenosis
Labial synechiae
Phimosis

mucosa to the tooth causing periodontitis and gingival hyperplasia starting in early childhood. Late-stage presentation of the periodontal disease includes alveolar bone resorption and premature loss of teeth. Dental caries risk is also heightened in Kindler syndrome.

Oral scarring and consequently obliteration of the oral vestibule, loss of lingual papillae, ankyloglossia, effacement of palatal rugae, microstomia, and other anatomical alterations can be prominent features in generalized recessive DEB. Scarring is also often seen in dominant DEB and the Dowling-Meara type of EBS, and microstomia is also present in the Herlitz type of JEB. Oral milia are commonly seen in all major categories of EB and are more frequent in DEB. Cutaneous and oral mucosal squamous cell carcinoma is a major concern in patients with severe generalized recessive DEB (Table 7.5).

Table 7.5 Oral presentations in EB

Oral blistering	All forms of EB
Oral milium	All forms of EB
Oral scarring	Recessive DEB, occasionally in Dominant DEB and Dowling-Meara-type EBS
Oral anatomical alterations	Recessive DEB
Microstomia	Recessive DEB, Herlitz-type JEB
Enamel defects	JEB, Kindler syndrome
Dental caries	JEB and DEB
Periodontal disease	JEB, Recessive DEB, Kindler syndrome
Oral cancer	Recessive DEB

Differential Diagnosis

In neonates with oral ulceration, acute herpetic gingivostomatitis should be ruled out. Most other blistering and erosive oral diseases can be differentiated from EB due to later onset, including pemphigus vulgaris, PNP/PAMS, MMP, DH, lichen planus, systemic lupus erythematosus, EM, and SJS/TEN.

Treatment Recommendations

No medical treatment or procedures are proven to be effective in treating the underlying cause of EB. Hence, management has been focused on symptomatic relief, supportive care, and preventive management. Patients should be made comfortable by effective pain management. Supportive care is needed when large areas of skin are affected, including adequate hydration, skin barrier creams, and temperature regulation. Preventive management is crucial, including meticulous oral hygiene to avoid infections, prevention of deformity thru measures such as finger bandaging, regular dental and skin examinations for caries, and cutaneous and oral malignancies. Severe recessive DEB patients may require soft diets that are high in calories. Given the intensive care required at home, detailed education of the parents is essential, and online resources as well as support groups also offer additional help. Gene therapy is currently under development for the treatment of EB [162–173].

Angina Bullosa Haemorrhagica

Epidemiology

Angina bullosa haemorrhagica (ABH) primarily affects middle-age to elderly populations, with a median age of 54 years [174].

Etiopathogenesis

The pathophysiology for ABH is unknown, but it is hypothesized to be subepithelial separation due to trauma, with concurrent capillary bleeding into the bulla. The connection to chronic inhalational corticosteroid therapy has been suggested [175].

Clinical Manifestations

ABH is characterized by rapidly resolving solitary hemorrhagic vesicles or bullae with an ecchymotic halo, in the absence of other causes such as immunobullous diseases, systemic diseases, and blood dyscrasias.

Oral Signs and Symptoms

ABH is abrupt in onset arising during or shortly after eating. A preceding stinging pain or burning sensation may be experienced. ABH is commonly found on the soft palate, where the mucosa is thin and friable, while other common locations include the buccal mucosa, lip, and lateral aspects of the tongue. ABH presents as an acute hemorrhagic vesicle or bulla surrounded by an ecchymotic halo. The typical blister is 1–3 cm in diameter. The blisters rupture spontaneously, leaving behind an erosion covered by a fibromembranous slough with surrounding diffuse erythema. Typically, the erosion will heal without scarring within a week. ABH lesions are most often solitary, but it may present with multiple lesions [176]. The disease is short-lived. Intermittent recurrence up to 25 years later has been reported [177].

ABH occurs in the absence of bleeding or ecchymosis when it affects the gingiva or extraoral locations. When the rapidly enlarging bulla is located on the posterior oropharynx or the epiglottic region, acute upper respiratory obstruction can result.

Systemic disease associations, though speculative, include hypertension, diabetes mellitus, chronic kidney disease on hemodialysis, asthma, rheumatoid arthritis, hyperuricemia, and systemic lupus erythematosus.

The histopathology is subepithelial separation with a large blister cavity containing red blood cells. Direct immunofluorescence testing is negative in ABH.

Differential Diagnosis

The differential diagnosis of ABH includes immunobullous diseases (bullous pemphigoid, MMP, LABD, DH, bullous systemic lupus erythematosus), systemic diseases, and blood dyscrasias. ABH is a diagnosis of exclusion. Hence, biopsy for histopathology, DIF, and laboratory investigation of platelet counts and coagulation tests are appropriate tests to consider.

Treatment Recommendations

When other disease conditions are excluded, ABH patients should be given reassurance. Treatment is focused on prevention of trauma and symptomatic amelioration. Short courses of topical corticosteroids have been suggested, but more aggressive treatment is generally not needed. Large bullae should be incised and drained [174–178].

Vitiligo

Epidemiology

The global prevalence of vitiligo is estimated at 1% of the general population, but the prevalence of oral mucosal involvement is far less recognized than skin [179]. Oral vitiligo is seen in both genders, with a slight female predominance. Age range is wide for the onset of vitiligo, and there is no known racial or regional predilection.

Etiopathogenesis

Microscopically, there is a complete absence of melanocytes. The mechanism for disappearance of the melanocytes is unknown. Several theories predominate, including autoimmune destruction, altered intrinsic melanocytic survival, and neural connection, as well as defective defense against hypoxia, toxins, and oxidative stress. Multifactorial and polygenic genetic factors appear to be contributory, with 20–30% of vitiligo patients having a positive family history. X-box-binding protein 1 is associated with vitiligo in the Han Chinese [179]. HLA-A2, DR4, DR7, and DQB1*0303 are among the many HLA haplotypes linked to vitiligo [179].

Clinical Manifestations

Depigmentation of the oral mucosa is commonly seen with facial, neck, and acral cutaneous vitiligo. The lips are most frequently affected, followed by the palate, buccal mucosa, gingiva, and labial mucosa.

Oral Signs and Symptoms

Oral discoloration can play a significant role in cosmetic appearance, and the associated visual disfigurement can be emotionally challenging for many afflicted individuals. Mucosal depigmentation is most common on the lip, followed by the palate, buccal mucosa, gingiva, and labial mucosa (Fig. 7.14). Involvement of multiple oral sites is common; however, depigmentation of the entire oral mucosa is infrequent [180]. Areas of leukoderma are well demarcated, with a geographic border. Most patients with oral vitiligo also have cutaneous involvement and are commonly found to have acral and facial involvement [181]. Wood's lamp is a device that aids in the identification of leukoderma that may not be readily visible otherwise. Individually, the course of vitiligo is unpredictable. Typically, vitiligo occurs in a stepwise fashion with long periods of inactive disease between episodes of progression. Mucosal vitiligo is associated with disease progression, and other risk factors include a positive family history, Koebner phenomenon, and non-segmental distribution. Spontaneous regression and complete repigmentation are uncommon. Aside from cosmetic alteration and the psychosocial impact thereof, vitiligo is otherwise asymptomatic.

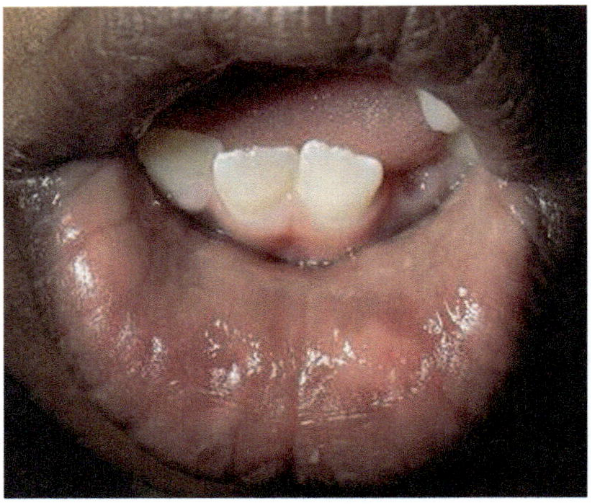

Fig. 7.14 Vitiligo. Complete loss of pigment on the mucosal lower lip

Associated systemic disease is predominantly thyroid disorders. Other autoimmune diseases are also seen, including diabetes mellitus, alopecia areata, rheumatoid arthritis, psoriasis, lupus erythematosus, pernicious anemia, and Addison's disease [179, 182]. On rare occasions, gastric cancer can also occur in the setting of vitiligo. When vitiligo and ocular disease coexist, Vogt-Koyanagi-Harada syndrome, ocular fundus depigmentation, and Alezzandrini syndrome should be considered. Alezzandrini syndrome is known to include depigmentation of the upper lip, with leukotrichia and ipsilateral visual changes. Quality of life assessment, a thorough review of systems, thyroid function tests, antinuclear antibody screening, and a hemoglobin A1C level should be considered in the work-up for vitiligo patients.

Histopathology demonstrates absence of melanocytes and suprabasilar vacuolar changes. Suprabasilar clear cells, perivascular mononuclear inflammation, epidermal thinning and effacement, sweat gland degeneration, and follicular degeneration are additional features that can be observed on histopathology.

Differential Diagnosis

In contrast to the depigmentation of vitiligo, white discoloration is seen in leukoplakia, leukoedema, and white sponge nevus. Albinism also results in depigmentation within the oral cavity, but it is accompanied by a lack of pigmentation through the entire body. Other causes of leukoderma include post-inflammatory hypopigmentation, chemical- or trauma-induced leukoderma, lichen sclerosus, sarcoidosis, discoid lupus erythematosus, corticosteroid- and hydroquinone-induced hypopigmentation, and amelanotic melanoma.

Treatment Recommendations

Patient education is quintessential in the management of vitiligo. Sun protection can help to reduce the contrast between areas of leukoderma and their surrounding normally pigmented skin, and sun protection is also important in skin cancer prevention. Trauma avoidance aids in the prevention of Koebner phenomenon that could induce further discoloration. Cosmetic cover-up with lipsticks and tattooing are available for the lips, although tattooing risks further development of vitiligo due to trauma. The psychosocial impact of vitiligo should be considered, and resources such as support groups are helpful (Vitiligo Support International, https://www.vitiligosupport.org). Due to a lack of melanocyte reservoirs from the absence of hair follicles, oral vitiligo is expected to be more resistant to treatment when compared to its cutaneous counterpart. Younger patients, recent onset of disease and darker skin types are the factors that increase the likelihood of a favorable therapeutic response.

Treatment is guided by the degree in which vitiligo impacts the patient's quality of life. The no-treatment option should be discussed, because there is no known treatment that can alter the natural disease process. Medically, topical corticosteroids, calcineurin inhibitors, or a combination of betamethasone and calcipotriol are common choices for oral mucosal therapy [183–186]. When potent topical corticosteroids are used, the risk of atrophy is a consideration. For the external component of the lips, narrowband UVB light therapy, excimer laser, and helium-neon laser therapy are options [183, 187]. Responders to excimer laser were found with Fitzpatrick skin types III or above. Systemic and surgical treatments are not common practice for isolated disease. Minocycline, antioxidants, folic acid and vitamin B12 supplementation, as well as ginkgo have been reported to arrest disease progression, although convincing validation is currently lacking [179–194].

References

1. Ahmed AR, Graham J, Jordon RE, Provost TT. Pemphigus: current concepts. Ann Intern Med. 1980;92(3):396–405.
2. Becker BA, Gaspari AA. Pemphigus vulgaris and vegetans. Dermatol Clin. 1993;11(3):429–52.
3. Ahmed AR, Nguyen T, Kaveri S, Spigelman ZS. First line treatment of pemphigus vulgaris with a novel protocol in patients with contraindications to systemic corticosteroids and immunosuppressive agents: preliminary retrospective study with a seven year follow-up. Int Immunopharmacol. 2016;34:25–31.
4. Sagi L, Sherer Y, Trau H, Shoenfeld Y. Pemphigus and infectious agents. Autoimmun Rev. 2008;8(1):33–5.
5. Krain LS. Pemphigus. Epidemiologic and survival characteristics of 59 patients, 1955–1973. Arch Dermatol. 1974;110(6):862–5.
6. Helander SD, Rogers RS 3rd. The sensitivity and specificity of direct immunofluorescence testing in disorders of mucous membranes. J Am Acad Dermatol. 1994;30(1):65–75.
7. Shamim T, Varghese VI, Shameena PM, Sudha S. Pemphigus vulgaris in oral cavity: clinical analysis of 71 cases. Med Oral Patol Oral Cir Bucal. 2008;13(10):E622–6.

8. Ahmed AR, Spigelman Z, Cavacini LA, Posner MR. Treatment of pemphigus vulgaris with rituximab and intravenous immune globulin. N Engl J Med. 2006;355(17):1772–9.
9. Robinson JC, Lozada-Nur F, Frieden I. Oral pemphigus vulgaris: a review of the literature and a report on the management of 12 cases. Oral Surg Oral Med Oral Pathol Oral Radiol Endod. 1997;84(4):349–55.
10. Ding X, Aoki V, Mascaro JM Jr, Lopez-Swiderski A, Diaz LA, Fairley JA. Mucosal and mucocutaneous (generalized) pemphigus vulgaris show distinct autoantibody profiles. J Invest Dermatol. 1997;109(4):592–6.
11. Atzmony L, Hodak E, Gdalevich M, Rosenbaum O, Mimouni D. Treatment of pemphigus vulgaris and pemphigus foliaceus: a systematic review and meta-analysis. Am J Clin Dermatol. 2014;15(6):503–15.
12. Harman KE, Seed PT, Gratian MJ, Bhogal BS, Challacombe SJ, Black MM. The severity of cutaneous and oral pemphigus is related to desmoglein 1 and 3 antibody levels. Br J Dermatol. 2001;144(4):775–80.
13. Scully C, Paes De Almeida O, Porter SR, Gilkes JJ. Pemphigus vulgaris: the manifestations and long-term management of 55 patients with oral lesions. Br J Dermatol. 1999;140(1):84–9.
14. Mignogna MD, Lo Muzio L, Galloro G, Satriano RA, Ruocco V, Bucci E. Oral pemphigus: clinical significance of esophageal involvement: report of eight cases. Oral Surg Oral Med Oral Pathol Oral Radiol Endod. 1997;84(2):179–84.
15. Dagistan S, Goregen M, Miloglu O, Cakur B. Oral pemphigus vulgaris: a case report with review of the literature. J Oral Sci. 2008;50(3):359–62.
16. Meurer M, Millns JL, Rogers RS 3rd, Jordon RE. Oral pemphigus vulgaris. A report of ten cases. Arch Dermatol. 1977;113(11):1520–4.
17. Sirois D, Leigh JE, Sollecito TP. Oral pemphigus vulgaris preceding cutaneous lesions: recognition and diagnosis. J Am Dent Assoc. 2000;131(8):1156–60.
18. Vinay K, Kanwar AJ, Mittal A, Dogra S, Minz RW, Hashimoto T. Intralesional rituximab in the treatment of refractory oral pemphigus vulgaris. JAMA Dermatol. 2015;151(8):878–82.
19. Carson PJ, Hameed A, Ahmed AR. Influence of treatment on the clinical course of pemphigus vulgaris. J Am Acad Dermatol. 1996;34(4):645–52.
20. Rogers RS 3rd, Van Hale HM. Immunopathologic diagnosis of oral mucosal inflammatory diseases. Australas J Dermatol. 1986;27(2):51–7.
21. Harman KE, Albert S, Black MM, British Association of Dermatologists. Guidelines for the management of pemphigus vulgaris. Br J Dermatol. 2003;149(5):926–37.
22. Michailidou EZ, Belazi MA, Markopoulos AK, Tsatsos MI, Mourellou ON, Antoniades DZ. Epidemiologic survey of pemphigus vulgaris with oral manifestations in northern Greece: retrospective study of 129 patients. Int J Dermatol. 2007;46(4):356–61.
23. Tabrizi MN, Chams-Davatchi C, Esmaeeli N, Noormohammadpoor P, Safar F, Etemadzadeh H, et al. Accelerating effects of epidermal growth factor on skin lesions of pemphigus vulgaris: a double-blind, randomized, controlled trial. J Eur Acad Dermatol Venereol. 2007;21(1):79–84.
24. Anhalt GJ, Kim SC, Stanley JR, Korman NJ, Jabs DA, Kory M, et al. Paraneoplastic pemphigus. An autoimmune mucocutaneous disease associated with neoplasia. N Engl J Med. 1990;323(25):1729–35.
25. Czernik A, Camilleri M, Pittelkow MR, Grando SA. Paraneoplastic autoimmune multiorgan syndrome: 20 years after. Int J Dermatol. 2011;50(8):905–14.
26. Poot AM, Diercks GF, Kramer D, Schepens I, Klunder G, Hashimoto T, et al. Laboratory diagnosis of paraneoplastic pemphigus. Br J Dermatol. 2013;169(5):1016–24.
27. Yong AA, Tey HL. Paraneoplastic pemphigus. Australas J Dermatol. 2013;54(4):241–50.
28. Poot AM, Siland J, Jonkman MF, Pas HH, Diercks GF. Direct and indirect immunofluorescence staining patterns in the diagnosis of paraneoplastic pemphigus. Br J Dermatol. 2016;174(4):912–5.
29. Joly P, Richard C, Gilbert D, Courville P, Chosidow O, Roujeau JC, et al. Sensitivity and specificity of clinical, histologic, and immunologic features in the diagnosis of paraneoplastic pemphigus. J Am Acad Dermatol. 2000;43(4):619–26.
30. Helou J, Allbritton J, Anhalt GJ. Accuracy of indirect immunofluorescence testing in the diagnosis of paraneoplastic pemphigus. J Am Acad Dermatol. 1995;32(3):441–7.
31. Murrell DF. Blistering diseases: clinical features, pathogenesis, treatment. New York: Springer; 2015. p. XXI.. 752
32. Schoen H, Foedinger D, Derfler K, Amann G, Rappersberger K, Stingl G, Volc-Platzer B. Immunoapheresis in paraneoplastic pemphigus. Arch Dermatol. 1998;134(6):706–10.
33. Jansen T, Plewig G, Anhalt GJ. Paraneoplastic pemphigus with clinical features of erosive lichen planus associated with Castleman's tumor. Dermatology. 1995;190(3):245–50.
34. Bech R, Baumgartner-Nielsen J, Peterslund NA, Steiniche T, Bang K, Deleuran M, et al. Alemtuzumab (ALZ) is an effective treatment for both primary and relapsed severe paraneoplastic pemphigus (PNP) associated to B-cell chronic lymphocytic leukemia (CLL). Blood. 2007;110(11):1.
35. Horn TD, Anhalt GJ. Histologic features of paraneoplastic pemphigus. Arch Dermatol. 1992;128(8):1091–5.
36. Nousari HC, Brodsky RA, Jones RJ, Grever MR, Anhalt GJ. Immunoablative high-dose cyclophosphamide without stem cell rescue in paraneoplastic pemphigus: report of a case and review of this new therapy for severe autoimmune disease. J Am Acad Dermatol. 1999;40(5 Pt 1):750–4.

37. Kaplan I, Hodak E, Ackerman L, Mimouni D, Anhalt GJ, Calderon S. Neoplasms associated with paraneoplastic pemphigus: a review with emphasis on non-hematologic malignancy and oral mucosal manifestations. Oral Oncol. 2004;40(6):553–62.
38. Ghigliotti G, Di Zenzo G, Cozzani E, Rongioletti F, De Col E, Pastorino C, et al. Paraneoplastic autoimmune multi-organ syndrome: association with retroperitoneal Kaposi's sarcoma. Acta Derm Venereol. 2016;96(2):261–2.
39. Anhalt GJ. Paraneoplastic pemphigus. J Investig Dermatol Symp Proc. 2004;9(1):29–33.
40. Kimyai-Asadi A, Jih MH. Paraneoplastic pemphigus. Int J Dermatol. 2001;40(6):367–72.
41. Mutasim DF, Pelc NJ, Anhalt GJ. Paraneoplastic pemphigus. Dermatol Clin. 1993;11(3):473–81.
42. Zhu X, Zhang B. Paraneoplastic pemphigus. J Dermatol. 2007;34(8):503–11.
43. Namba C, Tohyama M, Hanakawa Y, Murakami M, Shirakata Y, Matsumoto T, et al. Paraneoplastic pemphigus associated with fatal bronchiolitis obliterans and intractable mucosal erosions: treatment with cyclosporin in addition to steroid, rituximab and intravenous immunoglobulin. J Dermatol. 2016;43(4):419–22.
44. Ghandi N, Ghanadan A, Azizian MR, Hejazi P, Aghazadeh N, Tavousi P, et al. Paraneoplastic pemphigus associated with inflammatory myofibroblastic tumour of the mediastinum: a favourable response to treatment and review of the literature. Australas J Dermatol. 2015;56(2):120–3.
45. Camisa C, Helm TN. Paraneoplastic pemphigus is a distinct neoplasia-induced autoimmune disease. Arch Dermatol. 1993;129(7):883–6.
46. Didona D, Paolino G, Richetta A, Cantisani C, Moliterni E, Calvieri S, et al. Paraneoplastic pemphigus: a trait d'union between dermatology and oncology. Adv Mod Oncol Res. 2015;1(2):7.
47. Descamps V, Belaich S. Paraneoplastic pemphigus. Presse Med. 1999;28(7):363–7.
48. Martel P, Joly P. Paraneoplastic pemphigus. Ann Dermatol Venereol. 2001;128(11):1256–9.
49. Preisz K, Karpati S. Paraneoplastic pemphigus. Orv Hetil. 2007;148(21):979–83.
50. Wang R, Li J, Wang M, Hao H, Chen X, Li R, et al. Prevalence of myasthenia gravis and associated autoantibodies in paraneoplastic pemphigus and their correlations with symptoms and prognosis. Br J Dermatol. 2015;172(4):968–75.
51. Leger S, Picard D, Ingen-Housz-Oro S, Arnault JP, Aubin F, Carsuzaa F, et al. Prognostic factors of paraneoplastic pemphigus. Arch Dermatol. 2012;148(10):1165–72.
52. Heizmann M, Itin P, Wernli M, Borradori L, Bargetzi MJ. Successful treatment of paraneoplastic pemphigus in follicular NHL with rituximab: report of a case and review of treatment for paraneoplastic pemphigus in NHL and CLL. Am J Hematol. 2001;66(2):142–4.
53. Kitagawa C, Nakajima K, Aoyama Y, Fujioka A, Nakajima H, Tarutani M, et al. A typical case of paraneoplastic pemphigus without detection of malignancy: effectiveness of plasma exchange. Acta Derm Venereol. 2014;94(3):359–61.
54. Williams JV, Marks JG Jr, Billingsley EM. Use of mycophenolate mofetil in the treatment of paraneoplastic pemphigus. Br J Dermatol. 2000;142(3):506–8.
55. Kershenovich R, Hodak E, Mimouni D. Diagnosis and classification of pemphigus and bullous pemphigoid. Autoimmun Rev. 2014;13(4–5):477–81.
56. Schmidt E, Zillikens D. Pemphigoid diseases. Lancet. 2013;381(9863):320–32.
57. Laskaris G, Nicolis G. Immunopathology of oral mucosa in bullous pemphigoid. Oral Surg Oral Med Oral Pathol. 1980;50(4):340–5.
58. Chuah SY, Tan SH, Chua SH, Tang MB, Lim YL, Neoh CY, et al. A retrospective review of the therapeutic response with remission in patients with newly diagnosed bullous pemphigoid. Australas J Dermatol. 2014;55(2):149–51.
59. Hodge L, Marsden RA, Black MM, Bhogal B, Corbett MF. Bullous pemphigoid: the frequency of mucosal involvement and concurrent malignancy related to indirect immunofluorescence findings. Br J Dermatol. 1981;105(1):65–9.
60. Lo Schiavo A, Ruocco E, Brancaccio G, Caccavale S, Ruocco V, Wolf R. Bullous pemphigoid: etiology, pathogenesis, and inducing factors: facts and controversies. Clin Dermatol. 2013;31(4):391–9.
61. Person JR, Rogers RS 3rd. Bullous and cicatricial pemphigoid. Clinical, histopathologic, and immunopathologic correlations. Mayo Clin Proc. 1977;52(1):54–66.
62. Shklar G, Meyer I, Zacarian SA. Oral lesions in bullous pemphigoid. Arch Dermatol. 1969;99(6):663–70.
63. Venning VA, Frith PA, Bron AJ, Millard PR, Wojnarowska F. Mucosal involvement in bullous and cicatricial pemphigoid. A clinical and immunopathological study. Br J Dermatol. 1988;118(1):7–15.
64. Williams DM. Vesiculo-bullous mucocutaneous disease: benign mucous membrane and bullous pemphigoid. J Oral Pathol Med. 1990;19(1):16–23.
65. Ghohestani RF, Nicolas JF, Rousselle P, Claudy AL. Identification of a 168-kDa mucosal antigen in a subset of patients with cicatricial pemphigoid. J Invest Dermatol. 1996;107(1):136–9.
66. Carrozzo M, Dametto E, Fasano ME, Broccoletti R, Carbone M, Rendine S, et al. Interleukin-4RA gene polymorphism is associated with oral mucous membrane pemphigoid. Oral Dis. 2014;20(3):275–80.
67. Oyama N, Setterfield JF, Powell AM, Sakuma-Oyama Y, Albert S, Bhogal BS, et al. Bullous pemphigoid antigen II (BP180) and its soluble extracellular domains are major autoantigens in mucous membrane pemphigoid: the pathogenic relevance to HLA class II alleles and disease severity. Br J Dermatol. 2006;154(1):90–8.

68. Rabelo DF, Nguyen T, Caufield BA, Ahmed AR. Mucous membrane pemphigoid in two half-sisters. The potential roles of autoantibodies to beta4 integrin subunits and HLA-DQbeta1*0301. J Dermatol Case Rep. 2014;8(1):9–12.
69. Xu HH, Werth VP, Parisi E, Sollecito TP. Mucous membrane pemphigoid. Dent Clin N Am. 2013;57(4):611–30.
70. Shklar G, McCarthy PL. Oral lesions of mucous membrane pemphigoid. A study of 85 cases. Arch Otolaryngol. 1971;93(4):354–64.
71. Grattan CE, Small D, Kennedy CT, Scully C. Oral herpes simplex infection in bullous pemphigoid. Oral Surg Oral Med Oral Pathol. 1986;61(1):40–3.
72. Maley A, Warren M, Haberman I, Swerlick R, Kharod-Dholakia B, Feldman R. Rituximab combined with conventional therapy versus conventional therapy alone for the treatment of mucous membrane pemphigoid (MMP). J Am Acad Dermatol. 2016;74(5):835–40.
73. Chan LS, Ahmed AR, Anhalt GJ, Bernauer W, Cooper KD, Elder MJ, et al. The first international consensus on mucous membrane pemphigoid: definition, diagnostic criteria, pathogenic factors, medical treatment, and prognostic indicators. Arch Dermatol. 2002;138(3):370–9.
74. Setterfield J, Shirlaw PJ, Kerr-Muir M, Neill S, Bhogal BS, Morgan P, et al. Mucous membrane pemphigoid: a dual circulating antibody response with IgG and IgA signifies a more severe and persistent disease. Br J Dermatol. 1998;138(4):602–10.
75. Ali S, Kelly C, Challacombe SJ, Donaldson AN, Dart JK, Gleeson M, et al. Salivary IgA and IgG antibodies to bullous pemphigoid 180 noncollagenous domain 16a as diagnostic biomarkers in mucous membrane pemphigoid. Br J Dermatol. 2016;174(5):1022–9.
76. Sacher C, Hunzelmann N. Cicatricial pemphigoid (mucous membrane pemphigoid): current and emerging therapeutic approaches. Am J Clin Dermatol. 2005;6(2):93–103.
77. Canizares MJ, Smith DI, Conners MS, Maverick KJ, Heffernan MP. Successful treatment of mucous membrane pemphigoid with etanercept in 3 patients. Arch Dermatol. 2006;142(11):1457–61.
78. Rogers RS 3rd. Mucous membrane pemphigoid. Dermatology at the millennium. Nashville: Parthenon Publishing; 1999. p. 5.
79. Hanson RD, Olsen KD, Rogers RS 3rd. Upper aerodigestive tract manifestations of cicatricial pemphigoid. Ann Otol Rhinol Laryngol. 1988;97(5 Pt 1):493–9.
80. Darling MR, Daley T. Blistering mucocutaneous diseases of the oral mucosa – a review: part 1. Mucous membrane pemphigoid. J Can Dent Assoc. 2005;71(11):851–4.
81. Di Zenzo G, Carrozzo M, Chan LS. Urban legend series: mucous membrane pemphigoid. Oral Dis. 2014;20(1):35–54.
82. Hayakawa T, Furumura M, Fukano H, Li X, Ishii N, Hamada T, et al. Diagnosis of oral mucous membrane pemphigoid by means of combined serologic testing. Oral Surg Oral Med Oral Pathol Oral Radiol. 2014;117(4):483–96.
83. Messmer EM, Hintschich CR, Partscht K, Messer G, Kampik A. Ocular cicatricial pemphigoid. Retrospective analysis of risk factors and complications. Ophthalmologe. 2000;97(2):113–20.
84. Murrell DF, Marinovic B, Caux F, Prost C, Ahmed R, Wozniak K, et al. Definitions and outcome measures for mucous membrane pemphigoid: recommendations of an international panel of experts. J Am Acad Dermatol. 2015;72(1):168–74.
85. Rogers RS 3rd, Mehregan DA. Dapsone therapy of cicatricial pemphigoid. Semin Dermatol. 1988;7(3):201–5.
86. Rogers RS, Sheridan PJ, Jordon RE. Desquamative gingivitis. Clinical, histopathologic, and immunopathologic investigations. Oral Surg Oral Med Oral Pathol. 1976;42(3):316–27.
87. Rogers RS 3rd, Sheridan PJ, Nightingale SH. Desquamative gingivitis: clinical, histopathologic, immunopathologic, and therapeutic observations. J Am Acad Dermatol. 1982;7(6):729–35.
88. Scully C, Lo Muzio L. Oral mucosal diseases: mucous membrane pemphigoid. Br J Oral Maxillofac Surg. 2008;46(5):358–66.
89. Serrano TL, et al. Mucous membrane pemphigoid: diagnosis and sequel. Int Arch Otorhinolaryngol. 2014;18(S 01):1.
90. Shetty S, Ahmed AR. Critical analysis of the use of rituximab in mucous membrane pemphigoid: a review of the literature. J Am Acad Dermatol. 2013;68(3):499–506.
91. Taylor J, McMillan R, Shephard M, Setterfield J, Ahmed R, Carrozzo M, et al. World Workshop on Oral Medicine VI: a systematic review of the treatment of mucous membrane pemphigoid. Oral Surg Oral Med Oral Pathol Oral Radiol. 2015;120(2):161–71 e20.
92. Yeh SW, Usman AQ, Ahmed AR. Profile of autoantibody to basement membrane zone proteins in patients with mucous membrane pemphigoid: long-term follow up and influence of therapy. Clin Immunol. 2004;112(3):268–72.
93. Greer RO, McDowell JD, Hoernig G. Oral lichen planus: a premalignant disease? Pro Pathol Case Rev. 1999;4:7.
94. Nagao T, Ikeda N, Fukano H, Hashimoto S, Shimozato K, Warnakulasuriya S. Incidence rates for oral leukoplakia and lichen planus in a Japanese population. J Oral Pathol Med. 2005;34(9):532–9.
95. Farhi D, Dupin N. Pathophysiology, etiologic factors, and clinical management of oral lichen planus, part I: facts and controversies. Clin Dermatol. 2010;28(1):100–8.
96. Porter SR, Kirby A, Olsen I, Barrett W. Immunologic aspects of dermal and oral lichen planus: a review.

Oral Surg Oral Med Oral Pathol Oral Radiol Endod. 1997;83(3):358–66.
97. Lodi G, Scully C, Carrozzo M, Griffiths M, Sugerman PB, Thongprasom K. Current controversies in oral lichen planus: report of an international consensus meeting. Part 2. Clinical management and malignant transformation. Oral Surg Oral Med Oral Pathol Oral Radiol Endod. 2005;100(2):164–78.
98. Au J, Patel D, Campbell JH. Oral lichen planus. Oral Maxillofac Surg Clin N Am. 2013;25(1):93–100.. vii
99. Ismail SB, Kumar SK, Zain RB. Oral lichen planus and lichenoid reactions: etiopathogenesis, diagnosis, management and malignant transformation. J Oral Sci. 2007;49(2):89–106.
100. Laeijendecker R, Dekker SK, Burger PM, Mulder PG, Van Joost T, Neumann MH. Oral lichen planus and allergy to dental amalgam restorations. Arch Dermatol. 2004;140(12):1434–8.
101. Olson MA, Rogers RS 3rd, Bruce AJ. Oral lichen planus. Clin Dermatol. 2016;34(4):495–504.
102. Parashar P. Oral lichen planus. Otolaryngol Clin N Am. 2011;44(1):89–107.. vi
103. Pavlovsky L, Israeli M, Sagy E, Berg AL, David M, Shemer A, et al. Lichen planopilaris is associated with HLA DRB1*11 and DQB1*03 alleles. Acta Derm Venereol. 2015;95(2):177–80.
104. Sugerman PB, Savage NW, Zhou X, Walsh LJ, Bigby M. Oral lichen planus. Clin Dermatol. 2000;18(5):533–9.
105. Wetter DA, Davis MD. Recurrent erythema multiforme: clinical characteristics, etiologic associations, and treatment in a series of 48 patients at Mayo Clinic, 2000 to 2007. J Am Acad Dermatol. 2010;62(1):45–53.
106. Huff JC, Weston WL, Tonnesen MG. Erythema multiforme: a critical review of characteristics, diagnostic criteria, and causes. J Am Acad Dermatol. 1983;8(6):763–75.
107. Scully C, Bagan J. Oral mucosal diseases: erythema multiforme. Br J Oral Maxillofac Surg. 2008;46(2):90–5.
108. Ayangco L, Rogers RS 3rd. Oral manifestations of erythema multiforme. Dermatol Clin. 2003;21(1):195–205.
109. Lozada-Nur F, Gorsky M, Silverman S Jr. Oral erythema multiforme: clinical observations and treatment of 95 patients. Oral Surg Oral Med Oral Pathol. 1989;67(1):36–40.
110. Sokumbi O, Wetter DA. Clinical features, diagnosis, and treatment of erythema multiforme: a review for the practicing dermatologist. Int J Dermatol. 2012;51(8):889–902.
111. Leaute-Labreze C, Lamireau T, Chawki D, Maleville J, Taïeb A. Diagnosis, classification, and management of erythema multiforme and Stevens-Johnson syndrome. Arch Dis Child. 2000;83(4):347–52.
112. Bakis S, Zagarella S. Intermittent oral cyclosporin for recurrent herpes simplex-associated erythema multiforme. Australas J Dermatol. 2005;46(1):18–20.
113. Assier H, Bastuji-Garin S, Revuz J, Roujeau JC. Erythema multiforme with mucous membrane involvement and Stevens-Johnson syndrome are clinically different disorders with distinct causes. Arch Dermatol. 1995;131(5):539–43.
114. Bastuji-Garin S, Rzany B, Stern RS, Shear NH, Naldi L, Roujeau JC. Clinical classification of cases of toxic epidermal necrolysis, Stevens-Johnson syndrome, and erythema multiforme. Arch Dermatol. 1993;129(1):92–6.
115. Brown RS. Oral erythema multiforme: trends and clinical findings of a large retrospective: European case series. Oral Surg Oral Med Oral Pathol Oral Radiol. 2016;121(6):681.
116. Canavan TN, Mathes EF, Frieden I, Shinkai K. Mycoplasma pneumoniae-induced rash and mucositis as a syndrome distinct from Stevens-Johnson syndrome and erythema multiforme: a systematic review. J Am Acad Dermatol. 2015;72(2):239–45.
117. Celentano A, Tovaru S, Yap T, Adamo D, Aria M, Mignogna MD. Oral erythema multiforme: trends and clinical findings of a large retrospective European case series. Oral Surg Oral Med Oral Pathol Oral Radiol. 2015;120(6):707–16.
118. Joseph RH, Haddad FA, Matthews AL, Maroufi A, Monroe B, Reynolds M. Erythema multiforme after orf virus infection: a report of two cases and literature review. Epidemiol Infect. 2015;143(2):385–90.
119. Joseph TI, Vargheese G, George D, Sathyan P. Drug induced oral erythema multiforme: a rare and less recognized variant of erythema multiforme. J Oral Maxillofac Pathol. 2012;16(1):145–8.
120. Kishore BN, Ankadavar NS, Kamath GH, Martis J. Varicella zoster with erythema multiforme in a young girl: a rare association. Indian J Dermatol. 2014;59(3):299–301.
121. Patil B, Hegde S, Naik S, Sharma R. Oral blistering – report of two cases of erythema multiforme & literature review. J Clin Diagn Res. 2013;7(9):2080–3.
122. Rogers RS 3rd. Pseudo-Behcet's disease. Dermatol Clin. 2003;21(1):49–61.
123. Samim F, Auluck A, Zed C, Williams PM. Erythema multiforme: a review of epidemiology, pathogenesis, clinical features, and treatment. Dent Clin N Am. 2013;57(4):583–96.
124. Schwartz RA, McDonough PH, Lee BW. Toxic epidermal necrolysis: part I. Introduction, history, classification, clinical features, systemic manifestations, etiology, and immunopathogenesis. J Am Acad Dermatol. 2013;69(2):173 e1–13.. quiz 185–6
125. Mittmann N, Knowles SR, Koo M, Shear NH, Rachlis A, Rourke SB. Incidence of toxic epidermal necrolysis and Stevens-Johnson Syndrome in an HIV cohort: an observational, retrospective case series study. Am J Clin Dermatol. 2012;13(1):49–54.
126. Bastuji-Garin S, Fouchard N, Bertocchi M, Roujeau JC, Revuz J, Wolkenstein P. SCORTEN: a severity-of-illness score for toxic epidermal necrolysis. J Invest Dermatol. 2000;115(2):149–53.

127. Lu N, Rai SK, Terkeltaub R, Kim SC, Menendez ME, Choi HK. Racial disparities in the risk of Stevens-Johnson syndrome and toxic epidermal necrolysis as urate-lowering drug adverse events in the United States. Semin Arthritis Rheum. 2016;46(2):253–8.
128. Miliszewski MA, Kirchhof MG, Sikora S, Papp A, Dutz JP. Stevens-Johnson syndrome and toxic epidermal necrolysis: an analysis of triggers and implications for improving prevention. Am J Med. 2016;129(11):1221–5.
129. Schwartz RA, McDonough PH, Lee BW. Toxic epidermal necrolysis: part II. Prognosis, sequelae, diagnosis, differential diagnosis, prevention, and treatment. J Am Acad Dermatol. 2013;69(2):187 e1–16.. quiz 203–4
130. Stern RS. Recurrence of Stevens-Johnson syndrome and toxic epidermal necrolysis. JAMA. 2014;312(15):1590–1.
131. Salmi TT, Hervonen K, Kautiainen H, Collin P, Reunala T. Prevalence and incidence of dermatitis herpetiformis: a 40-year prospective study from Finland. Br J Dermatol. 2011;165(2):354–9.
132. Bolotin D, Petronic-Rosic V. Dermatitis herpetiformis. Part I. Epidemiology, pathogenesis, and clinical presentation. J Am Acad Dermatol. 2011;64(6):1017–24; quiz 1025–6
133. Smith JB, Tulloch JE, Meyer LJ, Zone JJ. The incidence and prevalence of dermatitis herpetiformis in Utah. Arch Dermatol. 1992;128(12):1608–10.
134. Karpati S. Dermatitis herpetiformis: close to unravelling a disease. J Dermatol Sci. 2004;34(2):83–90.
135. Bolotin D, Petronic-Rosic V. Dermatitis herpetiformis. Part II. Diagnosis, management, and prognosis. J Am Acad Dermatol. 2011;64(6):1027–33; quiz 1033–4
136. Peters MS, McEvoy MT. IgA antiendomysial antibodies in dermatitis herpetiformis. J Am Acad Dermatol. 1989;21(6):1225–31.
137. Dieterich W, Laag E, Bruckner-Tuderman L, Reunala T, Kárpáti S, Zágoni T, et al. Antibodies to tissue transglutaminase as serologic markers in patients with dermatitis herpetiformis. J Invest Dermatol. 1999;113(1):133–6.
138. Griffiths CE, Leonard JN, Fry L. Dermatitis herpetiformis exacerbated by indomethacin. Br J Dermatol. 1985;112(4):443–5.
139. Bardella MT, Fredella C, Saladino V, Trovato C, Cesana BM, Quatrini M, et al. Gluten intolerance: gender- and age-related differences in symptoms. Scand J Gastroenterol. 2005;40(1):15–9.
140. Economopoulou P, Laskaris G. Dermatitis herpetiformis: oral lesions as an early manifestation. Oral Surg Oral Med Oral Pathol. 1986;62(1):77–80.
141. Fraser NG, Kerr NW, Donald D. Oral lesions in dermatitis herpetiformis. Br J Dermatol. 1973;89(5):439–50.
142. Sansaricqa FC, Petronic-Rosic V. Dermatitis herpetiformis: what practitioners need to know. Pract Gastr. 2012;111:39–44.
143. Hietanen J, Reunala T. IgA deposits in the oral mucosa of patients with dermatitis herpetiformis and linear IgA disease. Scand J Dent Res. 1984;92(3):230–4.
144. Katz SI. Dermatitis herpetiformis. Clinical, histologic, therapeutic and laboratory clues. Int J Dermatol. 1978;17(7):529–35.
145. Nicolas ME, Krause PK, Gibson LE, Murray JA. Dermatitis herpetiformis. Int J Dermatol. 2003;42(8):588–600.
146. Nisengard RJ, Chorzelski T, Maciejowska E, Kryst L. Dermatitis herpetiformis: IgA deposits in gingiva, buccal mucosa, and skin. Oral Surg Oral Med Oral Pathol. 1982;54(1):22–5.
147. Sawant P, Kshar A, Byakodi R, Paranjpe A. Immunofluorescence in oral mucosal diseases –a review. Oral Surg Oral Med Oral Radiol. 2014;2(1):5.
148. Chan LS, Regezi JA, Cooper KD. Oral manifestations of linear IgA disease. J Am Acad Dermatol. 1990;22(2 Pt 2):362–5.
149. Kelly SE, Frith PA, Millard PR, Wojnarowska F, Black MM. A clinicopathological study of mucosal involvement in linear IgA disease. Br J Dermatol. 1988;119(2):161–70.
150. Leonard JN, Wright P, Williams DM, Gilkes JJ, Haffenden GP, McMinn RM, et al. The relationship between linear IgA disease and benign mucous membrane pemphigoid. Br J Dermatol. 1984;110(3):307–14.
151. Porter SR, Bain SE, Scully CM. Linear IgA disease manifesting as recalcitrant desquamative gingivitis. Oral Surg Oral Med Oral Pathol. 1992;74(2): 179–82.
152. O'Regan E, Bane A, Flint S, Timon C, Toner M. Linear IgA disease presenting as desquamative gingivitis: a pattern poorly recognized in medicine. Arch Otolaryngol Head Neck Surg. 2004;130(4):469–72.
153. Fine JD, Neises GR, Katz SI. Immunofluorescence and immunoelectron microscopic studies in cicatricial pemphigoid. J Invest Dermatol. 1984;82(1): 39–43.
154. Coelho S, Tellechea O, Reis JP, Mariano A, Figueiredo A. Vancomycin-associated linear IgA bullous dermatosis mimicking toxic epidermal necrolysis. Int J Dermatol. 2006;45(8):995–6.
155. Cohen DM, Bhattacharyya I, Zunt SL, Tomich CE. Linear IgA disease histopathologically and clinically masquerading as lichen planus. Oral Surg Oral Med Oral Pathol Oral Radiol Endod. 1999;88(2):196–201.
156. Green ST, Natarajan S. Linear IgA disease and oesophageal carcinoma. J R Soc Med. 1987;80(1): 48–9.
157. Marinkovich MP, Taylor TB, Keene DR, Burgeson RE, Zone JJ. LAD-1, the linear IgA bullous dermatosis autoantigen, is a novel 120-kDa anchoring filament protein synthesized by epidermal cells. J Invest Dermatol. 1996;106(4):734–8.

158. McEvoy MT, Connolly SM. Linear IgA dermatosis: association with malignancy. J Am Acad Dermatol. 1990;22(1):59–63.
159. Ongole R, Praveen BN, editors. Textbook of oral medicine, oral diagnosis and oral radiology. 2nd ed. New Delhi: Elsevier India; 2014. p. 924.
160. Sago J, Hall RP. Dapsone. Dermatol Ther. 2002;15:11.
161. Yomada M, Komai A, Hashimato T. Sublamina densa-type linear IgA bullous dermatosis successfully treated with oral tetracycline and niacinamide. Br J Dermatol. 1999;141(3):608–9.
162. Fine JD, Eady RA, Bauer EA, Bauer JW, Bruckner-Tuderman L, Heagerty A, et al. The classification of inherited epidermolysis bullosa (EB): report of the Third International Consensus Meeting on Diagnosis and Classification of EB. J Am Acad Dermatol. 2008;58(6):931–50.
163. Intong LR, Murrell DF. Inherited epidermolysis bullosa: new diagnostic criteria and classification. Clin Dermatol. 2012;30(1):70–7.
164. Youssefian L, Vahidnezhad H, Uitto J. Kindler syndrome. In: Pagon RA, et al., editors. GeneReviews (R). Seattle: University of Washington; 1993.
165. Murauer EM, Koller U, Pellegrini G, De Luca M, Bauer JW. Advances in gene/cell therapy in epidermolysis bullosa. Keio J Med. 2015;64(2):21–5.
166. Osborn MJ, Starker CG, McElroy AN, Webber BR, Riddle MJ, Xia L, et al. TALEN-based gene correction for epidermolysis bullosa. Mol Ther. 2013;21(6):1151–9.
167. Tolar J, McGrath JA, Xia L, Riddle MJ, Lees CJ, Eide C, et al. Patient-specific naturally gene-reverted induced pluripotent stem cells in recessive dystrophic epidermolysis bullosa. J Invest Dermatol. 2014;134(5):1246–54.
168. Aberdam D, Aguzzi A, Baudoin C, Galliano MF, Ortonne JP, Meneguzzi G. Developmental expression of nicein adhesion protein (laminin-5) subunits suggests multiple morphogenic roles. Cell Adhes Commun. 1994;2(2):115–29.
169. Asaka T, Akiyama M, Domon T, Nishie W, Natsuga K, Fujita Y, et al. Type XVII collagen is a key player in tooth enamel formation. Am J Pathol. 2009;174(1):91–100.
170. Kudva P, Jain R. Periodontal manifestation of epidermolysis bullosa: looking through the lens. J Indian Soc Periodontol. 2016;20(1):72–4.
171. Siegel DH, Ashton GH, Penagos HG, Lee JV, Feiler HS, Wilhelmsen KC, et al. Loss of kindlin-1, a human homolog of the *Caenorhabditis elegans* actin-extracellular-matrix linker protein UNC-112, causes Kindler syndrome. Am J Hum Genet. 2003;73(1):174–87.
172. Wright JT. Oral manifestations in the epidermolysis bullosa spectrum. Dermatol Clin. 2010;28(1):159–64.
173. Wright JT, Fine JD, Johnson LB. Oral soft tissues in hereditary epidermolysis bullosa. Oral Surg Oral Med Oral Pathol. 1991;71(4):440–6.
174. Stephenson P, Lamey PJ, Scully C, Prime SS. Angina bullosa haemorrhagica: clinical and laboratory features in 30 patients. Oral Surg Oral Med Oral Pathol. 1987;63(5):560–5.
175. High AS, Main DM. Angina bullosa haemorrhagica: a complication of long-term steroid inhaler use. Br Dent J. 1988;165(5):176–9.
176. Kurban M, Kibbi AG, Ghosn S. Expanding the histologic spectrum of angina bullosa hemorrhagica: report of one case. Am J Dermatopathol. 2007;29(5):477–9.
177. Shashikumar B, Reddy RR, Harish M. Oral hemorrhagic blister: an enigma. Indian J Dermatol. 2013;58(5):407.
178. Shoor H, Mutalik S, Pai KM. Angina bullosa haemorrhagica. BMJ Case Rep. 2013;2013:bcr2013200352.
179. Alikhan A, Felsten LM, Daly M, Petronic-Rosic V. Vitiligo: a comprehensive overview Part I. Introduction, epidemiology, quality of life, diagnosis, differential diagnosis, associations, histopathology, etiology, and work-up. J Am Acad Dermatol. 2011;65(3):473–91.
180. Nagarajan A, Masthan MK, Sankar LS, Narayanasamy AB, Elumalai R. Oral manifestations of vitiligo. Indian J Dermatol. 2015;60(1):103.
181. Lawoyin D, Brown R, Reid E, Sam F, Obayomi T. Concurrent presentation of cutaneous and oral soft tissue vitiligo: a case report and literature review. Int J Dent Sci. 2007;5:5.
182. Dawber RP. Clinical associations of vitiligo. Postgrad Med J. 1970;46(535):276–7.
183. Bordere AC, Lambert J, van Geel N. Current and emerging therapy for the management of vitiligo. Clin Cosmet Investig Dermatol. 2009;2: 15–25.
184. Felsten LM, Alikhan A, Petronic-Rosic V. Vitiligo: a comprehensive overview Part II: treatment options and approach to treatment. J Am Acad Dermatol. 2011;65(3):493–514.
185. Gawkrodger DJ, Ormerod AD, Shaw L, Mauri-Sole I, Whitton ME, Watts MJ, et al. Guideline for the diagnosis and management of vitiligo. Br J Dermatol. 2008;159(5):1051–76.
186. Whitton ME, Ashcroft DM, Gonzalez U. Therapeutic interventions for vitiligo. J Am Acad Dermatol. 2008;59(4):713–7.
187. Al-Otaibi SR, Zadeh VB, Al-Abdulrazzaq AH, Tarrab SM, Al-Owaidi HA, Mahrous R, et al. Using a 308-nm excimer laser to treat vitiligo in Asians. Acta Dermatovenerol Alp Pannonica Adriat. 2009;18(1):13–9.
188. Ashok N, Karunakaran A, Singh P, Rodrigues J, Ashok N, Tarakji B, et al. Gingival vitiligo: report of a case and review of the literature. Case Rep Dent. 2014;2014:874025.
189. Juhlin L, Olsson MJ. Improvement of vitiligo after oral treatment with vitamin B12 and folic acid and the importance of sun exposure. Acta Derm Venereol. 1997;77(6):460–2.

190. Parsad D, Pandhi R, Juneja A. Effectiveness of oral *Ginkgo biloba* in treating limited, slowly spreading vitiligo. Clin Exp Dermatol. 2003;28(3):285–7.
191. Parsad D, Kanwar A. Oral minocycline in the treatment of vitiligo – a preliminary study. Dermatol Ther. 2010;23(3):305–7.
192. Dave S, Thappa DM, Dsouza M. Clinical predictors of outcome in vitiligo. Indian J Dermatol Venereol Leprol. 2002;68(6):323–5.
193. McHepange UO, Gao XH, Liu YY, Liu YB, Ma L, Zhang L, Chen HD. Vitiligo in North-Eastern China: an association between mucosal and acrofacial lesions. Acta Derm Venereol. 2010;90(2):136–40.
194. Powell FC, Dicken CH. Psoriasis and vitiligo. Acta Derm Venereol. 1983;63(3):246–9.

8 Oral Signs of Viral Disease

Danielle N. Brown, Ramya Kollipara, and Stephen Tyring

Herpes Simplex Infections

Viral disease of the soft tissues of the mouth, oral pharynx, and salivary glands is often encountered in practice in both children and adults. The clinical manifestations and implications dramatically vary depending on the specific virus involved (Table 8.1). The prevalence of herpes simplex virus 1 (HSV-1) infection increases with age, with rates as high as 90% in the seventh decade of life. In contrast, since HSV-2 is primarily sexually transmitted, prevalence does not increase linearly with age. In the US, HSV-2 prevalence is estimated to be around 22% for people aged 12–70 years. HSV-2 is much more prevalent in women and among groups who engage in high-risk sexual behavior [1].

The *Herpesviridae* family contains over 80 herpes viruses [2]. HSV-1 and HSV-2 are enveloped, double-stranded DNA viruses [3]. HSV-1 is referred to as causing disease "above the belt," while HSV-2 classically causes disease "below the belt." Primary inoculation with the virus leads to local replication in epithelial cells. Following the primary disease, the virus travels in a retrograde fashion and becomes dormant in sensory ganglia [4]. HSV-1 typically resides in the trigeminal ganglia, and HSV-2 typically resides in the sacral ganglia [2]. Recurrence of disease occurs when the virus travels in an anterograde fashion from the sensory ganglia back to the epithelium and causes an outbreak of grouped vesicles. Any type of physiological stress can lead to reactivation of the virus. HSV-1 is primarily transmitted through oral secretions, and HSV-2 is primarily transmitted through genital secretions [2].

D. N. Brown
Department of Pediatrics, Massachusetts General Hospital for Children, Boston, MA, USA

R. Kollipara (✉)
Dermatology, Cosmetic Laser Dermatology, San Diego, CA, USA
e-mail: rkollipara@clderm.com

S. Tyring
Department of Dermatology, University of Texas Health Sciences Center at Houston, Houston, TX, USA

Primary Acute Herpetic Gingivostomatitis

Primary herpetic gingivostomatitis (PHGS) occurs as a result of initial exposure to the herpes virus. Clinical manifestations can include general malaise, fever, nausea, vomiting, and lymphadenopathy. Following these symptoms, vesiculoulcerative lesions appear on the palate, tongue, lips, gingiva, or buccal mucosa (Fig. 8.1) [4]. The initial lesions rupture and coalesce to form painful round, superficial ulcers. The gingiva will appear edematous and inflamed. PHGS occurs most commonly in young children and young adults [4]. The differential diagnosis for PHGS includes impetigo, hand-foot-mouth disease, herpangina,

N. Fazel (ed.), *Oral Signs of Systemic Disease*, https://doi.org/10.1007/978-3-030-10863-2_8

Table 8.1 The salient features, clinical characteristics, differential diagnoses, and treatments of oral manifestations of viral diseases

	Virus	Oral signs	Other signs and symptoms	Differential diagnosis	Treatment
Primary acute herpetic gingivostomatitis	HSV	Vesiculoulcerative lesions on the palate, tongue, lips, gingiva, buccal mucosa; superficial, painful ulcers; inflamed gingiva	Malaise, fever, nausea, vomiting, lymphadenopathy	Impetigo, HFMD, herpangina, EM, pemphigus vulgaris, acute necrotizing ulcerative gingivitis	Oral antivirals, antipyretics; topical anesthetics
Herpes labialis and recurrent intraoral herpes	HSV	Grouped vesicles that rupture and coalesce to form ulcers	Prodrome of tingling, burning, and pain	Aphthous ulcers, intraoral herpes zoster	Oral or topical antivirals; topical anesthetics
Herpes zoster	VZV	Unilateral painful macular, papular, vesicular; V2: lesions can involve malar region, temporal region, lateral nose, upper lip, upper palate; V3: tongue, buccal mucosa, lower lip, and lower third of the face	Unilateral dermatomal pain	EM, lupus, insect bites, rosacea, linear IgA bullous dermatosis	Oral antivirals, topical or oral anesthetics
Varicella	VZV	Vesicles and ulcers on the tongue, palate, gingiva, buccal mucosa, or oropharynx	Constitutional symptoms, maculopapular then vesicular exanthem ("dew drops on rose petal"	*Staphylococcus aureus* infection, contact dermatitis, insect bite, enterovirus infection	Oral acyclovir
Hand, foot, and mouth disease	Typically, coxsackievirus A16 and enterovirus 71	Vesicles on the palate, tongue, and buccal mucosa that rupture and form shallow ulcers with a pseudomembrane and pink halo	Erythematous macules that form white vesicles on hands, feet, and buttocks	Aphthous ulcers, HSV gingivostomatitis, herpangina, oral varicella	Symptomatic treatment
Herpangina	Coxsackievirus group A serotypes, less commonly coxsackie B, echovirus, and enterovirus	Vesicles on soft palate, tonsillar pillars, uvula, posterior oropharynx, fauces progressing to ulcers with a pseudomembrane and pink halo	Constitutional symptoms, encephalitis, aseptic meningitis	Aphthous ulcers, HSV-1 infection	Supportive care
Molluscum contagiosum	Poxvirus	Pale or erythematous papules on the lips, buccal mucosa, gingiva, palatal mucosa, or retromolar region	Asymptomatic, skin-colored papules with central depression	None reported in literature	Cryotherapy, curettage, cantharidin, podophyllotoxin
Common warts	HPV genotypes 1, 2, 4, and 7	White, firm papules or nodules on the hard palate, vermillion border, gingiva, anterior tongue, or lips	Verrucous papules involving the skin	Squamous cell papillomas or condyloma acuminata	Surgical excision, podophyllin

Condyloma acuminatum	HPV genotypes 6, 11	Pink or white sessile or pendunculated papules or cauliflower-like lesions involving the palate, lips, labial mucosa, or tongue	Lesions similar in morphology involving the genital mucosa	Leukoplakia	Cryosurgery, electrocautery, surgical excision, laser excision
Focal epithelial hyperplasia	HPV genotypes 13, 32	Intraoral papules on the tongue, labial mucosa, buccal mucosa	None	Verruca vulgaris, condyloma acuminata	Surgical excision, cryotherapy, CO2 laser therapy
Infectious mononucleosis	EBV	Pharyngitis, petechial hemorrhages of the soft palate and oropharynx, gray-green or white tonsillar exudates, mucosal edema, lymphoid hyperplasia	Posterior cervical lymphadenopathy, hepatitis, eyelid edema, sore throat, fever, chills, malaise	HIV, CMV infection, toxoplasmosis, streptococcal pharyngitis	Antipyretics
Oral hairy leukoplakia	HIV	Painless, "hairy" gray or white plaque on the tongue, soft palate, oropharynx, buccal mucosa	None	Lichen planus, hyperplastic candidiasis, white sponge nevus	Antiretroviral therapy, high-dose ganciclovir or acyclovir
Aphthous ulcers	HIV	Well-circumscribed ulcerations with central necrosis and erythematous halo; minor aphthous ulcers on floor of mouth, buccal, or labial mucosa; major aphthous ulcers can also involve the gingiva and hard palate	None	CMV infection, HSV, squamous cell carcinoma, fungal, bacterial, or protozoan infection	Topical analgesics, sucrasulfate, potent topical steroids, intralesional or systemic steroids, thalidomide
Immune thrombocytopenic purpura	HIV	Petechiae and bleeding of the gingiva or tongue	Cutaneous petechiae and bleeding	Other platelet deficiency disorders	Antiviral therapy, IVIG, anti-D immunoglobulin, corticosteroids, splenectomy
Salivary gland disease with xerostomia	HIV	Bilateral enlargement of parotid glands, xerostomia	None	Kaposi's sarcoma, lymphoma, Sjögren's disease	Antiretroviral therapy, oral corticosteroids
Kaposi's sarcoma	HHV-8	Non-blanching, deep red to purple, macules, plaques, or exophytic nodules most commonly on dorsal tongue, hard palate, and gingiva	Cutaneous violaceous red-purple patches, plaques, and nodules; dissemination to lymph nodes, GI tract, or lungs	Bacillary angiomatosis, hemangioma, angiosarcoma, pyogenic granuloma, melanoma	Excision, sclerotherapy, intralesional vincristine, radiotherapy, systemic chemotherapy
Cytomeglaovirus	CMV	Painful, punched-out ulcers on the labial mucosa, tongue, buccal mucosa, gingiva, or oropharynx	Retinitis, GI or CNS disease, congenital CMV, hepatomegaly, leukopenia	Aphthous ulcers, neoplasm, protozoan, bacterial, fungal, or viral infection	Oral antivirals

(continued)

Table 8.1 (continued)

	Virus	Oral signs	Other signs and symptoms	Differential diagnosis	Treatment
Rubella	*Rubivirus*	Red macules or petechiae on the soft palate (Forscheimer's spots)	Erythematous maculopapular rash, postauricular, cervical, suboccipital lymphadenopathy, constitutional symptoms	Measles, mononucelosis	Symptomatic therapy
Mumps	*Paramyxoviridae*	Painful unilateral or bilateral parotitis (ear lobe elevation that conceals angle of mandible), edematous and inflamed opening of Stensen's duct, bilateral submandibular or sublingual salivary gland inflammation	Constitutional symptoms, epididymo-orchitis, bilateral orchitis, oophoritis, encephalitis, deafness, pancreatitis	EBV, parainfluenza types 1 and 3, influenza A, coxsackievirus, adenovirus, parvovirus B19, lymphocytic choriomeningitis virus, HIV, drugs, malnutrition	Analgesics, antipyretics, hot or cold compresses
Measles	*Morbillivirus*	Koplik spots (white-gray papules) at the posterior buccal mucosa	Cough, coryza, conjunctivitis, erythematous, maculopapular exanthem	Parovirus B19 infection	Vitamin A

Abbreviations: *HSV* herpes simplex virus, *VZV* varicella zoster virus, *HPV* human papillomavirus, *EBV* Epstein-Barr virus, *HIV* human immunodeficiency virus, *HHV-8* human herpesvirus 8, *CMV* cytomegalovirus, *HFMD* hand, foot, and mouth disease, *EM* erythema multiforme

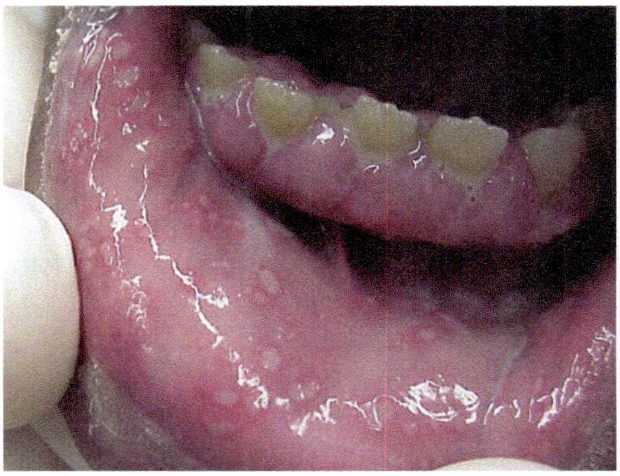

Fig. 8.1 Pediatric patient presenting with multiple round ulcers on the labial mucosa and associated inflammation of the gingiva due to primary acute herpetic gingivostomatitis. (Reprinted from Fatahzadeh [2], with permission from Elsevier)

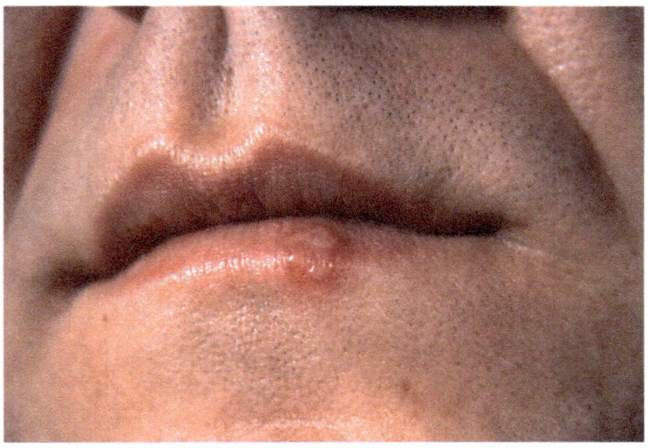

Fig. 8.2 Herpes simplex lesion on the lower lip 2 days after onset. (Courtesy of CDC/Dr. Hermann)

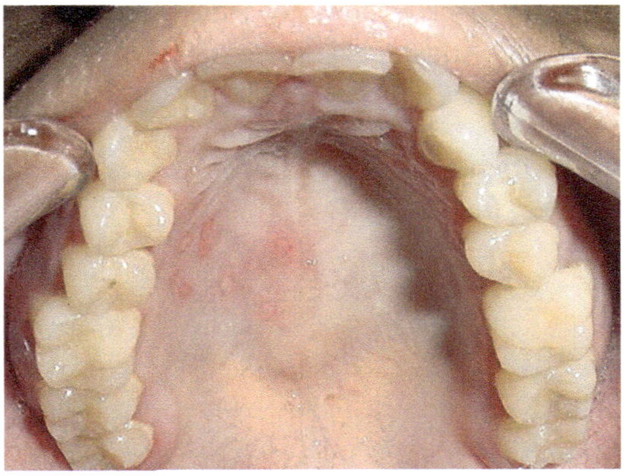

Fig. 8.3 Recurrent intraoral herpes manifesting as a group of small, painful ulcers caused by rupture of transient vesicles on keratinized tissue of right palate. (Reprinted from Fatahzadeh [2], with permission from Elsevier)

erythema multiforme (EM), pemphigus vulgaris, and acute necrotizing ulcerative gingivitis [2].

The diagnosis of PHGS is based on clinical findings. The age of the patient, prodromal symptoms, a history of vesicular lesions, and the presence of multiple painful, round, superficial ulcers help differentiate PHGS from other diagnoses. The "gold standard" of diagnosis is tissue culture and isolation of the HSV virus [5]. Other methods of diagnosis include a cytologic smear (Tzanck smear) of fluid from the vesicle, immunologic assays, or serologic studies. Treatment for PHGS is supportive with antipyretics and topical anesthetics. Oral antiviral medications reduce symptomatology and disease shedding, if initiated within the first 72 h of oral disease manifestation, and can be used for patients with severe symptomatology. Typically, PHGS is self-limited, and patients recover from the primary disease within 14 days [5, 6].

Herpes Labialis and Recurrent Intraoral Herpes

While PHGS is caused by primary infection with HSV-1, reactivation of HSV-1 or HSV-2 latent infection presents as recurrent herpes labialis (RHL), or a cold sore. RHL is preceded by prodromal signs of tingling, burning, and pain at the localized perioral region [7]. Following the prodromal stage, macules appear on the outer vermillion border. These macules become vesicular lesions that coalesce and breakdown to form a painful, crusted lesion (Fig. 8.2) [4]. RHL is diagnosed based on clinical morphology and can be differentiated from aphthous ulcers, which occur on nonkeratinized epithelium [8].

Recurrent intraoral herpes (RIH) is more commonly found in immunosuppressed patients. Rarely, recurrent intraoral herpes can occur in immunocompetent hosts. It is most common unilaterally on the upper hard palate (Fig. 8.3) but can be found on any mucosal surface of the mouth (such as the tongue) [2]. Initially RIH presents as small grouped vesicles, which rupture and coalesce to form superficial ulcers. The differential diagnosis for RIH includes aphthous ulcers and intraoral herpes zoster [2]. Aphthous ulcers do not have a vesicular stage and are most commonly found on nonkeratinized epithelium [8]. To differentiate herpes zoster infection from RIH, immunohistochemical studies, direct immunofluorescence studies, or HSV-1 and HSV-2 PCR analysis must be conducted [2].

Treatment for both RHL and RIH in immunocompetent individuals is largely based on reducing symptomatology through the use of ice or topical anesthetics [6]. Antiviral therapy may reduce viral shedding and the duration of disease [9]. FDA-approved therapies for RHL include topical acyclovir, penciclovir, and docosanol as well as oral acyclovir, famciclovir, and valacyclovir [10].

Herpes Zoster

Herpes zoster, an infection caused by varicella zoster virus (VZV), is commonly referred to as shingles. Prior to the introduction of Zostavax, after 45 years of age, incidence linearly increased to reach a rate of about 10.7 per 1000 in 80-year-old individuals [11]. Zostavax has been FDA approved for individuals over the age of 50 and is currently recommended by the Advisory Committee on Immunization Practices for all individuals over the age of 60. Vaccination has been shown to reduce zoster incidence of disease by over 60% in individuals 65 years or older, bringing the incidence to 5.42 per 1000 [12].

VZV, also classified as human herpes virus 3 (HHV-3), is an enveloped, double-stranded DNA virus. VZV, like HSV1 and HSV2, is an alphaherpesvirus and, thus, initially infects mucoepithelial cells before residing latent in neurons. The virus is responsible for causing chicken pox in primary infection [13]. After primary infection, the virus travels to remain latent in sensory and cranial nerve ganglia. Reactivation of the virus causes herpes zoster infection, a painful rash typically limited to 1–3 dermatomes [14].

Herpes zoster manifests with a 2–3-day prodromal stage of localized tingling and burning pain prior to development of a rash. The rash evolves through the following stages: macular, papular, vesicular, and pustular. The pustules eventually crust over. The rash is located in a unilateral dermatomal distribution. The lesions typically cause intense burning pain but may also cause dysesthesia or itching [15].

Herpes zoster infection of the trigeminal nerve, specifically the maxillary or mandibular branches, occurs in roughly 20% of cases [16]. Patients may initially present with tooth pain or unilateral dermatomal pain. When infection of the left or right maxillary nerve (V2) occurs, lesions may appear unilaterally on the mid-face to include the temporal region, malar region, lateral nose, upper lip, and upper palate [17]. Infection of the mandibular branch of the trigeminal nerve (V3) will result in unilateral lesions on the tongue, buccal mucosa, lower lip, and lower third of the face (Fig. 8.4) [18].

The differential diagnosis for herpes zoster includes EM, lupus, insect bites, rosacea, or linear IgA bullous dermatosis [19]. Biopsy can be performed to differentiate when clinical evaluation is not diagnostic [19]. PCR analysis or direct immunofluorescence studies can be used to differentiate herpes zoster from HSV-1 or -2 infections. Herpes zoster involving the face should be treated with antiviral medications. FDA-approved medications for the treatment of herpes zoster include acyclovir, valacyclovir, and famciclovir

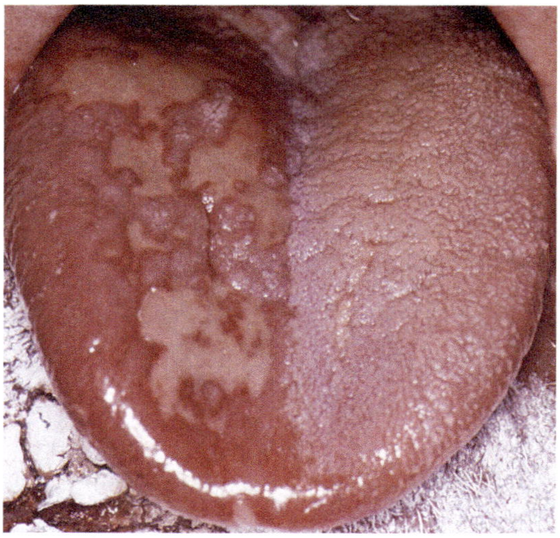

Fig. 8.4 Pathologic changes seen on right unilateral side of elderly male patient's tongue and chin, representing a herpes outbreak due to varicella zoster virus (VZV). (Courtesy of CDC/Robert E. Sumpter)

[15]. Treatment reduces the duration of symptoms and viral shedding [15]. When given in addition to antiviral medications, glucocorticoids may hasten healing [20]. Antivirals plus gabapentin (acutely) reduce the intensity and duration of postherpetic neuralgia [21]. Treatment of acute pain associated with herpes zoster should be based on the severity of symptoms. Pain medications used include NSAIDS, analgesics, gabapentin, lidocaine patches, or tricyclic antidepressants [15].

Varicella (Chicken Pox)

Varicella, or chicken pox, is the primary disease caused by VZV. Prior to universal vaccination, four million cases of chicken pox occurred each year, and it was estimated that 99.5% of the US population over age 20 had VZV antibodies [22, 23]. Greater than 90% of infections with varicella occurred before the age of 15, and the highest incidence was from 3 to 6 years of age [24]. Single-dose administration of the varicella vaccine, beginning in 1995, decreased disease incidence by 80–85% [25]. In 2006, a second dose of the vaccine was recommended, and the two-dose schedule prevents over 98% of disease [26].

HHV-3 or VZV is a double-stranded DNA virus that infects mucoepithelial cells. VZV is transmitted through the inhalation of infected respiratory droplets or through contact with infected lesions [27]. After a 14- to 16-day viral incubation period, patients will present with constitutional symptoms, which include fever, malaise, and abdominal pain. The constitutional symptoms will remain for the primary phase of the chicken pox rash. Within 48 h of the onset of the prodromal symptoms, itchy, erythematous, and maculopapular lesions appear. The rash of primary varicella evolves from maculopapular to vesicular to crusted lesions. The vesicular lesions are described as "dew drops on a rose petal," due to the zone of erythema that surrounds each vesicle. Initially, the rash begins on the face and trunk, but new crops of lesions may subsequently present on the extremities [27].

Varicella may present as oral vesicular lesions on the tongue, palate, gingival, buccal mucosa, or oropharynx (Fig. 8.5) [28]. Oral varicella is not usually painful. These vesicular lesions rupture to form ulcers 2–3 mm in diameter [29]. The prevalence of oral lesions directly correlates with the severity of the varicella infection. Oral lesions have been reported to always be present in severe infection [30].

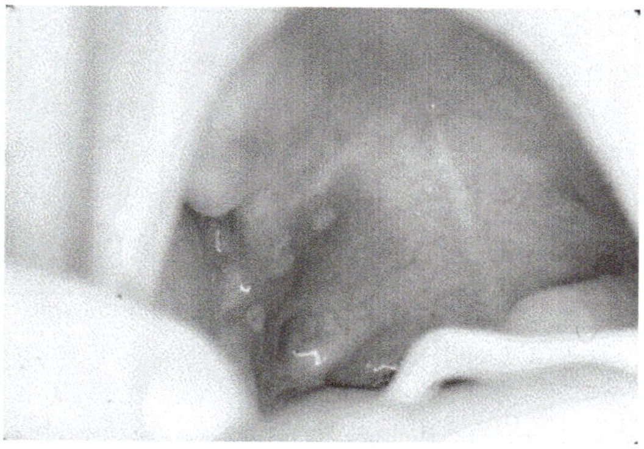

Fig. 8.5 Palatal mucosal lesions of varicella (chicken pox) in a pediatric patient due to primary infection with varicella zoster virus (VZV). (Courtesy of CDC)

Staphylococcus aureus infection, contact dermatitis, insect bite, or enterovirus infection may be confused with primary varicella infection. However, the presence of constitutional symptoms and a history of an infectious contact should aid in diagnosing varicella [27]. Hand, foot, and mouth disease, EM, and pemphigoid are distinguished from oral VZV by serum VZV IgM antibody testing or a Tzanck smear of vesicular fluid [29].

In healthy children under age 12, treatment of varicella can be symptomatic with acetaminophen as an antipyretic and antihistamines for pruritus, but oral acyclovir will result in faster healing of lesions, allowing the child to return to school sooner [31, 32]. For all individuals over 12 years of age or immunocompromised individuals, oral acyclovir is indicated. Acyclovir should be initiated within 24 h of the rash appearing but can be beneficial as late as 72 h [33].

Hand, Foot, and Mouth Disease

Hand, foot, and mouth disease (HFMD) is a common and highly contagious viral disease that occurs around the world. Outbreaks occur in the spring, summer, and fall. Most symptomatic cases are in children under 10 years old but can also occur in older children and in adults exposed to children in child care [34]. Approximately 11% of exposed adults are infected with HFMD, and 1% of these adults are symptomatic [35]. In the last 16 years, there have been several large outbreaks in China and in the United States [34].

HFMD is caused by viruses in the enterovirus genus, typically coxsackievirus A16 and enterovirus 71, and sometimes A5, A6, A7, A9, A10, B2, and B5 [36]. Of note, in recent years, there have been outbreaks of HFMD in adults caused by coxsackievirus A6 (CVA6). Outbreaks have occurred in Europe, Asia, and the United States [35]. HFMD is spread via orofecal and respiratory routes [37]. The incubation period is 3–5 days [34].

HFMD begins with a prodromal phase of fever, malaise, abdominal pain, and myalgia. Oral lesions on the palate, tongue, and buccal mucosa appear at the same time or a short time before cutaneous lesions. Mucosal lesions begin as vesicles that eventually rupture, leading to the development of shallow ulcers (Fig. 8.6). These ulcers have a pseudomembrane and are encircled by an erythematous halo [6]. Cutaneous lesions on the hands, feet, and buttocks present as 3–7 mm erythematous, elliptical macules that rapidly transform into pale, white, oval vesicles. These lesions can be asymptomatic, tender, or painful. The vesicles ulcerate/encrust over 2–3 days and heal without any scarring in 1 week [37]. CVA6 tends to cause more severe disease with widespread vesicubullous eruption, "eczema coxsackium," purpuric lesions, or an eruption similar to Gianotti-Crosti and has a higher incidence of onychomadesis [35].

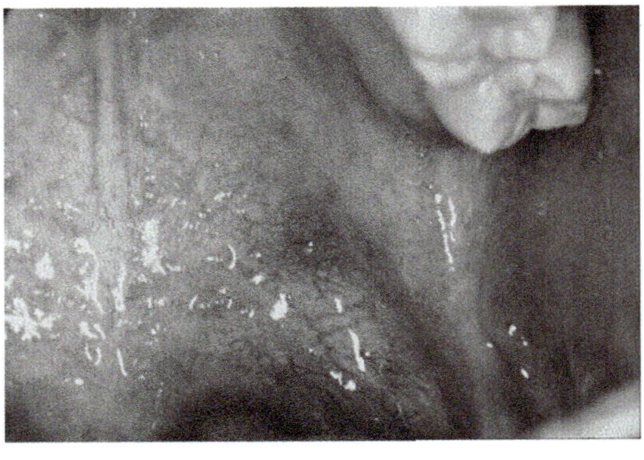

Fig. 8.6 Oropharyngeal ulcers associated with hand, foot, and mouth disease due to infection with coxsackievirus. (Reprinted from Silverman and Miller [124], with permission from Elsevier)

If cutaneous lesions are not present, then the oral HFMD lesions could be mistaken for aphthous ulcers, HSV gingivostomatitis, herpangina, or oral varicella [37]. The diagnosis of HFMD is primarily clinical, but laboratory confirmation can be used in severe or atypical cases. Laboratory testing options include viral culture, PCR analysis to detect viral RNA, and IgM-capture enzyme linked immunosorbent assay (ELISA). Samples can be collected from the serum, stool, throat, or vesicles. HFMD is self-limited and treatment is symptomatic. The CDC recommends frequent handwashing after toileting, disinfecting used surfaces, and avoiding contact with infected utensils to prevent spread of HFMD [34].

Herpangina

Herpangina is a benign viral illness with primarily oral manifestations. It is caused by many of the coxsackievirus group A serotypes (1–6, 8, 10, and 22) and uncommonly by coxsackievirus group B, echovirus, and enterovirus 71 [6, 38]. These viruses are transmitted via contaminated droplets of saliva, but fecal-oral transmission can also occur. After oral infection, the virus multiplies within the cells of the lower gastrointestinal tract and eventually viremia ensues [38]. Herpangina commonly occurs in the summer and fall months [6]. It affects children less than 5 years old and, rarely, adults [38]. Outbreaks have occurred in daycare centers, military communities, schools, and summer camps.

In the prodromal phase of herpangina, patients manifest high fever, malaise, headache, pharyngitis, and dysphagia. Soon after, small vesicles appear on the soft palate, tonsillar pillars, uvula, posterior oropharynx, and fauces and eventually ulcerate (Fig. 8.7). These ulcers are topped by a pseudomembrane and with an erythematous halo. Symptoms resolve in 1 week. Complications of herpangina are rare including encephalitis and aseptic meningitis [6, 38].

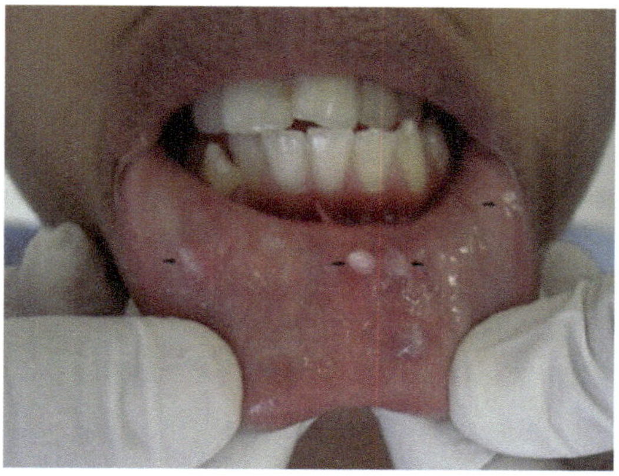

Fig. 8.7 Ulcerative lesions on the soft palate and oral pharynx associated with herpangina. (Reprinted from Lynch [6], with permission from Elsevier)

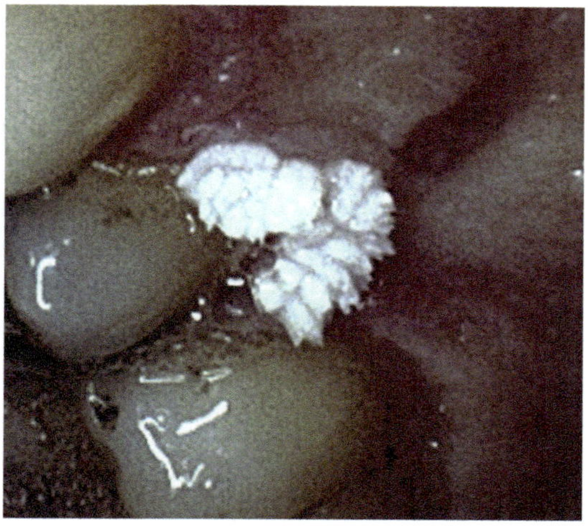

Fig. 8.8 Intraoral appearance of molluscum contagiosum lesions showing flesh-colored exophytic papules on the lower labial mucosa (Reprinted from de Carvalho et al. [39], with permission from Elsevier)

The differential diagnoses for the oral signs of herpangina are recurrent aphthous ulcers and HSV-1 infection. Unlike aphthous ulcers, herpangina has constitutional signs and is localized to the posterior mouth and pharynx. Also, herpangina differs from HSV-1 infection in that it does not affect the gingiva or labial mucosa. Herpangina is a clinical diagnosis. However, serum antibodies and viral cultures of the oral lesions can be performed in atypical cases. Supportive care with mouth rinses and gargles is recommended [6].

Molluscum Contagiosum

Molluscum contagiosum is a prevalent childhood infection and causes 8.6% of skin infections in children less than 16 years old [39]. It can occur in healthy adults as well and is viewed as a sexually transmitted infection, if it presents in the genital region [40]. Risk factors for molluscum contagiosum include inherited immunodeficiency states, HIV infection, and the use of immunosuppressive medications [41]. The role of atopic dermatitis as a predisposing factor is a subject of debate.

Molluscum contagiosum is caused by a poxvirus, which is a double-stranded DNA virus. Although there are four genotypes of poxvirus, 90% of molluscum infections in the United States are caused by genotype 1 [40]. The poxvirus is spread via direct skin-to-skin contact, autoinoculation (scratching or shaving), and fomites (bath sponges and towels) [42]. The poxvirus infects the epidermis, triggers mitosis in the basal cellular layer, and replicates in the spinous and granular epidermal cells. The incubation period lasts from 2 weeks to 3 months [39].

Molluscum contagiosum presents with 2–5 mm, asymptomatic, skin-colored papules with central depressions. Complications include secondary bacterial infection and foreign body reaction. Oral mucosal involvement is very rare. In the few cases reported, pale or erythematous papules presented on the lips, buccal mucosa, gingiva, palatal mucosa, or retromolar region (Fig. 8.8) [39]. Given the rarity of oral molluscum contagiosum, a differential diagnosis or treatment plan is not reported in the literature. Cutaneous molluscum contagiosum is diagnosed clinically or via biopsy. It is often treated with cryotherapy, curettage, cantharidin, or podophyllotoxin.

Human Papillomavirus

The human papillomavirus (HPV) infects the oropharynx and genital tract. The prevalence of oral infection in American males and females is estimated to be 4.5%, while cervical infection in American females is estimated to range from 27% to 43% [43, 44].

HPV is a non-enveloped, double-stranded DNA virus in the *Papillomaviridae* family. The alpha genus of HPV preferentially infects the mucosa, while the beta genus preferentially infects the skin [45]. There are over 40 genotypes of HPV that infect human epithelial cells. These genotypes are further classified as high risk, if infection leads to high-grade dysplasia and carcinoma, or low risk, if infection leads to low-grade or no dysplasia [46]. Genotypes 16 and 18 are the most prevalent high-risk genotypes, while genotypes 6 and 11 are the most prevalent low-risk genotypes [45]. Direct contact with HPV-infected lesions allows for transmission of the virus, which infects and replicates in the basal epithelial cells [46]. Oral manifestations of HPV include common warts, condyloma acuminata, focal epithelial hyperplasia, and oral carcinomas, e.g., tonsils and larynx.

Common Warts

While verruca vulgaris, or common warts, are most commonly found on the extremities, they can rarely be found in the oral cavity. Common warts are caused by infection with HPV genotypes 1, 2, 4, and 7, all of which are in the β-HPV genus [45]. Oral warts are most commonly found in children. Infection of the oral cavity typically occurs via autoinoculation of the virus from the hands. Intraoral common warts may be found on keratinized squamous epithelium such as the hard palate, vermillion border, gingiva, anterior tongue, or lips (Fig. 8.9) [47]. Oral common warts range in size from 0.5 to 1.0 cm. They are white, firm, and well circumscribed. Their morphology is that of nodules or papules, and they may appear in isolation or in groups [46, 48]. Oral warts are painless. A diagnostic clue for oral verruca vulgaris may be that the patient has these lesions located on other areas of the body, such as the hands. Oral common warts may be confused with squamous cell papillomas or condyloma acuminata. The diagnosis can be made histologically or by genotyping the HPV virus [47]. Recommended treatment is surgical excision of the warts, and the lesions can be pretreated with podophyllin prior to excision [48].

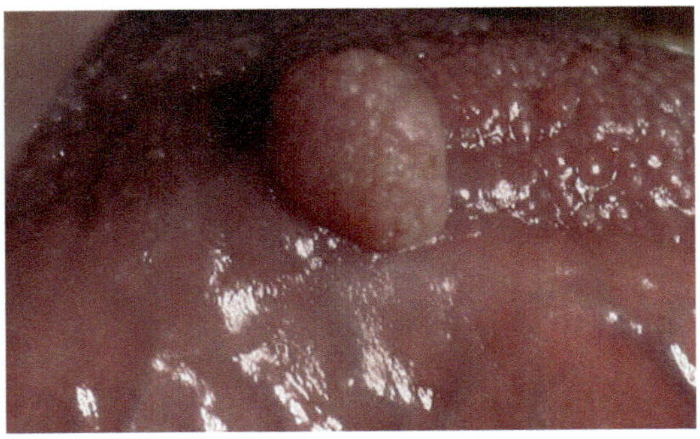

Fig. 8.9 Oral verruca vulgaris on the palatal gingiva presenting as well-circumscribed, white, highly keratinized lesions. (Reprinted from Pringle [46], with permission from Elsevier and Thomas Daley, DDS, MSc, London, Ontario, Canada)

Condyloma Acuminatum

Condyloma acuminata, or venereal warts, are spread through sexual transmission. These lesions are caused by infection with alpha-HPV, primarily genotypes 6 and 11 [45]. Rarely, they may be caused by infection with high-risk HPV genotypes 16 and 18 [46]. Over 75% of condyloma acuminata cases occur in patients who are HIV-positive [49]. While these lesions are most commonly found on genital mucosal surfaces, they can also be found in the oral cavity. In the oral cavity, condyloma acuminata appear as pink or white lesions. Their morphology is sessile or pedunculated, and they may coalesce to form a cauliflower-like mass (Fig. 8.10) [46, 50]. Oral venereal warts grow slowly and range in size from 0.5 to 3 cm [28]. Condyloma acuminata occur orally on the palate, lips, labial mucosa, and the dorsal or ventral surfaces of the tongue [49]. When oral condyloma acuminata are diagnosed in childhood, sexual abuse should be suspected, and a full risk assessment and exam should be conducted. Oral condyloma acuminata may be confused with leukoplakia, and a punch biopsy can differentiate between the two

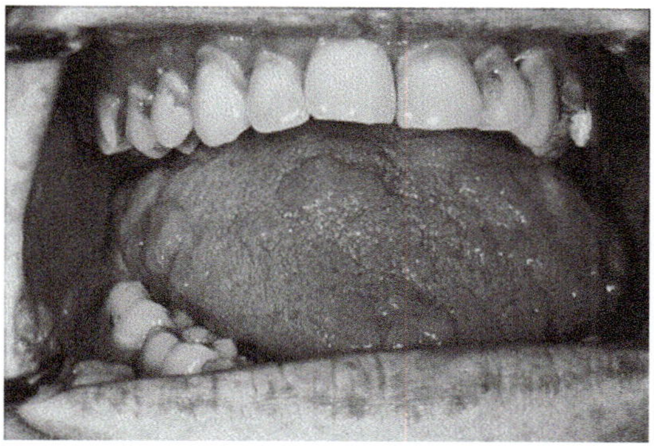

Fig. 8.10 Condyloma acuminata found on the lateral border of the tongue. (Reprinted from Pringle [46], with permission from Elsevier and Thomas Daley, DDS, MSc, London, Ontario, Canada)

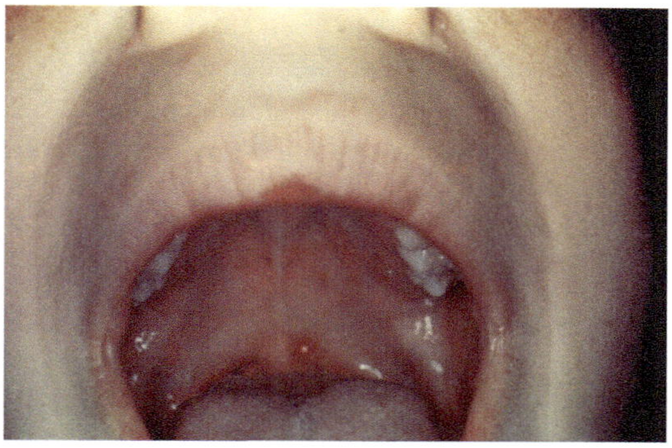

Fig. 8.11 Focal epithelial hyperplasia (Heck's disease) manifesting as multiple mucosal-colored papules on the tongue. (Reprinted from Lynch [6], with permission from Elsevier)

diagnoses [50]. The development of squamous cell carcinoma has been associated with condyloma acuminata when the lesions contain high-risk HPV genotypes. Oral condyloma acuminata should be removed via cryosurgery, electrocautery, surgical excision, or laser excision [49]. Patients must be monitored for recurrence [50].

Focal Epithelial Hyperplasia (Heck's Disease)

Focal epithelial hyperplasia (FEH), or Heck's disease, is caused by infection with members of the alpha-HPV genus, specifically genotypes 13 and 32 [45]. Transmission of the virus is most likely via direct contact with the oral mucosa [51]. It is most prevalent in the Native American, Mexican, and Eskimo populations, specifically in children with the HLA-DR4 allele [52]. FEH is found in children and young adults and is more prevalent in females than males [53]. While other disease manifestations of HPV can be found on numerous epithelial surfaces, FEH is specific to the oral cavity and is asymptomatic. The disease manifests as intraoral papules that give the mucosa a cobblestoned appearance (Fig. 8.11) [46]. Each individual lesion varies in diameter from 0.3 to 1 cm; however, FEH typically manifests as multiple, grouped lesions of varying size [28]. The papules are similar in color to that of the oral mucosa. FEH is found on the tongue, labial mucosa, and buccal mucosa [46, 47].

The differential diagnosis for FEH includes both verruca vulgaris and condyloma acuminata. The clinician should screen for HPV 6 and 11 via an in vitro nucleic acid hybridization assay to rule out condyloma acuminata. Condyloma acuminata, if diagnosed in childhood, should raise suspicion for sexual abuse [54]. In children, a full physical exam should be conducted to look for signs of sexual abuse. If the exam does not reveal signs of sexual abuse or infection with sexually transmitted HPV genotypes, and the child's ethnicity is one known to have a high prevalence of the disease, then the diagnosis of FEH can be made [54]. Lesions will naturally regress in an average of 18 months, and, typically, treatment is unnecessary [54]. The lesions may be removed through surgical excision, cryotherapy, or CO2 laser therapy. Additionally, there are reports in the literature of the use of topical interferon, imiquimod, electrocoagulation, and electrodessication for the treatment of FEH [51].

Epstein Barr Virus (Infectious Mononucleosis)

Ninety-five percent of adults worldwide are seropositive for Epstein-Barr virus (EBV), the etiologic agent of infectious mononucleosis. In developed countries, half of the population is infected between ages 1 and 5 years. Another large portion of the population acquires EBV in the second decade of life. In third world countries and lower socioeconomic groups, EBV is acquired during early childhood [55]. Annually, there are 500 cases of infectious mononucleosis per 100,000 persons in the United States, and the group with the highest incidence rate is individuals aged 15–24 years. Infectious mononucleosis manifests in 30–50% of people exposed to EBV [56]. When infected with EBV, young children are typically asymptomatic, and adults typically exhibit the disease manifestations of infectious mononucleosis [57].

EBV is a double-stranded DNA virus and part of the *Herpesviridae* family. Infectious mononucleosis is acquired via transfer of EBV-infected saliva, typically through kissing and uncommonly through sexual transmission [58]. Once EBV is transferred into the mouth, it replicates in the oropharyngeal secretions and infects B lymphocytes in the lymphoid-rich areas of the mouth. B lymphocyte infection leads to EBV spread into the lymphoid tissue triggering CD4+ and CD8+ T lymphocyte responses, which contribute to infectious mononucleosis symptoms [59]. These replicating CD8+ cells are atypical and are called Downey cells [57]. Viral salivary shedding decreases over the 1st year but persists throughout life. The incubation period is 30–50 days [55].

Clinically, infectious mononucleosis presents with malaise, fever, chills, sore throat, posterior cervical lymphadenopathy, hepatitis, and fatigue. Some patients also experience eyelid edema, myalgias, and sore throat. Symptoms last 16 days on average and recovery might take months [57]. Oral manifestations of infectious mononucleosis are pharyngitis and petechial hemorrhages of the soft palate and oropharynx (Fig. 8.12). Gray-green or white tonsillar exudates can also occur [6]. A rare oral complication of infectious mononucleosis is upper airway obstruction due to lymphoid hyperplasia and mucosal edema [60].

The differential diagnoses for the malaise, lymphadenopathy, and pharyngitis associated with infectious mononucleosis are HIV infection, cytomegalovirus (CMV) infection, toxoplasmosis, and streptococcal pharyngitis [55]. Diagnostic testing is required to differentiate infectious mononucleosis from these clinical entities. The presence of the classical symptoms and signs in the setting of atypical lymphocytosis points to infectious mononucleosis. Laboratory testing includes the rapid monospot test and EBV-specific antibodies. The rapid monospot test detects heterophile antibodies or IgM antibodies against viral antigens that also react to antigens on horse or sheep erythrocytes [61]. Infectious mononucleosis requires only symptomatic treatment (antipyretics), and oral symptoms eventually regress.

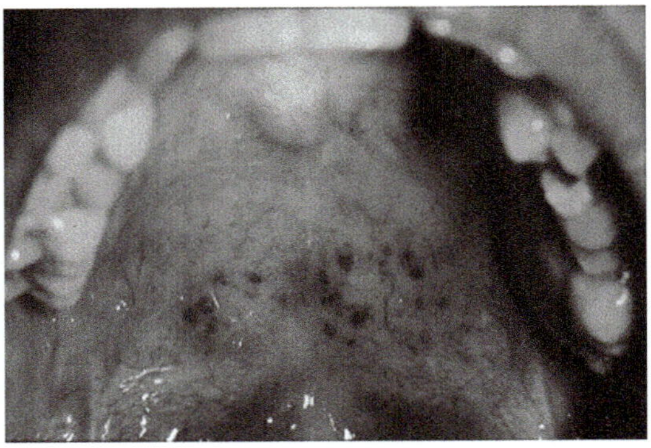

Fig. 8.12 Petechiae on the soft palate and oral pharynx due to infectious mononucleosis caused by Epstein-Barr virus (Reprinted from Lynch [6], with permission from Elsevier)

HIV Disease

Worldwide, 35 million people are infected with human immunodeficiency virus (HIV). This number includes 24.7 million individuals in sub-Saharan Africa and over 1 million individuals in the United States [62, 63]. HIV can be transmitted through blood, sexual fluids, or breast milk. It can be transmitted vertically from mother to child during childbirth. HIV mainly infects CD4+ T cells, and without treatment, CD4 + T cells are progressively destroyed [64]. To diagnose HIV, a fourth-generation antigen/antibody immunoassay should be ordered, and if positive, it must be followed with a HIV-1/HIV-2 antibody test. If this second immunoassay is not definitive, an HIV-1 nucleic acid test can be conducted [65].

It is recommended that all HIV-positive individuals receive antiretroviral therapy (ART) to prevent transmission and progression of the disease. Oral manifestations of HIV disease include oral hairy leukoplakia, aphthous ulcers, immune thrombocytopenic purpura, salivary gland disease, and Kaposi's sarcoma.

Oral Hairy Leukoplakia

Oral hairy leukoplakia (OHL), found in up to 43% of HIV-positive adults, is considered to be strongly associated with HIV infection [66, 67]. Within 5 years of HIV diagnosis, 42% of individuals develop OHL. Mean CD4+ cell count in individuals with OHL is 468 cells/μL [68]. It is an indicator of a high degree of immune suppression. OHL presents as intraoral gray or white plaques that cannot be removed with scraping (Fig. 8.13). The plaques of OHL have a grooved and "hairy" appearance and can be large as to cover the entire surface of the tongue [69]. While OHL is most commonly painless, it may present with burning or discomfort [70]. OHL is usually found on the lateral, ventral, or dorsal surface of the tongue but may rarely present on the soft palate, oropharynx, buccal mucosa, or ventral tongue [70]. It is caused by infection of epithelial cells with EBV [71]. The differential diagnosis for OHL includes lichen planus, hyperplastic candidiasis, and white sponge nevus. OHL is typically a clinical diagnosis; however, definitive diagnostic methods include exfoliative cytology via scraping or biopsy of the lesion. Following obtainment of tissue, EBV is detected from cells through PCR, immunohistochemistry, or in situ hybridization [72]. OHL is a chronic condition in which the plaques heal and reappear over time. Treatment is unnecessary; however, the plaques may regress with initiation of ART or with high-dose acyclovir or ganciclovir [73].

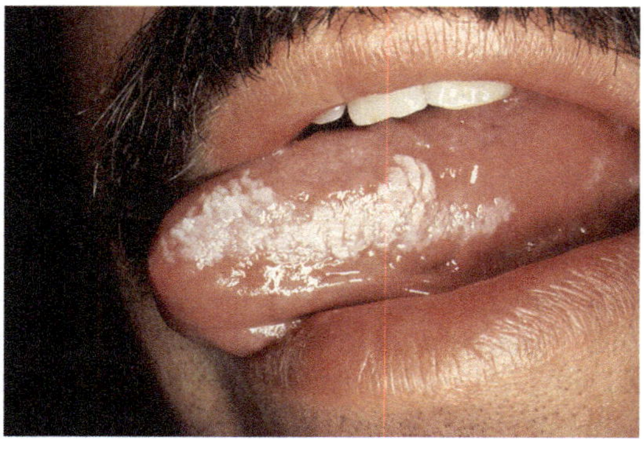

Fig. 8.13 Advanced oral hairy leukoplakia on the lateral border of the tongue in an HIV-positive patient. (Courtesy of CDC/J.S. Greenspan, B.D.S., University of California, San Francisco; Sol Silverman, Jr., D.D.S.)

Aphthous Ulcers

Severe aphthous ulcers are found in up to 7% of children and 3.1% of adults with HIV [69, 74]. Major aphthous ulcer development correlates with a severe degree of immunosuppression in HIV-positive individuals. In contrast to minor aphthous ulcers, major aphthous ulcers are usually multiple and measure greater than 1 cm in diameter (Fig. 8.14) [75]. They are well-circumscribed ulcerations with a surrounding halo of erythema and a necrotic central focus [76]. While minor aphthous ulcers most commonly present on the nonkeratinized mucosa of the oral cavity, such as the floor of the mouth and buccal and labial mucosa, major aphthous ulcers can also present on keratinized epithelium of the oral cavity, such as the gingiva and hard palate [76]. Therefore, in HIV-positive populations, major aphthous ulcers may present on any oral surface [74]. Major aphthous ulcers are extremely

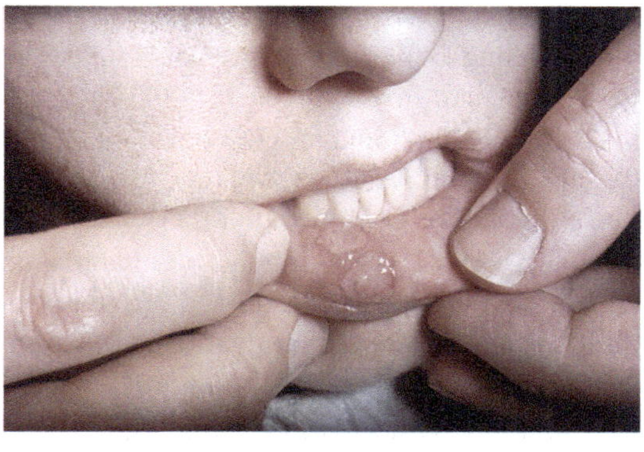

Fig. 8.14 Depiction of a mucosal ulceration, diagnosed as a major aphthous ulcer, on the lower lip of a female patient. (Courtesy of CDC/Robert E. Sumpter)

painful lesions that may be present for months. The differential diagnosis for aphthous ulcers in the immunocompromised population includes CMV infection, HSV infection, squamous cell carcinoma, fungal infections, bacterial infections, or protozoan infections [77]. In contrast to major aphthous ulcers, ulcers secondary to HSV typically present as clustered lesions on nonkeratinized epithelium and are associated with prodromal burning and pain. When an HIV-positive patient presents with a non-healing ulcer that has been present for 7–14 days duration, a biopsy should be performed for definitive diagnosis [76]. Treatment of aphthous ulcers involves reduction of symptoms and therapy to improve healing. Topical analgesic therapy with lidocaine should be used to relieve the pain associated with major aphthous ulcers. Sucralfate may also be used as a topical layer of protection over the ulcer. Potent topical corticosteroids are used to hasten healing. If topical steroid therapy is ineffective and the lesion has been identified as a recurrent major aphthous ulcer via biopsy, therapy with intralesional or systemic steroids may be considered. The next line of therapy is thalidomide [76]. Treatment is desired in most patients to avoid complications such as weight loss secondary to difficulty with oral intake as a result of the associated pain. Residual mucosal scarring may occur after ulcers heal.

Immune Thrombocytopenic Purpura

Immune thrombocytopenic purpura (ITP) is a diagnosis of exclusion. It is defined by bleeding in the presence of isolated thrombocytopenia [78]. In HIV, thrombocytopenia can occur through both destruction and reduced production of platelets. In HIV-related ITP, antibodies against HIV GP160/120 cross-react to bind with GPIIb/IIIa on platelets, leading to autoimmune destruction of platelets through molecular mimicry [79]. Additionally, HIV may infect megakaryocytes and lead to decreased platelet production [80]. In a 2012 study analyzing the incidence of severe ITP in HIV-positive patients, it was found that 0.6% of these patients had HIV-related ITP, and two-thirds of these cases occurred in individuals with CD4+ cell counts greater than 200 cells/μl. However, thrombocytopenia, defined as less than 100,000 platelets/μL, was present in 26% of this population [81]. Mild manifestations of ITP include easy bruising or petechiae on the skin. Severe ITP presents clinically with oral mucocutaneous bleeding, once platelet levels drop below 10,000 cells/μl. Petechiae and bleeding commonly involve the gingiva or tongue (Fig. 8.15). Antiviral therapy is the primary treatment for HIV-related ITP. Treatments such as IVIG, anti-D immunoglobulin, or corticosteroids may be used in patients with significant bleeding. If treatment is unsuccessful, splenectomy can be performed [78].

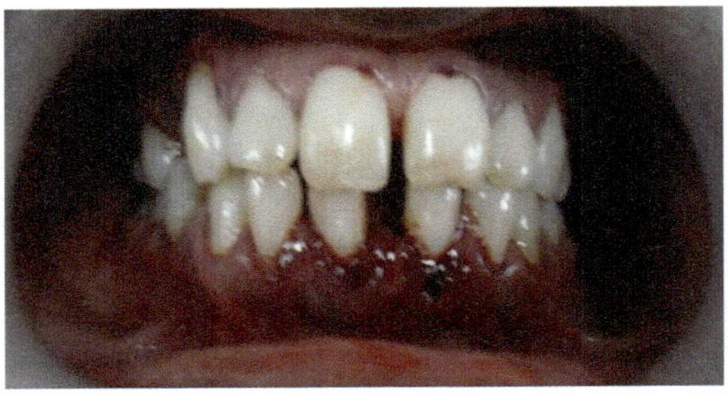

Fig. 8.15 Inflamed, bleeding gingiva secondary to immune thrombocytopenic purpura. (Reprinted from Kayal et al. [125])

Salivary Gland Disease with Xerostomia

HIV-associated salivary gland disease presents as diffuse enlargement of the salivary glands and can occur with xerostomia, or decreased saliva production [82]. It is present in up to 50% of HIV-positive children [66]. Salivary gland disease, secondary to diffuse infiltrative lymphocytosis syndrome (DILS), occurs in HIV when CD8+ T cells infiltrate the parotid gland. Over time, the gland is destroyed leading to xerostomia [69] and the development of cystic lesions. HIV-associated salivary gland disease presents as bilateral enlargement of the parotid glands (Fig. 8.16), with or without symptoms of

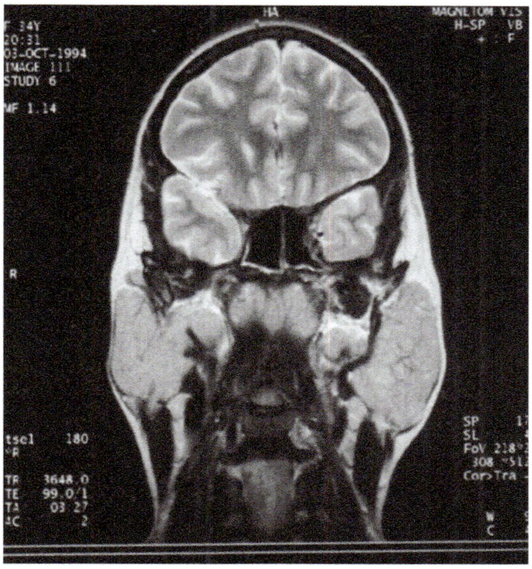

Fig. 8.16 MRI showing parotid gland enlargement secondary to HIV-associated salivary gland disease. (Reproduced from Chapple and Hamburger [82], with permission from BMJ Publishing Group Ltd)

decreased salivary production. The differential diagnosis for parotid gland enlargement includes Kaposi's sarcoma (KS), lymphoma, and Sjögren's disease. Imaging and biopsy are required to accurately diagnose salivary gland disease with xerostomia [82]. Antiretroviral therapy or oral corticosteroids are primary treatments for DILS [83]. Patients should be monitored for the development of dental caries secondary to xerostomia.

Kaposi's Sarcoma

KS is strongly associated with HIV infection and is the most prevalent neoplasm in this patient population [67, 84]. In a 2012 study of HIV-positive individuals in South Africa, the incidence of KS was 1.682% for individuals not on antiretroviral therapy and 0.138% for individuals on antiretroviral medication [85]. Previous studies have reported KS incidence rates up to 38% in HIV-positive individuals [66]. KS risk factors include male gender and CD4+ cell count less than 350 cells/μl [85]. Incidence is highest in individuals aged 20–40 years [86].

KS is caused by infection with human herpes virus 8 (HHV-8), a herpes gamma virus. Transmission can occur sexually or nonsexually, as the virus can be transmitted through genital and oral secretions [87, 88]. After infection, HHV-8, like all herpes viruses, remains latent in the body [86].

KS is a multicentric cancer of endothelial cells that presents as numerous lesions on the skin, viscera, and mucocutaneous surfaces. Skin lesions arise as variably sized violaceous red-purple patches before evolving into plaques and then nodules [86]. Other variations of KS include ecchymotic, keloidal, telangiectatic, and lymphadenopathic subtypes [86]. In AIDS, the nodules of KS first appear on the upper body before disseminating widely on the skin and then spreading to the viscera [89]. The most commonly infected viscera are lymph nodes, gastrointestinal organs, and the lungs [90]. Mortality associated with KS in this population is due to visceral involvement.

Oral KS is a World Health Organization (WHO) clinical stage IV disease of HIV/AIDS [91]. In 22% of patients with HIV-associated KS, the first lesions appear in the oral cavity [92]. KS manifests orally as non-blanching macules or nodules. Oral lesions evolve from patches to plaques to exophytic nodules. If the lesions progress to erythematous, exophytic nodules, they are frequently painful. Oral KS lesions are quite diverse ranging in color from deep red to purple, in number from singular to multiple, and in size from millimeters to centimeters [93]. KS can present anywhere within the oral cavity; however, these red-purple lesions are most commonly found on the dorsal tongue, hard palate, and gingiva (Fig. 8.17) [94]. Complications of oral KS include periodontal disease, bone resorption, and the inability to masticate leading to malnutrition and significant weight loss [94]. KS can be differentiated from bacillary angiomatosis, hemangioma, angiosarcoma, pyogenic granuloma, or melanoma via histopathology [89].

Treatment of KS is based on the stage, rate of progression of the disease, and the presence of visceral involvement. A workup for patients with KS includes HIV serology, a full physical exam (including an oral and rectal exam), imaging, and

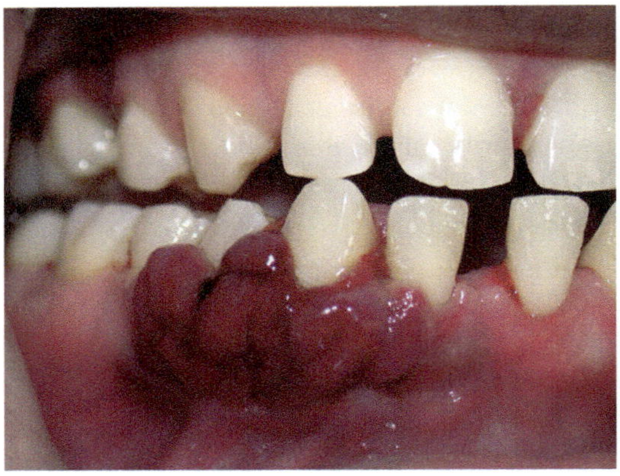

Fig. 8.17 Kaposi's sarcoma manifesting as a lobulated and nodular purple mass on the gingiva. (Reprinted from Restrepo and Ocazionez [126], with permission from Elsevier)

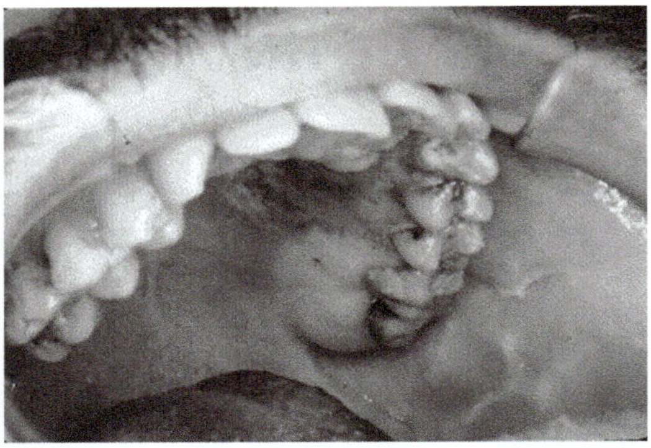

Fig. 8.18 Painful palatal ulceration of 1-month duration in an HIV-positive patient. Biopsy showed lesion to be CMV-induced, and it responded to high-dose antiviral medications. (Reprinted from Silverman and Miller [124], with permission from Elsevier)

subsequent studies such as bronchoscopy or chest CT based on the patient's symptoms. KS is not curable but may regress with HAART treatment [95]. Intraoral lesions may be treated via excision, sclerotherapy, intralesional vincristine, or radiotherapy [94]. Systemic chemotherapy with interferon, sirolimus, or liposomal anthracyclines has been FDA approved for the treatment of KS and is reserved for severe, progressive disease and cases with symptomatic involvement of the viscera or lungs [95].

Cytomegalovirus

The prevalence of CMV ranges from 50% to 100% in the general population [96]. In immunocompetent individuals, the majority of these infections are asymptomatic; however, in neonates and the immunosuppressed, CMV infection causes significant morbidity and mortality [96]. CMV is the leading infectious cause of congenital abnormalities and of nongenetic deafness. Congenital infection with CMV may lead to mortality or severe neurologic impairment [97].

CMV is a member of the *Herpesviridae* family. Viral transmission can occur through blood, genital fluid, breast milk, or saliva [98]. After primary infection, the virus remains dormant in lymphocytes and salivary glands. Infection in healthy individuals is typically asymptomatic but may present similarly to EBV mononucleosis, with flu-like symptoms, cervical lymphadenopathy, and low-grade hepatitis [5].

In the immunocompromised, specifically transplant recipients, cancer patients, or individuals with HIV/AIDS, CMV infection can manifest as retinitis, gastrointestinal, and CNS disease [99]. Transplant patients may present with "CMV syndrome," or hepatomegaly, fever, leukopenia, and arthralgias [100]. CMV is the most common cause of infection in transplant recipients [101]. In these patients, CMV can infect any organ [99]. In HIV-positive individuals, the highest risk of CMV infection occurs when the CD4+ cell count drops below 50 cells/μL. The most common CMV-associated infection in this population is retinitis [102]. CMV prophylaxis is not currently standard of care, but may be used for HIV-positive patients with CD4 <50 [103]. HAART is the most effective method of preventing CMV in this population [102]. Finally, CMV is the most common infectious cause of fetal abnormalities. Congenital CMV causes pneumonia and gastrointestinal, ocular, and neurologic disease via maternal transmission.

Oral lesions of CMV in the immunocompromised present as painful, punched-out lesions on various oral surfaces (Fig. 8.18) [104]. These ulcerations appear as well-circumscribed lesions without induration. Unlike aphthous ulcers, CMV ulcers do not have a surrounding erythematous halo. CMV lesions are most commonly found on the labial mucosa, tongue, buccal mucosa, gingiva, or oropharynx [69]. In the immunosuppressed, the presence of oral ulcers should always raise suspicion for CMV infection. Oral ulceration in the immunocompromised may be secondary to neoplasm, aphthous ulcer, or protozoan, bacterial, fungal, and viral (including HSV and CMV) infections [77].

Diagnosis based on clinical findings is insufficient. Histopathology, revealing characteristic cells with intranuclear "owl's eye" inclusions, is the most sensitive diagnostic method [104, 105]. Diagnosis of oral CMV infection is pertinent as it may be the initial presentation of systemic CMV infection in the immunocompromised individual [104]. In the HIV/AIDS population, oral ulcers are commonly coinfected with both HSV and CMV [105]. Additionally, in HIV-positive individuals, oral CMV lesions are highly suggestive of very low CD4+ counts and may allow for a diagnosis of AIDS. Antiviral medications, primarily ganciclovir, valganciclovir, and cidofovir, are used to treat CMV infection [101]. Immunosuppressed patients may benefit from prophylactic antiviral therapy.

Rubella

Rubella, alternatively known as German measles or 3-day measles, is typically a mild, uncomplicated, postnatal infection but can be devastating, if it is acquired in utero [106]. Prior to the introduction of the rubella vaccine in 1969, rubella epidemics occurred every 7 years, and the reported rubella incidence was 58 cases per 100,000 people. By 1983, the rubella incidence rate was less than 0.5 cases per 100,000 people [107]. In 2005, rubella was declared eliminated in the United States, per the CDC [106]. However, rare outbreaks do occur in countries with immunization programs [108].

Rubella is caused by the *Rubivirus*, a single-stranded, enveloped RNA virus, which is part of the *Togaviridae* family. It is spread via aerosolized nasopharyngeal secretions from infected patients [109]. It infects the respiratory tract and then disseminates to multiple organs via the lymphatic system [106]. The incubation period for rubella is 14–15 days prior to the onset of fever and rash. The rubella virus is shed for 2 weeks, starting 1 week prior to onset of the rash [109]. Infection rates are highest in the late winter and early spring [106].

Fifty percent of postnatal infections do not have clinical manifestations. In those with clinical manifestations, a prodromal phase with headache, sore throat, anorexia, nausea, fever, lethargy, and eye pain may be present. Postauricular, cervical, and suboccipital lymphadenopathy develops 1–5 days before the exanthem appears. The exanthem, described as an erythematous maculopapular rash, begins on the face and then spreads to the rest of the body in 24 h. The rash recedes on the 3rd day [106]. An enanthem, consisting of red macules or petechiae on the soft palate (Forschheimer spots), may be present (Fig. 8.19) [110].

Rubella can be diagnosed via IgM antibody detection assay (most common) or demonstration of a fourfold increase in IgG antibody or viral culture of a nasopharyngeal specimen. The IgM antibody can be detected by assays 4 days after the exanthem appears and can remain in the serum for 6–8 weeks [111]. Rubella is treated symptomatically [106].

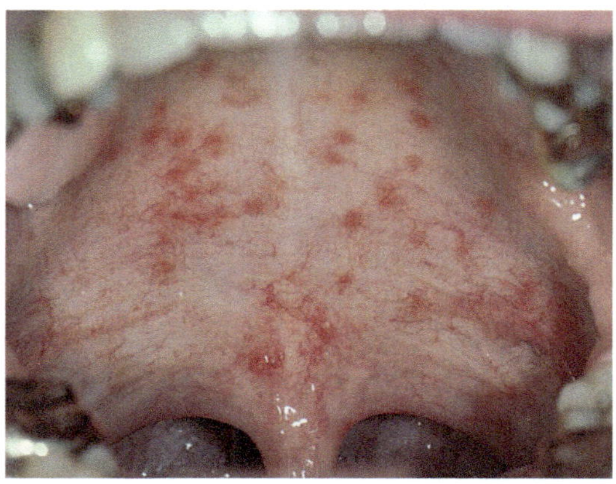

Fig. 8.19 Forschheimer sign of rubella, red macules on the palate. (This figure was published in Textbook of Physical Diagnosis: History and Examination, Mark Swartz, Review of Systems and Examination of the Young Child, 727, Copyright Elsevier (2014))

Mumps

Prior to the introduction of the vaccine in 1967, mumps was a common childhood illness. However, the US MMR vaccination program reduced mumps incidence by greater than 99% when comparing pre-vaccination and 2005 incidence rates [112]. However, outbreaks have continued to occur in the United States due to two-dose MMR vaccine failure in preventing mumps or due to non-vaccination [113]. High-risk settings for mumps are schools and college campuses [114].

Mumps is caused by an enveloped, single-stranded RNA virus that is part of the genus Rubulavirus in the family *Paramyxoviridae*. It is transmitted by direct contact, droplet spread, or contaminated fomites. Once transmitted, the virus replicates in the nasopharyngeal mucosa, and viremia leads to spread to other organs. The incubation period is between 15 and 24 days [115]. Infected patients are most contagious 1–2 days before symptoms occur to several days thereafter [116].

One-third of mumps infections are asymptomatic. In the prodromal stage of mumps, patients experience low-grade fever, anorexia, malaise, and headache. The hallmark manifestation of mumps is parotitis, but other signs include epididymo-orchitis (with possible testicular atrophy and sterility), bilateral orchitis, oophoritis, meningitis, encephalitis, permanent unilateral deafness, spontaneous abortion, and pancreatitis [114].

The classical oral manifestation of mumps is parotitis, which occurs in 95% of patients with symptoms. Parotitis occurs 48 h after the onset of prodromal symptoms. Inflammation and swelling of the parotid gland elevates the earlobe outward and conceals the angle of the mandible over the course of 2–3 days and lasts for 1 week [114, 117]. Severe pain is often present. The opening of Stensen's duct is usually edematous and inflamed [114]. In 90% of parotitis cases, contralateral parotitis also arises within several days [114, 117]. Bilateral submandibular and sublingual salivary gland inflammation may be present in 10% of cases. Rare complications of parotitis include sialectasia with recurrent sialadenitis and presternal or supraglottic edema from obstruction of lymphatic drainage [114].

The differential diagnosis of parotitis is EBV, parainfluenza virus types 1 and 3, influenza A virus, coxsackievirus, adenovirus, parvovirus B19, lymphocytic choriomeningitis virus, HIV, staphylococcus, atypical mycobacteria, drugs (phenothiazines, iodides, thiouracil, phenylbutazone), starch, malnutrition, metabolic disorders, cyst, salivary tumor, Sjögren's syndrome, or sialolithiasis [114]. Mumps is primarily a clinical diagnosis. In atypical cases, laboratory confirmation with IgM antibody detection, fourfold increase in IgG antibody titer, viral culture of saliva, or viral nucleic acid detection can be done. Treatment of mumps is symptomatic with analgesics, antipyretics, and hot or cold compresses.

Measles

Measles is one of the most contagious viral diseases known to man. It is estimated that more than 200 million people have died globally in the last five centuries from measles. However, measles incidence fell with the introduction of the measles vaccine in 1963 and subsequently the combined measles-rubella vaccine in 1971 [118]. Measles was declared to be eliminated in the United States in 2000 but is becoming more common as a result of refusal of vaccination [119]. However, despite this public health achievement, an estimated 20 million cases of measles occur yearly worldwide, and some of these outbreaks are in regions with access to the MMR vaccine [119].

Measles is caused by the *Morbillivirus*, a spherical, enveloped, single-stranded RNA virus that is part of the *Paramyxoviridae* family. It is spread via respiratory droplets over short distances [120]. A recent systematic review indicated that the incubation period of the virus is 12.5 days. Specifically, the incubation period to onset of fever and rash is 10 and 14 days, respectively [121]. However, patients are infectious a few days prior to onset of the rash, which is the period when the virus is present at high levels in body fluids and symptoms of coryza, cough, and sneezing are the most severe [122].

The clinical manifestations of measles can be grouped into the prodromal and exanthemous phases. Signs and symptoms of the prodromal phase include fever of 39–40 °C, malaise, anorexia, coryza, conjunctivitis, rhinitis, cough, pharyngitis, and tracheitis. These symptoms worsen progressively until the classic erythematous, maculopapular rash of measles appears. The rash begins on the face and behind the ears and then spreads to the trunk and extremities before resolving in 3–5 days [122].

The oral sign of measles is Koplik spots, which are white-gray papules that begin on the posterior buccal mucosa and spread to the rest of the oral mucosa (Fig. 8.20). Occasionally, the mucosal lips may be involved. Koplik spots appear in the prodromal stage, but it is unclear if they appear at the beginning of the prodromal phase or just 1 or 2 days before the exanthemous phase. They are noted to last until the onset of the exanthemous phase [123]. Of note, although Koplik spots are considered pathognomonic for measles, they have also been noted in parvovirus B19 infection [123].

Physicians should consider measles, if a patient demonstrates the classical signs and symptoms, especially if there is an outbreak in the region. Detection of serum measles IgM antibody or a fourfold increase in serum measles IgG antibody titer can confirm the diagnosis of measles [122]. The WHO recommends daily vitamin A therapy for children with measles [120].

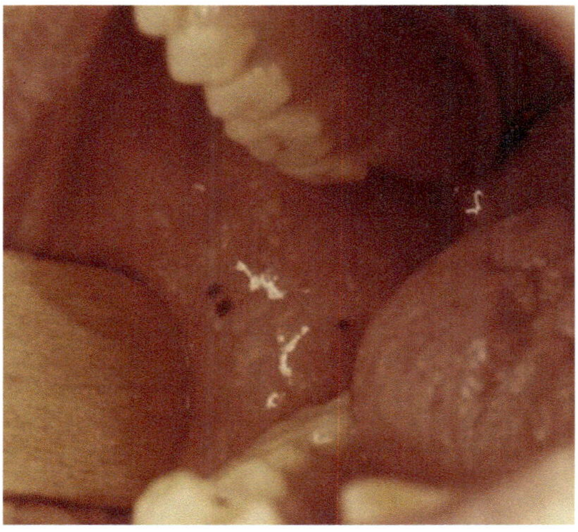

Fig. 8.20 Koplik spots of measles shown as white-gray papules on the buccal mucosa. (Reprinted from Patel et al. [127], with permission from Elsevier)

This chapter has provided an overview of the epidemiology, pathogenesis, differential diagnosis, diagnostic studies, and treatment for viral etiologies causing oral disease manifestations. Clinical criteria for the diagnosis of oral viral disease include the precise location, size, color, and morphology of the oral lesions. The specific population group and the presence or absence of both systemic and localized prodromal symptoms associated with each viral disease serve as diagnostic clues. As described in this chapter, subtle differentiating characteristics of viral oral disease manifestations serve as tools for diagnosis.

References

1. Smith J, Robinson N. Age specific prevalence of infection with herpes simplex virus types 2 and I: a global review. J Infect Dis. 2002;186(Suppl 1):3–28.
2. Fatahzadeh M. Human herpes simplex virus infections: epidemiology, pathogenesis, symptomatology, diagnosis and management. J Am Acad Dermatol. 2007;57(5):737–63.
3. Roizman B. The organization of the herpes simplex virus genome. Ann Rev Genet. 1979;13:25–7.
4. Arduino P, Porter S. Herpes simplex virus type 1 infection: overview on relevant clinico-pathologic features. J Oral Pathol Med. 2008;37:107–21.
5. Stoopler E. Oral herpetic infections (HSV 1-8). Dent Clin N Am. 2005;49(1):15–29.
6. Lynch D. Oral viral infections. Clin Dermatol. 2000;18(5):619–28.
7. Simmons A. Clinical manifestations and treatment considerations of herpes simplex virus infection. J Infect Dis. 2002;186(Suppl 1):71–7.
8. Eisen D. The clinical characteristics of intraoral herpes simplex virus infections in 52 immunocompetent patients. Oral Surg Oral Med Oral Pathol Oral Radiol Endod. 1998;86:432–7.
9. Leflore S, Anderson P, Fletcher C. A risk-benefit evaluation of acyclovir for the treatment and prophylaxis of herpes simplex infections. Drug Saf. 2000;23(2):131–42.
10. Brady R, Bernstein D. Treatment of herpes simplex infections. Antivir Res. 2004;61:73–81.
11. Yawn BP, Saddier P, Wollan PC, St Sauver JL, Kurland MJ, Sy LS. A population-based study of the incidence and complication rates of herpes zoster

before zoster vaccine introduction. Mayo Clin Proc. 2007;82:1341–9.
12. Oxman M, Levin MJ, Johnson GR, Schmader KE, Straus SE, Gelb LD, et al. A vaccine to prevent herpes zoster and postherpetic neuralgia in older adults. N Engl J Med. 2005;352:2271–84.
13. Gringe B. Herpesviruses: latency and reactivation-viral strategies and host response. J Oral Microbiol. 2013;25(5). https://doi.org/10.3402/jom.v5i0.22766.
14. Gilden D, Cohrs R, Mahalingam R. Clinical and molecular pathogenesis of varicella virus infection. Viral Immunol. 2004;16(3):243–58.
15. Cohen J. Herpes zoster. N Engl J Med. 2013;369:255–63.
16. Greenberg MS. Ulcerative, vesicular, and bullous lesions. In: Greenberg MS, Glick M, editors. Burket's oral medicine: diagnosis and treatment. 10th ed. Ontario: Decker; 2003. p. 50–84.
17. Manjunath BR, Chidambar YS, Telkar S, Japatti S, Choudary L, Dodamani A. Oral complications of herpes zoster infection- report of 3 cases. Int J Dent Clin. 2010;2(4):70–3.
18. Srikrishna K, Prabhat MPV, Balmuri P, Sudhakar S, Ramaraju D. Herpes zoster: report of a treated case with review of literature. J Ind Acad Oral Med Radiol. 2012;24(1):51–5.
19. Hoyt B, Bhawan J. Histological spectrum of cutaneous herpes infections. Am J Dermatopathol. 2014;36(8):609–19.
20. Wood M, Johnson R, McKendrick M, Taylor J, Mandal B, Crooks J. A randomized trial of acyclovir for 7 days or 21 days with and without prednisolone for treatment of acute herpes zoster. N Engl J Med. 1994;330:896–900.
21. Lapolla W, Digiorgio C, Haitz K, Magel G, Grady J, Lu W, Tyring S. Incidence of postherpetic neuralgia after combination treatment with gabapentin and valacylcovir in patients with acute herpes zoster: open-label study. Arch Dermatol. 2011;147(8):901–7.
22. Wharton M. The epidemiology of varicella-zoster virus infections. Infect Dis Clin N Am. 1996;10(3):571–81.
23. Kilgore PE, Kruszon-Moran D, Seward JF, Jumaan A, Van Loon FP, Forghani B, et al. Varicella in Americans from NHANES III: implications for control through routine immunization. J Med Virol. 2003;70(Suppl 1):111–8.
24. Finger R, Hughes JP, Meade BJ, Pelletier AR, Palmer CT. Age-specific incidence of chickenpox. Public Health Rep. 1994;109(6):750–5.
25. Marin M, Meissner HC, Seward JF. Varicella prevention in the United States: a review of successes and challenges. Pediatrics. 2008;122(3):e744–51.
26. Shapiro ED, Vazquez M, Esposito D, Holabird N, Steinberg SP, Dziura J, et al. Effectiveness of 2 doses of varicella vaccine in children. J Infect Dis. 2011;203(3):312–5.
27. Arvin A. Varicella-zoster virus. Clin Microbiol Rev. 1996;9(3):361–81.
28. Heerden V. Oral manifestations of viral infections. S A Fam Pract. 2006;48(8):20–4.
29. Na SY, Son YM, Lee HY, Baek JO, Roh JY, Lee JR. A case of varicella combined with hand-foot-mouth disease in a healthy child. Ann Dermatol. 2009;21(1):98–101.
30. Kolokotronis A, Louloudiadis K, Fotiou G, Matiais A. Oral manifestations of infections due to varicella zoster virus in otherwise healthy children. J Clin Pediatr Dent. 2001;25(2):107–12.
31. American Academy of Pediatrics Committee on Infectious Diseases. The use of oral acyclovir in otherwise healthy children with varicella. Pediatrics. 1993;91(3):674–6.
32. Belay ED, Bresee JS, Holman RC, Khan AS, Shahriari A, Schonberger LB. Reye's syndrome in the United States from 1981 through 1997. N Engl J Med. 1999;340:1377–82.
33. Wallace MR, Bowler WA, Murray NB, Brodine SK, Oldfield EC 3rd. Treatment of adult varicella with oral acyclovir: a randomized, placebo-controlled trial. Ann Intern Med. 1992;117(5):358–63.
34. Repass G, Palmer WC, Stancampiano FF. Hand, foot, and mouth disease: identifying and managing an acute viral syndrome. Cleve Clin J Med. 2014;8199:537–43.
35. Downing C, Ramirez-Fort MK, Doan HQ, Benoist F, Oberste MS, Khan F, et al. Coxsackievirus A6 associated hand, foot and mouth disease in adults: clinical presentation and review of the literature. J Clin Virol. 2014;60:381–6.
36. Stewart CL, Chu EY, Introcaso CE, Schaffer A, James WD. Coxsackievirus A6-induced hand-foot-mouth disease. JAMA Dermatol. 2013;149(12):1419–21.
37. Mehta KI, Mahajan VK. Hand foot and mouth disease. Indian Pediatr. 2010;46:345–6.
38. Slots J. Oral viral infections of adults. Periodontology. 2000;49:60–86.
39. De Carvalho CH, De Andrade AL, de Oliverira DH, Lima E, de Silveira EJ, de Medeiros AM. Intraoral molluscum contagiosum in a young immunocomputent patient. Oral Maxillofacial Pathol. 2012;114(1):e57–60.
40. Dohil MA, Lin P, Lee J, et al. The epidemiology of molluscum contagiosum in children. J Am Acad Dermatol. 2006;54:47–54.
41. Zhang Q, Davis JC, Lamborn IT, Freeman AF, Jing H, Favreau AJ, et al. Combined immunodeficiency associated with DOCK8 mutations. N Engl J Med. 2009;361:2046–55.
42. Braue A, Ross G, Varigos G, Kelly H. Epidemiology and impact of childhood molluscum contagiosum: a case series and critical review of the literature. Pediatr Dermatol. 2005;22:287–94.
43. Kreimer AR, Bhatia RK, Messeguer AL, González P, Herrero R, Giuliano AR. Oral human papillomavirus in healthy individuals: a systematic review of the literature. Sex Transm Dis. 2010;37:386–91.

44. Chung C, Bagheri A, Gypsyamber D. Epidemiology of oral human papillomavirus. Oral Oncol. 2014;50:364–9.
45. Grce M, Marinka M. Human papillomavirus-associated diseases. Clin Dermatol. 2014;32:253–8.
46. Pringle G. The role of human papillomavirus in oral disease. Dent Clin N Am. 2014;58:385–99.
47. Syrjanen S. Human papillomavirus infections and oral tumors. Med Microbiol Immunol. 2003;192:123–8.
48. Nguyen H, McNiece K, Duong A, Khan F. Human papillomavirus infections of the oral mucosa and upper respiratory tract. Curr Prob Dermatol. 2015;45:132–53.
49. Jaiswal R, Pandey M, Shukla M, Dip NB, Kumar M. Condyloma acuminatum of the buccal mucosa. Ear Nose Throat J. 2014;93(6):219–23.
50. Prabhu SR, Wilson DF. Human papillomavirus and oral disease- emerging evidence: a review. Aust Den J. 2013;58:2.
51. Said AK, Leao JC, Fedele S, Porter SR. Focal epithelial hyperplasia—an update. J Oral Pathol Med. 2013;42:435–42.
52. García-Corona C, Vega-Memije E, Mosqueda-Taylor A, Yamamoto-Furusho JK, Rodríguez-Carreón AA, Ruiz-Morales JA, et al. Association of HLA-DR4 (DRB1*0404) with human papillomavirus infection in patients with focal epithelial hyperplasia. Arch Dermatol. 2004;140(10):1227–31. https://doi.org/10.1001/archderm.140.10.1227.
53. González LV, Gaviria AM, Sanclemente G, Rady P, Tyring SK, Carlos R, et al. Clinical, histopathological and virological findings in patients with focal epithelial hyperplasia from Colombia. Int J Dermatol. 2005;44:274–9.
54. Bennett LK, Hinshaw M. Heck's disease: diagnosis and susceptibility. Pediatr Dermatol. 2009;26:87–9.
55. Luzuriaga K, Sullivan JL. Infectious mononucleosis. N Engl J Med. 2010;362(21):1993–2000.
56. Crawford DH, Macsween KF, Higgins CD, Thomas R, McAulay K, Williams H, et al. A cohort study among university students: identification of risk factors for Epstein-Barr virus seroconversion and infectious mononucleosis. Clin Infect Dis. 2006;43:276–82.
57. Odumade OA, Hogquist KA, Balfour HH. Progress and problems in understanding and managing primary Epstein-Barr virus infections. Clin Microbiol Rev. 2011;24(1):193–209.
58. Thorley-Lawson DA. Epstein-Barr virus: exploiting the immune system. Nat Rev Immunol. 2001;1:75–82.
59. Hadinoto V, Shapiro M, Greenough TC, Sullivan JL, Luzuriaga K, Thorley-Lawson DA. On the dynamics of acute EBV infection and the pathogenesis of infectious mononucleosis. Blood. 2008;111:1420–7.
60. Jenson HB. Acute complications of Epstein-Barr virus infectious mononucleosis. Curr Opin Pediatr. 2000;12:263–8.
61. Ebell MH. Epstein-Barr virus infectious mononucleosis. Am Fam Physician. 2004;70:1279–87.
62. World Health Organization. Core Epidemiological Slides: HIV/AIDS Estimates; 2014. Powerpoint presentation available from: http://www.who.int/hiv/data/en/. Accessed 19 Oct 2014.
63. Centers for Disease Control and Prevention. Monitoring selected national HIV prevention and care objectives by using HIV surveillance data—United States and 6 U.S. dependent areas—2011. In: HIV surveillance supplemental report, vol. 18(5); 2013.
64. Quinn TC. Acute primary HIV infection. JAMA. 1997;278:58.
65. Centers for Disease Control and Prevention and Association of Public Health Laboratories. Laboratory testing for the diagnosis of HIV infection: updated recommendations; 2014. http://stacks.cdc.gov/view/cdc/23447. Accessed 8 Oct 2014.
66. Patton LL, Phelan JA, Ramos-Gomez FJ, Nittayananta W, Shiboski CH, Mbuguye TL. Prevalence and classification of HIV- associated oral lesions. Oral Dis. 2002;8(Suppl 2):98–109.
67. Axell T, Azul AM, Challacombe S, Ficcara G, Flint S, Greenspan D. Classification and diagnostic criteria for oral lesions in HIV infection. EC-clearinghouse on oral problems related to HIV infection and WHO collaborating centre on oral manifestations of the immunodeficiency virus. J Oral Pathol Med. 1993;22(7):289–91.
68. Lifson AR, Hilton JF, Westenhouse JL, Canchola AJ, Samuel MC, Katz MH, et al. Time from HIV seroconversion to oral candidiasis or hairy leukoplakia among homosexual and bisexual men enrolled in three prospective cohorts. AIDS. 1994;8:73–9.
69. Patton LL, van der Horst C. Oral infections and other manifestations of HIV disease. Infect Dis Clin N Am. 1999;13(4):879–900.
70. Triantos D, Porter SR, Scully C, Teo CG. Oral hairy leukoplakia: clinicopathologic features, pathogenesis, diagnosis, and clinical significance. Clin Infect Dis. 1997;25:1392–6.
71. Bhandarkar SS, MacKelfresh J, Fried L, Arbiser JL. Targeted therapy of oral hairy leukoplakia with gentian violet. J Am Acad Dermatol. 2008;58:711–2.
72. Braz-Silva P, Santos R, Schussel J, Gallottini M. Oral hairy leukoplakia diagnosis by Epstein–Barr virus in situ hybridization in liquid-based cytology. Cytopathology. 2013;25(1):21–6. https://doi.org/10.1111/cyt.12053.
73. Greenspan JS, Greenspan D. HIV-related oral disease. Lancet. 1996;348:729–33.
74. Patton LL. Oral lesions associated with human immunodeficiency virus disease. Dent Clin N Am. 2013;57(4):673–98.
75. Tappuni AR, Kovacevic T, Shirlaw PJ, Challacombe SJ. Clinical assessment of disease severity in recurrent aphthous stomatitis. J Oral Pathol Med. 2013;42:635–41.

76. Kerr A, Ship J. Management strategies for HIV-associated aphthous stomatitis. Am J Clin Dermatol. 2003;4(10):669–80.
77. Reichart PA. Oral ulcerations in HIV infection. Oral Dis. 1997;3(Suppl 1):180–2.
78. American Society of Hematology. 2011 clinical practice guideline on the evaluation and management of immune thrombocytopenia; 2011. http://www.hematology.org. Accessed 21 Oct 2014.
79. Bettaieb A, Fromont P, Louache F, Osksenhendler E, Vainchenker W, Duédari N, et al. Presence of cross-reactive antibody between human immunodeficiency virus (HIV) and platelet glycoproteins in HIV-related immune thrombocytopenic purpura. Blood. 1992;80:162–9.
80. Reid E. Hematologic manifestations of acquired immunodeficiency syndrome. In: Lichtman MA, Kipps TJ, Seligsohn U, Kaushansky, editors. Williams hematology. 8th ed. China: McGraw-Hill; 2010. p. 1175–99.
81. Ambler K, Vickars L, Leger C, Foltz L, Montaner JS, Harris M, et al. Clinical features, treatment and outcome of HIV-associated immune thrombocytopenia in the HAART era. Adv Hematol. 2012;2012:910–54. https://doi.org/10.1155/2012/910954.
82. Chapple I, Hamburger J. The significance of oral health in HIV disease. Sex Transm Infect. 2000;76(4):236–43. https://doi.org/10.1136/sti.76.4.23.
83. Kazi S, Cohen PR, Williams F, Schempp R, Reveille JD. The diffuse infiltrative lymphocytosis syndrome: clinical and immunogenetic features in 35 patients. AIDS. 1996;10(4):385–91.
84. Dourmishev LA, Dourmishev AL, Palmeri D, Schwartz RA, Lukac DM. Molecular genetics of Kaposi's sarcoma associated herpesvirus (human herpesvirus-8) epidemiology and pathogenesis. Microbiol Mol Biol Rev. 2003;67:175–212.
85. Bohlius J, Valeri F, Maskew M, Prozesky H, Prozesky H, Garone D, Sengayi M, et al. Kaposi's sarcoma in HIV-infected patients in South Africa: multicohort study in the antiretroviral therapy era. Int J Cancer. 2014;135:2644–52. https://doi.org/10.1002/ijc.28894.
86. Schwartz R, Micali G, Nasca M, Scuderi L. Kaposi sarcoma: a continuing conundrum. J Am Acad Dermatol. 2008;59(2):179–206.
87. Russo JJ, Bohenzky RA, Chien MC, Chen J, Yan M, Maddalena D, et al. Nucleotide sequence of the Kaposi sarcoma-associated herpesvirus (HHV8). Proc Natl Acad Sci U S A. 1996;93:14862–7.
88. Cattani P, Capuano M, Cerimele F, La Parola IL, Santangelo R, Masini C, et al. Human herpesvirus 8 seroprevalence and evaluation of nonsexual transmission routes by detection of DNA in clinical specimens from human immunodeficiency virus-seronegative patients from central and southern Italy, with and without Kaposi's sarcoma. J Clin Microbiol. 1999;37:1150–3.
89. Schwartz RA. Kaposi's sarcoma: advances and perspectives. J Am Acad Dermatol. 1996;34:804–14.
90. Lemlich G, Schwam L, Lebwohl M. Kaposi's sarcoma and acquired immunodeficiency syndrome: postmortem findings in twenty-four cases. J Am Acad Dermatol. 1987;16:319–25.
91. World Health Organization. WHO case definitions of HIV for surveillance and revised clinical staging and immunological classification of HIV-Related disease in adults and children; 2006. http://www.who.int/hiv/pub/guidelines/HIVstaging150307.pdf. Accessed 19 Oct 2014.
92. Feller L, Jadwat Y, Raubenheimer EJ. Kaposi sarcoma and calcium channel blocker-induced gingival enlargement occurring simultaneously: review of the literature and report of a case. Oral Biosci Med. 2004;4:291–7.
93. Pantanowitz L, Khammissa R, Lemmer J, Feller L. Oral HIV-associated Kaposi sarcoma. J Oral Pathol Med. 2013;42:201–7.
94. Fatahzadeh M, Schwartz RA. Oral Kaposi's sarcoma: a review and update. Int J Dermatol. 2013;52:666–72.
95. Vanni T, Sprinz E, Machado MW, Santana Rde C, Fonseca BA, et al. Systemic treatment of AIDS-related Kaposi sarcoma: current status and perspectives. Cancer Treat Rev. 2006;32:445–55. https://doi.org/10.1016/j.ctrv.2006.06.001.
96. Doumas S, Vladikas A, Papagianni M, Kolokotronis A. Human cytomegalovirus-associated oral and maxillo-facial disease. Clin Microbiol Infect. 2007;13:557–9.
97. Lazzarotto T, Guerra B, Gabrielli L, Lanari M, Landini MP. Update on the prevention, diagnosis and management of cytomegalovirus infection during pregnancy. Clin Microbiol Infect. 2011;17:1285–93. https://doi.org/10.1111/j.1469-0691.2011.03564.x.
98. Stoopler ET, Greenberg MS. Update on herpesvirus infections. Dent Clin N Am. 2003;47(4):517–32.
99. Bruminhent J, Razonable R. Management of cytomegalovirus infection and disease in liver transplant recipients. World J Hepatol. 2014;6(6):370–83.
100. Taylor GH. Cytomegalovirus. Am Fam Physician. 2003;67(3):519–24.
101. Kotton CN. CMV: prevention, diagnosis and therapy. Am J Transplant. 2013;13:24–40.
102. Whitcup SM. Cytomegalovirus retinitis in the era of highly active antiretroviral therapy. JAMA. 2000;283:653–7.
103. Kaplan J, Masur H, Holmes K. Recommendations of the U.S. Public Health Service and the Infectious Diseases Society of America. MMWR Morb Mortal Wkly Rep. 2002;51(08):1–46.
104. Dauden E, Fernandez-Buezo G, Fraga J, Cardenoso L, Garcia-Diez A. Mucocutaneous presence of cytomegalovirus associated with human immunodeficiency virus infection. Arch Dermatol. 2000;137:443–8.
105. Flaitz C, Nichols M, Hicks M. Herpesviridae-associated persistent mucocutaneous ulcers in

acquired immunodeficiency syndrome. Oral Surg Oral Med Oral Pathol Oral Radiol Endod. 1996;81(4):433–41.
106. Drutz JE. Rubella. Pediatr Rev. 2010;31(3):129–30.
107. Castillo-Solorzano C, Matus CR, Flannery B, Marsigli C, Tambini G, Andrus JK. The Americas: paving the road toward global measles eradication. J Infect Dis. 2011;204(Suppl 1):270–8.
108. Centers for Disease Control and Prevention (CDC). Nationwide rubella epidemic – Japan, 2013. MMWR Morb Mortal Wkly Rep. 2013;62:457.
109. Banatvala JE, Brown DW. Rubella. Lancet. 2004;363:1127–37.
110. Baden H, Provan J. Oral lesion of rubella. Arch Dermatol. 1976;112(12):1973.
111. Thomas HI, Morgan-Capner P, Cradock-Watson JE, Enders G, Best JM, O'Shea S. Slow maturation of IgG1 avidity and persistence of specific IgM in congenital rubella: implications for diagnosis and immunopathology. J Med Virol. 1993; 41:196.
112. Dayan GH, Quinlisk MP, Parker AA, Barskey AE, Harris ML, Schwartz JM, et al. Recent resurgence of mumps in the United States. N Engl J Med. 2008;358:1580–9.
113. Whitaker JA, Poland GA. Measles and mumps outbreaks in the United States: think globally, vaccinate locally. Vaccine. 2014;32:4703–4.
114. Hviid A, Rubin S, Muhlemann K. Mumps. Lancet. 2008;371:932–44.
115. Richardson M, Elliman D, Maguire H, Simpson J, Nicoll A. Evidence base of incubation periods, periods of infectiousness and exclusion policies for the control of communicable diseases in schools and preschools. Pediatr Infect Dis J. 2001;20: 380–91.
116. Ennis FA, Jackson D. Isolation of virus during the incubation period of mumps infection. J Pediatr. 1968;72:536–7.
117. Sallberg M. Oral viral infections of children. Periodontology. 2000;49:87–95.
118. Grabowsky M. The beginning of the end of the measles and rubella. Arch Pediatr Adolesc Med. 2014;168(2):108–9.
119. Centers for Disease Control and Prevention (CDC). Brief report: update: mumps activity – United States, January 1-October 7, 2006. MMWR Morb Mortal Wkly Rep. 2006;55(42):1152.
120. Duke T, Mgone CS. Measles: not just another viral exanthem. Lancet. 2003;361:763–73.
121. Lessler J, Reich NG, Brookmeyer R, Perl TM, Nelson KE, Cummings DA. Incubation periods of acute respiratory viral infections: a systematic review. Lancet Infect Dis. 2009;9:291–300.
122. Moss MJ, Griffin DE. Measles. Lancet. 2012;379:153–64.
123. Battegay R, Itin C, Itin P. Dermatological signs and symptoms of measles: a prospective case series and comparison with the literature. Dermatology. 2012;224:1–4.
124. Silverman S, Miller C. Diagnosis and treatment of viral infections. Oral Maxillofac Surg Clin N Am. 2003;15(1):79–89.
125. Kayal L, Jayachandran S, Singh K. Idiopathic thrombocytopenic purpura. Contemp Clin Dent. 2014;5(3):410–4.
126. Restrepo CS, Ocazionez D. Kaposi's sarcoma: imaging overview. Semin Ultrasound CT MRI. 2011;32(5):465–9.
127. Patel LM, Lambert PJ, Gagna CE, Maghari A, Clark Lambert W. Cutaneous signs of systemic disease. Clin Dermatol. 2011;28(5):511–2.

Oral Signs of Bacterial Disease

9

Emily W. Shelley and Rochelle R. Torgerson

The oral manifestations of bacterial diseases are varied ranging from nonspecific ulcers to the nearly pathognomonic strawberry tongue of scarlet fever. The bacterial diseases with oral manifestations range from the highly prevalent gingivitis/periodontitis to the much rarer diphtheria, a disease physicians in North America would not expect to encounter. This chapter covers the salient features of the following bacterial diseases with an emphasis upon oral manifestations: syphilis, gonorrhea, tuberculosis, acute necrotizing ulcerative gingivitis, scarlet fever, diphtheria, staphylococcal scalded skin, leprosy, gingivitis/periodontitis, granuloma inguinale, tularemia, and cat scratch disease.

Syphilis

Epidemiology

Syphilis, a bacterial infection caused by *Treponema pallidum*, is almost exclusively contracted through sexual intercourse but can also be acquired through contact with infectious lesions, needle sharing, or in utero. While found in all ages and races, incidence is highest in young men between the ages of 20 and 29. Rates are also higher in the African American population and in urban communities [1]. Since the nineteenth century, the worldwide presence of syphilis has been influenced by both political and medical factors. The first major decline in the prevalence of syphilis occurred after the introduction of penicillin. While rates have steadily declined for over a century, epidemics have been seen. In the 1970s–1980s, an increase in both syphilis and HIV was seen among men who had sex with men. Rates gradually declined with awareness of the diseases, antiretroviral therapy, and safer sex practices. Another rapid increase was seen between 1986 and 1990 primarily among heterosexuals and was thought to be associated with an increase in crack cocaine abuse [2, 3]. Despite falling to record low levels in 1999, 2.6 cases in 100,000, rates have since been slowly increasing, especially in women and among those in the southeastern USA [3].

Etiopathogenesis

T. pallidum, a motile, spiral-shaped organism, enters the body either directly through the mucous membranes or through minute abrasions in the skin. The organism cannot be cultured but can be detected via dark-field microscopy or serologic testing. After entering through epithelial surfaces, the bacteria multiply at the site of

E. W. Shelley
Cleveland Medical Center, University Hospitals, Cleveland, OH, USA

R. R. Torgerson (✉)
Departments of Dermatology and Obstetrics and Gynecology, Mayo Clinic, Rochester, MN, USA
e-mail: Torgerson.rochelle@mayo.edu

N. Fazel (ed.), *Oral Signs of Systemic Disease*, https://doi.org/10.1007/978-3-030-10863-2_9

inoculation and disseminate through blood and lymphatics via coordination of both adherence and inherent motility [4]. In primary syphilis, the presence of treponemes initiates a host inflammatory response of predominantly lymphocytes, plasma cells, and monocytes. These cells in turn activate macrophages. While this response does eliminate a large number of treponemes, it is believed that either resistance to phagocytosis or downregulation of the immune response allows the infection to spread in the absence of treatment [5]. If allowed to progress, secondary syphilis is characterized by hematologic dissemination of treponemes. It is the host inflammatory response of secondary and late syphilis that syphilologists now agree is the cause of the clinical manifestations of syphilis [4]. These responses include antibody formation, complement activation, and formation of circulating immune complexes with treponemal outer membrane proteins [5]. Granulomatous reaction is a hallmark of both secondary and late syphilis. These granulomas are histologically nonspecific and may be mistaken for other granulomatous processes such as sarcoidosis [4].

Clinical Manifestations

Clinical manifestations of syphilis depend on the stage. Primary syphilis is marked by the appearance of a chancre, often on the penis, cervix, or vulva. If left untreated, secondary syphilis develops 6–8 weeks after resolution of the chancre. Systemic symptoms of secondary syphilis present as a flu-like illness with malaise, anorexia, weight loss, fever, sore throat, and generalized, painful lymphadenopathy [6]. Skin manifestations of secondary syphilis include the characteristic papulosquamous rash of the trunk, extremities, and occasionally the palms and soles and a "moth-eaten" alopecia [7]. The clinical manifestations of secondary syphilis may resolve spontaneously without treatment. The infection then transitions to the latent phase where it may remain dormant in the liver or spleen for 3–30 years. If reactivated, tertiary syphilis is marked by the destruction of tissues, clinically manifested by the formation of gummas in the skin and mucosa. The central nervous system may be affected causing generalized paresis and tabes dorsalis. Cardiovascular involvement can lead to aortitis and heart failure [8].

Oral Signs and Symptoms

Oral manifestations may occur during all stages of syphilis. Leuci et al. (2013) performed a retrospective literature review that identified 34 patients reported to have oral syphilis. The manifestations among these patients included nonspecific ulcers (50%), gummas (17%), white patches (17%), blistering mucositis (8%), and necrosis of the dorsum of the tongue (8%) [9]. The chancre of primary syphilis, most often found in the genital area, can also arise in the oropharynx following oral sex (Fig. 9.1). Kent and Romanelli (2008) found that 40–70% of extragenital ulcers appear in the mouth [10]. The chancre is a raised, firm, and painless ulcer that can appear similar to an aphthous ulcer [11, 12]. Once eroded, the chancre heals, often without treatment, in 3–6 weeks. If allowed to spread hematogenously, secondary syphilis may present with oral lesions. These are characterized by cheilitis, also called syphilitic perlèche; gray patches on the palate, mucosa, and tongue in addition to erosions on the tongue with flattened papillae; and condyloma lata (Fig. 9.2) [7]. These manifestations are often nonspecific, however, making diagnosis difficult [13].

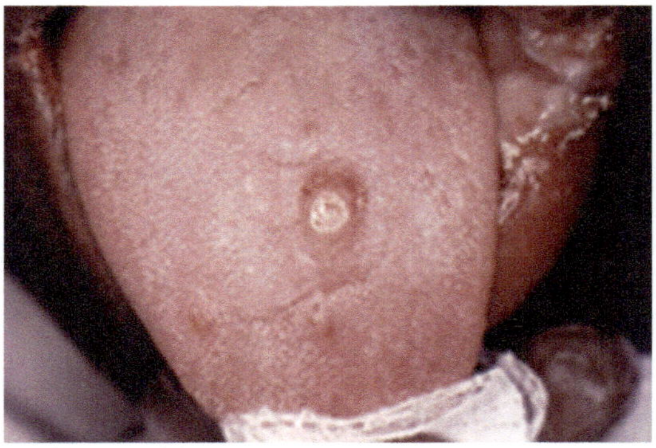

Fig. 9.1 Primary syphilis in the oral cavity. (Image courtesy of Centers for Disease Control and Prevention https://phil.cdc.gov/)

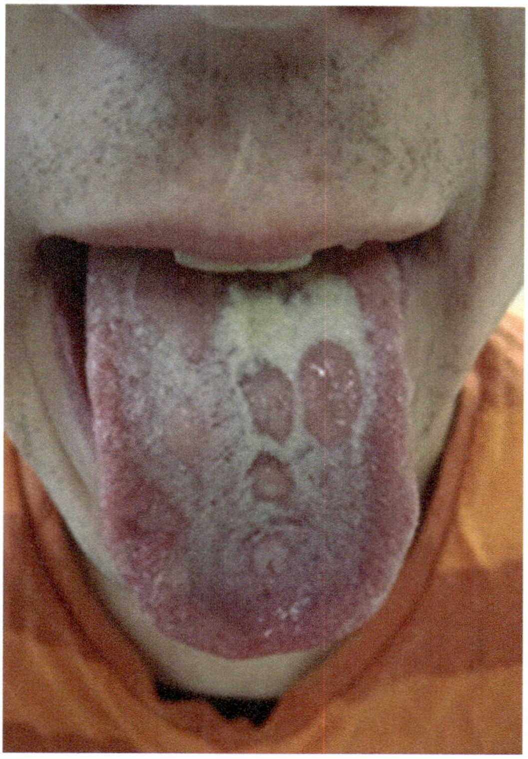

Fig. 9.2 Secondary syphilis of the tongue. (Image courtesy of Centers for Disease Control and Prevention https://phil.cdc.gov/)

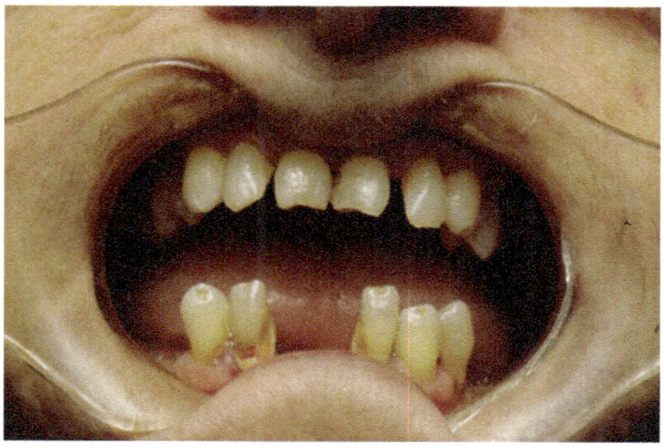

Fig. 9.3 Congenital syphilis. Hutchinson teeth

Tertiary syphilis is marked by granulomatous gummas. In the oral cavity, these gummas may occur on the palate, tongue, or tonsils and can cause tissue destruction and fistula formation. The tongue may also show interstitial glossitis [14]. Lastly, congenital syphilis presents with the characteristic Hutchinson teeth, widely spaced incisors with large notches, and mulberry molars (Figs. 9.3 and 9.4).

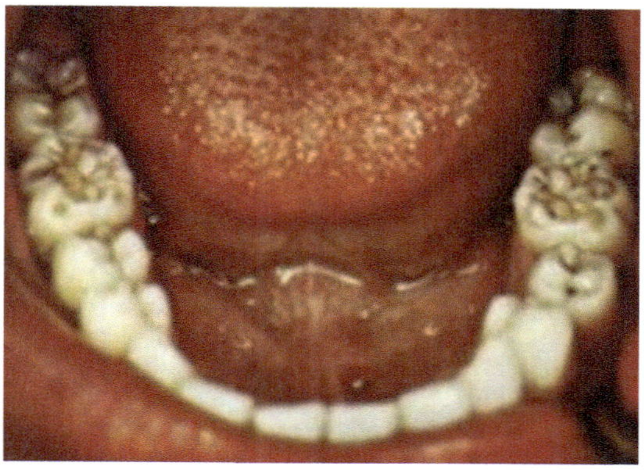

Fig. 9.4 Congenital syphilis. Mulberry molars

Differential Diagnosis

The differential diagnosis for oral lesions of syphilis may be broad owing to the nonspecific nature of many of the manifestations. Possibilities for the differential diagnosis of primary syphilis include aphthae, traumatic ulcers, drug-induced lesions, erosive oral lichen planus, oral squamous cell carcinoma, or lymphoma [12]. Secondary syphilis, as described above, may appear as plaques in the oral mucosa. The differential diagnoses for these oral lesions should include lichen planus, lupus erythematosus, erythroleukoplakia, and candidiasis. Other possibilities include autoimmune processes such as pemphigus/pemphigoid and other infectious causes such as tuberculosis, fungus, herpes, or oral hairy leukoplakia [9].

Histopathological examination may or may not be helpful in establishing a diagnosis of syphilis. Hertel et al. described case reports of three separate patients whose oral manifestations of syphilis were histologically nonspecific [12]. Epidermal changes of primary syphilis on histopathology include acanthosis and spongiosis as well as infiltration of neutrophils and lymphocytes [13]. Obliterative endarteritis is characteristic of these lesions and appears with dense perivascular and interstitial lymphocytes and plasma cells [5, 13]. These changes have also been found in lesions of secondary syphilis. Secondary syphilis may present with more prominent ulceration of the epidermis with a perivascular infiltrate containing plasma cells, a lichenoid infiltrate, and epithelial hyperplasia [5, 13]. Silver staining of lesions will also show the presence of spirochetes at the dermal-epidermal junction.

Treatment Recommendations

CDC guidelines from 2010 recommend the use of penicillin G for the treatment of syphilis due to its long history of effectiveness proven through clinical and observational trials. The preparation, dose, and length of treatment depend upon the stage of disease and clinical manifestations. For pregnant patients, the CDC states that the only therapy with proven effectiveness is penicillin G. Therefore, pregnant women who have a penicillin allergy must be desensitized and treated with the drug. Nonpregnant patients with primary or secondary syphilis who have a penicillin allergy may be treated with doxycycline. HIV-infected persons are also a special consideration. HIV-positive patients with primary or secondary syphilis can be effectively treated with penicillin G but must be monitored regularly for 2 years to detect possible treatment failure [15].

Gonorrhea

Epidemiology

Gonorrhea is the second most common sexually transmitted infection in the USA. Infection is caused by *N. gonorrhea*, a gram-negative diplococcus. The CDC estimates an incidence of 600,000–800,000 cases per year, although most cases are unreported. Peak incidence is seen in the 15- to 24-year-old age group. Women are more often affected than men and there is a 20-fold higher incidence in African Americans than Caucasians [16]. Incidence has waxed and waned over the years with a peak after World War I and II followed by subsequent decrease after the introduction of penicillins and antibiotics [5]. The HIV epidemic and subsequent introduction of safer sexual practices also lead to a rise and subsequent fall in the incidence of gonorrhea [5].

Etiopathogenesis

The primary mode of transmission for *N. gonorrhea* is by inoculation of mucous membranes during sexual contact. Other modes of transmission are less likely but include vertical transmission and contact with fomites. *N. gonorrhea* has several virulence factors that allow for penetration into the mucous membranes and adherence to cells allowing survival within the body. Pili and Opa ligands contribute to adherence and are vital for infectivity of the bacteria [5]. Pili also contribute to resistance to killing by neutrophils [6]. Unlike other sexually transmitted infections, *N. gonorrhea* can enter host cells where it can survive and multiply. Other Opa proteins and nonsialylated lipo-oligosaccharides (LOS) appear to be important for intracellular invasion. Once *N. gonorrhea* has entered the cell, it is able to evade host immune mechanisms. Once disseminated, the bacteria are able to use other virulence mechanisms such as phospholipase and peptidases to cause tissue damage.

Clinical Manifestations

The most common presenting symptoms of gonorrhea are urethritis in men and cervicitis in women. Extragenital infection can occur, and thus other areas should be examined in anyone presenting with gonococcal infection [17]. Extragenital infection involves rectal and oropharyngeal mucosa as well as the conjunctiva due to autoinoculation from the hands to the eyes. Vertical transmission is also possible resulting in gonococcal conjunctivitis in the newborn.

Acute gonococcal urethritis in men produces copious purulent discharge and dysuria in the majority of cases, while acute cervicitis in women is asymptomatic in 50% of cases [17]. Likewise, rectal involvement in men tends to produce symptoms of pruritus, tenesmus, constipation, and discharge, while women are largely asymptomatic. The symptomatology of gonorrheal conjunctivitis has no sexual predilection and produces purulent discharge with eyelid edema. Untreated gonorrheal infections can progress to upper genital tract infections including epididymitis and pelvic inflammatory disease [17].

Oral Signs and Symptoms

Oral gonorrhea is uncommon but can present with ulcers or fiery red mucosal patches with a white pseudomembrane [18]. Gonococcal lesions may range from asymptomatic to painful and may produce severe pharyngitis [19].

Differential Diagnosis

Oral manifestations of gonorrhea are often nonspecific and thus can be confused for other disease entities. The differential diagnosis should include HSV infection, erythema multiforme, and autoimmune bullous diseases [19].

Histopathological examination of gonococcal lesions shows epidermal changes with necrosis and pustules but, rarely, demonstrates any organisms [5]. Nucleic acid amplification tests (NAATs) have become the mainstay for diagnosis for many clinicians, because culturing and performing Gram stains can be technically difficult [1].

Treatment Recommendations

Treatment guidelines for *N. gonorrhea* have changed over the years due to growing resistance patterns. Current CDC recommendations from 2012 state that first-line monotherapy is a third-generation cephalosporin, specifically ceftriaxone 250 mg given once intramuscularly plus azithromycin 1 g orally or doxycycline 100 mg orally twice daily for 7 days [20]. The addition of doxycycline has been shown to have in vitro synergistic effects with ceftriaxone as well as treating concomitant chlamydial infection, if present [21]. Patients who are penicillin allergic may be given azithromycin [20]. Efforts should be made to treat sexual contacts and to follow up with patients to monitor for treatment failure.

Tuberculosis

Epidemiology

Tuberculosis (TB) is a chronic disease caused by three pathogens from the *M. tuberculosis* complex including the acid-fast bacilli *M. tuberculosis*, *M. africanum*, and *M. bovis*. The disease mainly affects the lung where it forms necrotizing granulomas. Extrapulmonary sites include lymph nodes, pleura, bones, and joints. While tuberculosis is a global problem, the highest percentage is seen in Asia and Africa with concentration in lower socioeconomic regions. Growing drug resistance is also an emerging concern making effective treatment a challenge.

Although rates of TB are at record low in the USA, identification and treatment still poses a problem. Outbreaks tend to occur in populations with limited access to healthcare resources such as the homeless and drug users [22, 23]. Tuberculosis tends to be more common in individuals over 65 years old and in those who have emigrated to the USA from areas with endemic TB. Worldwide, TB is more common in males than females and in the younger population. In 2011, there were 8.7 million new cases of TB with the largest number of cases occurring in India and China. Coinfection with HIV has been shown to encourage progression of latent TB into active disease [24]. Likewise, studies have shown that HIV-positive individuals with TB have a greater degree of immunodeficiency and mortality [25].

Etiopathogenesis

Tuberculosis is transmitted by inhalation of droplets. Once inhaled, bacteria reach the alveoli of the lung where they are taken up by alveolar macrophages. A Th-1 CD4+ response is initiated, which in turn activates alveolar macrophages. If unable to destroy the bacteria, continuous activation of these macrophages initiates the formation of granulomas [26]. While granuloma formation is intended to suppress the spread of bacteria, *M. tuberculosis* can use it as a way to spread to uninfected macrophages [26]. The primary focus of disease will eventually calcify forming the Ghon's complex located in the midlung fields. After initial exposure, the vast majority of people exposed to TB will enter a latent phase. During this time the body's immune system remains active against the disease.

Reactivation of TB can occur following immunosuppression, illness, or idiopathically. If a person has preexisting immunity to TB, reactivation of pulmonary disease will produce an aggressive immune response leading to caseating granulomatous disease of the lungs [1].

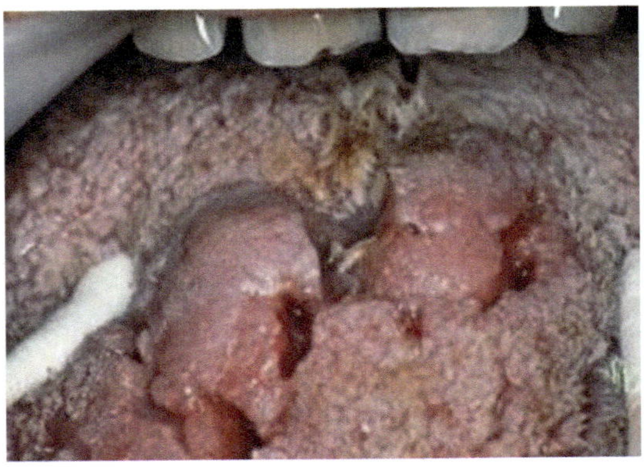

Fig. 9.5 Tuberculosis of the dorsal tongue. The Free Dictionary by Farlex

Clinical Manifestations

Clinical manifestations of TB are dependent upon the stage and organ involved. Primary TB may be asymptomatic or present with fever, shortness of breath, or nonproductive cough. Without a robust adaptive immune response, primary TB may develop into primary progressive TB. Manifestations include pulmonary TB, TB meningitis, and miliary TB. Pulmonary TB is the most common and presents as fever, night sweats, and productive cough. Extrapulmonary TB can affect any organ; some examples include pericarditis, lymphadenitis, peritonitis, and vertebral osteomyelitis.

Oral Signs and Symptoms

The oral form of TB is rare accounting for only 0.05–5% of total cases [27]. The inability of *M. tuberculosis* to penetrate intact oral and pharyngeal mucosa appears to be the reason why primary oral manifestations are so uncommon [28]. Primary lesions are more common in children and adolescents. Lesions usually involve the gingiva, gingival mucosa or extraction sites, and mucobuccal folds with associated cervical lymphadenitis [29, 30]. Case reports have also reported primary lesions of the lip, tongue, and uvula [31]. These lesions present as superficial ulcers, patches, nodules, fissures, plaques, granulomas, or verrucous proliferations [28].

Secondary lesions may be due to autoinoculation with infected sputum or due to spread of TB from another site [28]. These lesions tend to occur in middle-aged and older adults and appear as shallow-based ulcers affecting the dorsal surface of the tongue most often but also the palate, buccal mucosa, lips, salivary glands, tonsils, and uvula (Fig. 9.5) [28]. Secondary lesions also tend to be painful.

Differential Diagnosis

Oral TB ulcers can appear similar to aphthous ulcers, traumatic ulcers, syphilitic ulcers, and malignant conditions such as oral squamous cell carcinoma, lymphoma, and metastases [28]. Granulomatous diseases of the oropharynx should be considered as well including sarcoidosis, Crohn's disease, deep fungal diseases, cat scratch disease, tertiary syphilis, foreign body reactions, and Melkersson-Rosenthal syndrome [28]. Other alternative diagnoses include acute necrotizing ulcerative gingivitis and actinomycosis [31].

Treatment Recommendations

The newest treatment guidelines from the CDC for treatment of latent TB include either 12 weekly doses of isoniazid and rifapentine or 6–9 months of daily isoniazid for patients older than 12 years. Patients aged 2–11 years should receive 9 months of daily isoniazid [32].

There are many different approaches to the treatment of active TB. The CDC recommends that all patients with active TB should be started on a four-drug regimen of isoniazid, rifampin, pyrazinamide, and ethambutol for 2 months termed the initial phase. The patient then enters the continuation phase which should last for 4 or 7 months. Drug choice and duration of treatment are dependent on comorbidities such as HIV infection and severity of the disease. Drug susceptibility of the organisms should also be monitored to prevent and detect resistance [33].

Acute Necrotizing Ulcerative Gingivitis

Epidemiology

Acute necrotizing ulcerative gingivitis (ANUG), aka Vincent infection and trench mouth, is an uncommon periodontal disease that has been described for hundreds of years, especially among military recruits. A study done in 1988 found that the incidence of ANUG in the general population was 0.6% [34]. A literature review by Wade and Kerns (1998) found that ANUG is most common in young adults, with varying statistics on gender preference depending on the population studied. Additionally, incidence is higher among Caucasians and smokers [35]. Other risk factors associated with developing ANUG include poor oral hygiene, increased psychological stress, HIV infection, and malnutrition [34, 36].

Etiopathogenesis

The pathogenesis of ANUG seems to be multifactorial. Bacterial infection plays a role and is highlighted by an increase in ANUG among those with poor oral hygiene. However, it has been difficult to identify a causal relationship. One study showed evidence of spirochetes in gingival tissue by electron microscopy but did not show a causal relationship to ANUG [37]. Bacterial species that have been implicated including *Prevotella*, *Fusobacterium*, *Selenomonas*, and spirochetes such as *Treponema* and *Borrelia* [35].

Psychological stress and impaired immune function may also play a role in the pathogenesis of ANUG [38]. Elevated levels of norepinephrine caused by stress may increase vasoconstriction of the interdental papillae, leading to ischemia. Furthermore, excessive corticosteroids affect the immune response to inciting factors of ANUG [38]. Studies performed that evaluated leukocyte function found that people with ANUG had an impaired host immune response with depressed polymorphonuclear (PMN) cell responsiveness in both chemotaxis and phagocytosis [39, 40].

Smoking has also been shown to contribute to the pathogenesis of ANUG. Nicotine impairs the immune response and increases release of epinephrine from blood vessels. Increased epinephrine constricts blood vessels near the gingivae contributing to aseptic necrosis of the gingival mucosa [35].

Clinical Manifestations

In addition to the classic gingival manifestations of ANUG, patients may also present with fetor oris, lymphadenopathy, malaise, and fever [35]. Patients also report altered texture of the teeth, metallic taste, loose teeth, and ropy saliva [41].

Oral Signs and Symptoms

Signs and symptoms of ANUG are primarily oral. Lesions appear as ulcers, which may be solitary or multiple. Ulcerations appear on the gingival margin and are covered with a gray pseudomembrane [38]. In addition to ulcers, the gingival mucosa will appear erythematous and edematous and will bleed easily [42] (Fig. 9.6). A scale of seven stages of the disease has been devised and is described as follows: stage 1, necrosis of only the tip of the interdental papilla; stage 2, necrosis of the entire papilla; stage 3, necrosis also involving the marginal gingiva; stage 4, necrosis extending into the attached gingiva; stage

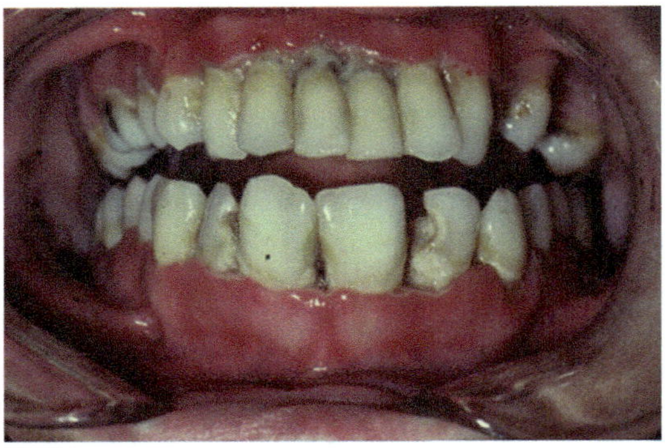

Fig. 9.6 Acute necrotizing ulcerative gingivitis. Erythematous and edematous gingiva. (Courtesy of Dr. Rochelle Torgerson)

5, necrosis extending into the buccal or labial mucosa; stage 6, necrosis exposing alveolar bone; and stage 7, necrosis perforating the skin of the cheek [43, 44].

Differential Diagnosis

The differential diagnosis for ANUG includes primary herpetic gingivostomatitis, leukemia-associated oral ulcers, desquamative gingivitis, mucous membrane pemphigoid, and HIV [35]. Additionally, ANUG may clinically resemble aphthous stomatitis, erythema multiforme, traumatic ulcers, infectious mononucleosis, agranulocytosis, secondary syphilis, and allergic stomatitis [36, 43].

The diagnosis of ANUG is based on the following clinical criteria: (1) acute necrosis and ulceration of the interdental papilla, (2) pain, and (3) bleeding [45].

Treatment Recommendations

A combination of antibacterial therapy and improved oral hygiene are recommended for the management of ANUG. Combination therapy with oral penicillin V and metronidazole for 5–10 days is recommended [38]. Tetracycline is a good alternative for patients who are penicillin-allergic. Pain can be managed with oral medication or topical viscous lidocaine. Optimizing oral hygiene, nutrition, and hydration are important in addition to eliminating inciting factors such as smoking and stress. For severe cases of ANUG, soft tissue debridement may be necessary.

Scarlet Fever

Epidemiology

Scarlet fever is caused by group A beta-hemolytic streptococcus (GAS). While infections can occur at any time in the year, incidence is highest during winter and spring. Children between the ages of 5 and 15 years of age are most commonly affected, although family members of infected children may develop the illness as well. The rash of scarlet fever occurs frequently in conjunction with streptococcal pharyngitis.

Etiopathogenesis

Infection is initiated through direct spread of large droplets and has an incubation period ranging from 12 h to 7 days. Development of the skin rash associated with scarlet fever is due to a delayed-type hypersensitivity reaction to a pyrogenic exotoxin (A, B, or C) produced by the bacteria [1]. Although antitoxin antibodies prevent recurrence of the scarlatiniform rash, the presence of three different types of exotoxin makes reinfection with GAS possible [46].

Clinical Manifestations

In addition to the characteristic rash, persons affected with scarlet fever also present with fever, sore throat, headache, vomiting, abdominal pain, and malaise. The rash of scarlet fever is characterized by confluent erythema with numerous small papules and a sandpaper-like texture. The rash begins at the head and moves downward to cover the trunk and extremities with sparing of the palms and soles. Circumoral pallor is also a feature. The rash eventually desquamates. Scarlet fever is also characterized by Pastia's lines, lin-

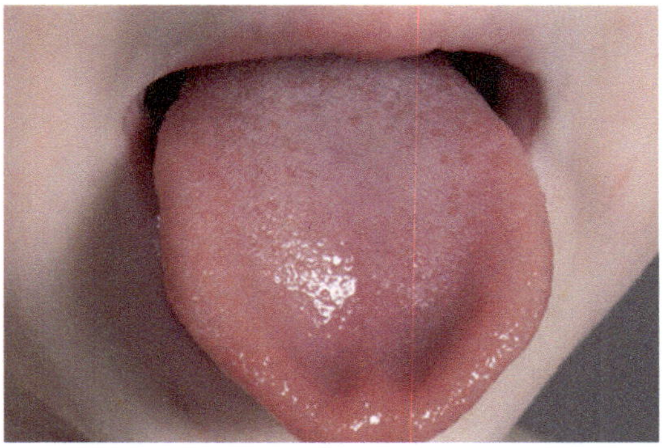

Fig. 9.7 Scarlet fever. Strawberry tongue. (Courtesy of Dr. Rochelle Torgerson)

ear petechial lesions present in the creases of the antecubital fossae and axillary lines [1].

Oral Signs and Symptoms

Oral manifestations of scarlet fever chiefly involve the tongue, although the entire mouth may be distinctively red. Initially, the tongue is coated with a yellowish white covering, which will subsequently be shed to reveal a bright red, raw appearing tongue with engorged papillae, also called "strawberry tongue." [47] (Fig. 9.7). Other oral findings include an enlarged uvula and tonsils with erythema and exudate as well as palatal erythema and petechiae [42].

Differential Diagnosis

Other causes of exanthems should be considered in the differential diagnosis of scarlet fever. Erythema infectiosum (fifth disease) is a viral exanthem that occurs in young children in the winter and spring. It causes an erythematous rash of the face and arms, and children have a "slapped cheek" appearance. Unlike scarlet fever, the rash does not concentrate in the skin folds or desquamate, and there is no oral involvement. Measles also appears as an erythematous maculopapular rash beginning on the head and moving toward the feet. Measles can be differentiated from scarlet fever by the presence of the characteristic Koplik spots in the oral mucosa. Rubella also causes a rash that can mimic scarlet fever. Again, the rash of rubella starts at the head and moves caudally. It can be differentiated from scarlet fever by the presence of palatal macules called Forchheimer spots [48]. Other viral causes of a similar exanthem include infectious mononucleosis, viral hepatitis, roseola infantum, and echovirus 14 [49]. A scarlatiniform rash may also be caused by staphylococcus. While the prodrome and exanthem may appear similarly, the rash of staphylococcal scarlet fever will be painful and will spare the tongue and palate [42]. Other bacterial causes that should be included in the differential diagnosis include staphylococcal scalded skin syndrome, secondary syphilis, toxic shock syndrome, rat-bite fever (caused by *Streptobacillus moniliformis*), and *Spirillum minus* [49].

Kawasaki disease should also be considered, which can cause a "strawberry tongue" similar to that seen in scarlet fever along with conjunctival injection and dry, cracked lips. The rash of Kawasaki disease has been described as polymorphous, urticarial-like lesions, which may appear similar to erythema multiforme [42]. Other considerations should include allergic drug reaction or juvenile rheumatoid arthritis.

The clinical signs of streptococcal infection are nonspecific, and diagnosis based on clinical findings alone is inadequate. Choices of diagnostic tests include rapid antigen detection tests, throat culture, and antistreptolysin O titer. Throat culture has a sensitivity of 90–95%; however, results are not quickly obtainable. Rapid antigen detection tests produce quicker results but have a lower sensitivity rate (80–90%). The use of antistreptolysin O titers has increased, and it is now the most commonly tested streptococcal antibody. These antibodies are not specific for GAS infection, however, and test results can be misinterpreted due to variability in age-related increases of the titers.

Treatment Recommendations

Penicillin orally remains the drug of choice for the treatment of GAS infections. Individuals who are allergic to penicillin may be given a cephalosporin, clindamycin, or a macrolide. A complete treatment course is important in order to prevent late sequelae of GAS infection including rheumatic fever.

Diphtheria

Epidemiology

Diphtheria is caused by *Corynebacterium diphtheriae*, a gram-positive pleomorphic rod. It is a disease found worldwide; however, it is concentrated in urban communities and in those with low vaccination rates such as Russia and Southeast Asia. Diphtheria is now an uncommon disease in the USA due in part to effective vaccination programs. In fact, there have been no reported cases of diphtheria in the USA since 2003 [50]. While vaccination prevents development of disease, the bacteria may still be carried in the nasopharynx allowing for continued transmission. Historically, diphtheria has been a pediatric disease; however, incidence is now higher in older age groups due in part to the institution of vaccination programs for children.

Etiopathogenesis

Spread of infection occurs either by inhalation of droplets or from contact with skin or respiratory secretions. Once transmitted, the bacteria will colonize the nasopharynx where it multiplies. The major virulence factor utilized by the bacteria is the A-B exotoxin, which interferes with elongation factor-2 (EF-2) thereby terminating host cell protein synthesis. The exotoxin causes tissue necrosis and the pseudomembrane that is characteristic of the disease [1]. The incubation period after inoculation with the bacteria is approximately 2–4 days.

Clinical Manifestations

Signs and symptoms of diphtheria infection depend on the patient's level of immunity and virulence of the organism. Diphtheria is chiefly a disease of the respiratory system and presents as sudden onset low-grade fever, sore throat, exudative pharyngitis, and malaise. A person who is partially immune will usually only experience mild respiratory symptoms, while disease in an unimmunized person may cause respiratory failure and death. The exotoxin may also cause swelling of the neck ("bull neck"), tender cervical lymphadenopathy, myocarditis, and neuritis (Fig. 9.8).

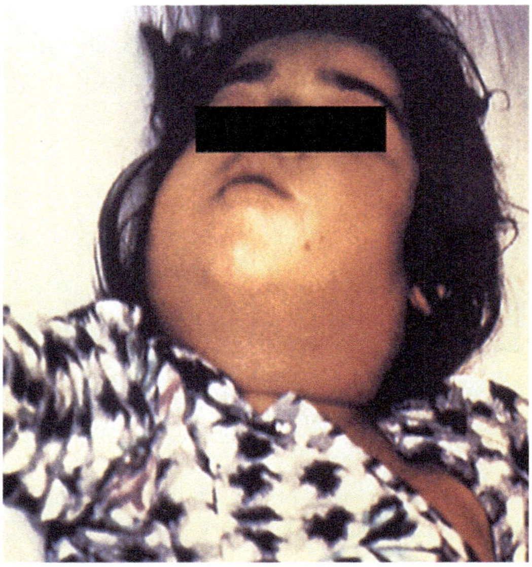

Fig. 9.8 Diphtheria. Bull neck. (Image courtesy of Centers for Disease Control and Prevention https://phil.cdc.gov/)

Oral Signs and Symptoms

The characteristic sign of diphtheria occurs in the oral cavity. The exudate produced due to the infection forms a thick gray-white pseudomembrane composed of bacteria, dead cells, and fibrin that covers the palate, uvula, and tonsils (Fig. 9.9). It adheres to the mucosa and will cause bleeding, if removed. This pseudomembrane can also spread into the nasopharynx or larynx and cause difficulty with swallowing and breathing.

Differential Diagnosis

The differential diagnosis for diphtheria includes candidiasis, ANUG, bacterial or viral pharyn-

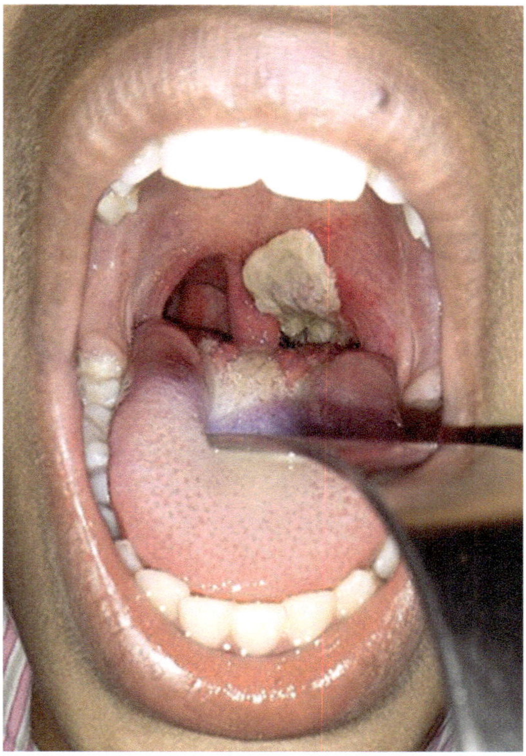

Fig. 9.9 Diphtheria. White pseudomembrane covering the hard palate. (Reprinted from Wikimedia Commons https://commons.wikimedia.org/wiki/File:Dirty_white_pseudomembrane_classically_seen_in_diphtheria_2013-07-06_11-07.jpg#filelinks)

gitis, tonsillitis, infectious mononucleosis, and acute epiglottitis [1].

Diagnosis can be made through culture of the nasopharynx and throat on a selective medium. Patients should also be tested for the presence of exotoxin. The gold standard test is Elek immunodiffusion assay but PCR analysis can also be done.

Treatment Recommendations

The mainstay of treatment continues to be diphtheria antitoxin to prevent toxin entry into cells where it will inevitably cause cell death. Antibiotic therapy includes penicillin (first-line) and erythromycin. The most effective measure, however, continues to be vaccination.

Staphylococcal Scalded Skin Syndrome

Epidemiology

Staphylococcal scalded skin syndrome (SSSS) is a potentially life-threatening disease caused by an exfoliative toxin produced by *S. aureus*. It is most commonly seen in infants and young children less than 5 years of age and carries an approximate 5% mortality rate due to significant volume loss, sepsis, and electrolyte imbalances [51]. The young tend to be disproportionately affected due to decreased renal clearance of the toxin and lack of antitoxin antibodies. However, adults with chronic renal insufficiency may be affected as well [5]. Outbreaks may occur in nurseries and daycare settings.

Etiopathogenesis

Cases of SSSS are generally caused by phage strains of *S. aureus* that produce one of two different epidermolytic exotoxins. Both toxins are serine proteases that cleave desmoglein-1 resulting in separation of the epidermal granular layer and, ultimately, bulla formation [5]. Unlike other causes of bullous disease which produce local disease, the exotoxin of SSSS spreads hematogenously causing diffuse skin involvement.

Clinical Manifestations

Clinical manifestations of SSSS appear within hours to days of infection. Prior to the onset of the exanthem, the disorder is usually mild and presents with nasopharyngitis, conjunctivitis, or impetigo. As the toxin spreads hematogenously, abrupt onset high fever and vomiting occur followed by generalized erythema spreading from head to toe. One to 3 days later, large, flaccid, bullous lesions appear that soon rupture and exhibit a positive Nikolsky sign. The toxin causes other areas of skin to cleave between the epidermis and the dermis resulting in shedding of large areas of skin. Complications of denudation include fluid loss and abnormalities of temperature regulation.

Oral Signs and Symptoms

Oral involvement is not characteristic for SSSS. Hyperemia may be present but mucosal lesions are generally not a feature.

Differential Diagnosis

The primary differential diagnosis is toxic epidermal necrolysis, which can produce a similar clinical picture to SSSS, but patients tend to be older and present with mucosal involvement. Toxic shock syndrome, also caused by staphylococcus, can appear similarly but favors adult patients, and exfoliation occurs weeks after infection [5]. Bullous variants of certain diseases should be considered including ichthyosis, pemphigus foliaceus, impetigo, epidermolysis bullosa, and bullous mastocytosis. Other differential diagnoses include sunburn, drug reaction, GVHD, or viral exanthem [5].

A diagnosis of SSSS can be made based on clinical presentation. Cultures from the bullae will generally be negative; however, cultures of the nasopharynx may be positive for *S. aureus*. Exotoxin identification may be done via latex agglutination, immunodiffusion assay, or ELISA. Histologic examination shows cleavage of the epidermis along the stratum granulosum and lack of inflammatory cells in both the bullae and the dermis.

Treatment Recommendations

New studies show that most cases of SSSS are caused by oxacillin-sensitive, clindamycin-resistant strains of *S. aureus* [52]. Despite this fact, recommendations now are for use of penicillinase-resistant antibiotics in combination with clindamycin as it has excellent skin penetration and inhibits toxin production [52]. Vancomycin is also commonly added as it has excellent coverage for MRSA [53]. Temperature regulation and volume resuscitation are an important part of supportive therapy.

Leprosy

Epidemiology

The global health burden of leprosy has decreased dramatically in recent history. The WHO reported that in 2013, there were 180,618 cases reported worldwide, a far cry from the millions of cases reported in the 1980s [54]. This dramatic decrease is due to multidrug therapy and institution of public health programs to combat the disease. The majority of cases (81%) are reported from Brazil, India, and Indonesia where the disease is endemic [54]. Because vaccines are not available, early detection and treatment are the main strategies for disease control.

Etiopathogenesis

Leprosy, also called Hansen's disease, is a chronic granulomatous disease caused by *Mycobacterium leprae*, an acid-fast, gram-positive bacillus. It is an obligate intracellular pathogen with affinity for macrophages and Schwann cells. The infection exhibits tropism for certain areas of the body such as the skin and peripheral nerves because the bacteria require cool temperatures to grow [55]. Transmissibility is poorly understood, but it is believed that patients with higher bacterial loads tend to be more infectious than others. Genetics are also thought to play a role in susceptibility to infection due to the fact that the disease is not highly contagious despite close contact with infected persons [5]. The bacilli are slow growing with a 2–12 year incubation period [56].

Clinical Manifestations

The Ridley-Jopling classification divides leprosy into categories based on clinical manifestations and bacterial load: lepromatous, tuberculoid, dimorphous, and indeterminate [56]. The WHO also developed a classification system separating the disease into paucibacillary and multibacillary based on the number of skin lesions present. Lepromatous leprosy is the most destructive and infectious form and is characterized by widespread, symmetrically distributed papules and nodules. The skin becomes thickened especially on the face and earlobes leading to coarsening of facial features called "leonine facies." Peripheral nerves are also preferentially affected causing anesthesia and a "glove and stocking" neuropathy. As the disease progresses, infiltration of the bacilli into the skin and peripheral nerves causes widespread tissue destruction leading to madarosis, lagophthalmos, saddle nose, contracture and shortening of the digits, acquired ichthyosis, and peripheral neuropathic ulcers [5] (Figs. 9.10a, b and 9.11).

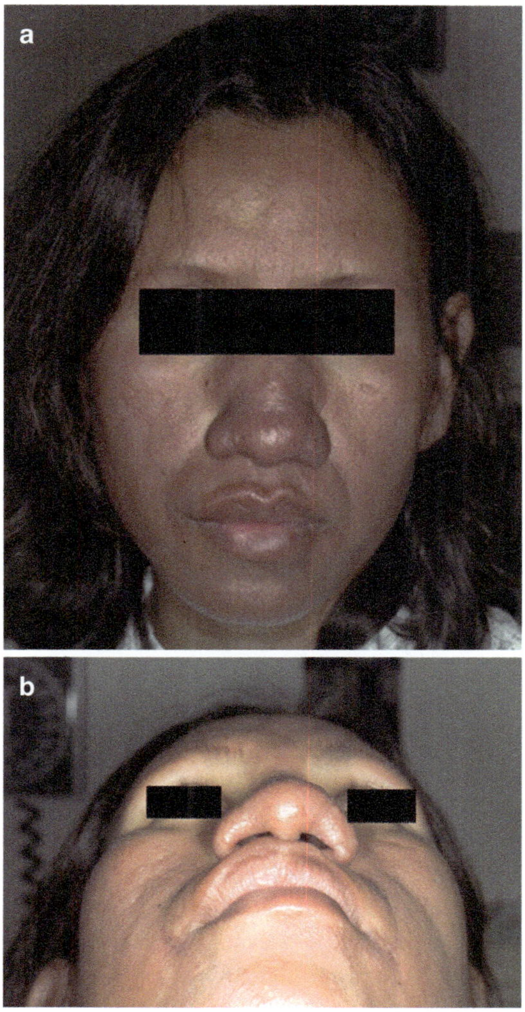

Fig. 9.10 Leprosy. Saddle nose deformity. (Courtesy of Dr. Rochelle Torgerson)

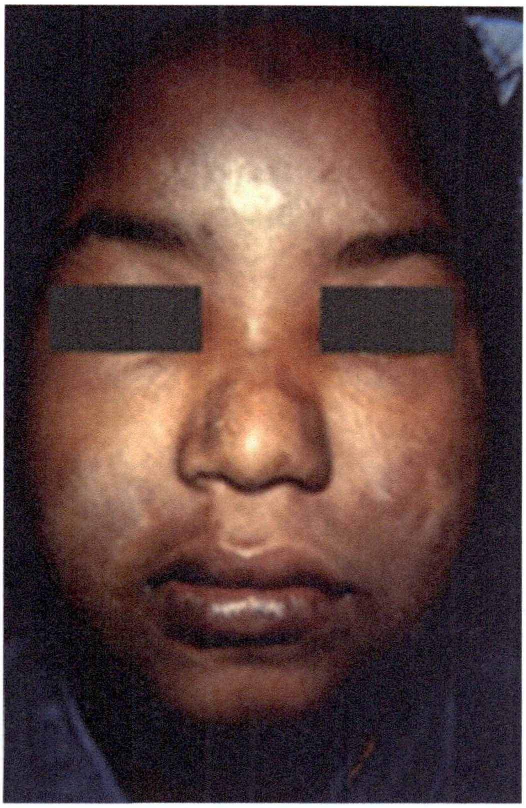

Fig. 9.11 Leprosy

The clinical manifestations of tuberculous leprosy are less severe, and lesions generally appear as scattered, well-demarcated plaques, which are often hypopigmented with an erythematous border. There will also be loss of sensation within the lesions and of the extremities as well.

Dimorphous leprosy is considered an intermediate form between lepromatous and tuberculoid and can present with features of either.

Oral Signs and Symptoms

Oral manifestations of leprosy are nonspecific and usually appear in the lepromatous form of the disease as ulcers [57, 58]. Case reports have found that the most commonly affected areas are the midline of the hard and soft palates, tongue, uvula, and gingivae [59–63]. Erythema nodosum leprosum (ENL), also referred to as a type 2 lepra reaction, is another cause of oral involvement. A lepra reaction is an immunologically mediated episode of acute or subacute inflammation. ENL has been reported to cause palatal destruction and perforation as well as bullous and necrotic lesions [64, 65].

Interestingly, isolation of bacilli from the oral cavity is difficult, and studies performed have had varying success in their ability to identify the bacteria via PCR and immunohistochemistry [58, 66].

Differential Diagnosis

The differential diagnosis for leprosy includes secondary or tertiary syphilis, cutaneous leishmaniasis, systemic lupus erythematosus, sarcoidosis, fungal infections, trauma, or malignancy [46, 67]. The presence of anesthesia within cutaneous lesions and peripheral nerve thickening should alert the examiner to the possibility of leprosy as peripheral nerve involvement is a characteristic feature.

Identification of characteristic skin lesions with sensory loss is virtually pathognomonic for leprosy. Peripheral nerve enlargement and the presence of acid-fast bacilli in the skin are not required for establishing a diagnosis and may or may not be present [46].

Treatment Recommendations

The WHO recommends multidrug therapy as the standard of treatment for anyone with leprosy. A combination of rifampicin and dapsone is used for paucibacillary disease, while patients with multibacillary disease receive combination therapy of rifampicin, dapsone, and clofazimine. Multidrug therapy helps to prevent resistance to dapsone and also to decrease the infectivity of the person being treated [68]. The WHO recommends 6 months of treatment for paucibacillary disease and 24 months of treatment for multibacillary disease [69]. Second-line agents are available and include ofloxacin, moxifloxacin, minocycline, and clarithromycin.

Gingivitis/Periodontitis

Epidemiology

Gingivitis is an extremely common condition. Reports state that most children and adults, 50–90%, have signs of the disease [70]. The incidence of severe periodontitis in adults worldwide is 5–20% [70]. It is more common in the older populations and those in lower socioeconomic groups. While development of a bacterial biofilm (plaque) is the major contributor to gingivitis, genetic and environmental factors such as smoking are also major risk factors for the development of periodontal disease [71, 72]. Gingivitis has also been shown to be exacerbated by pregnancy, diabetes mellitus, puberty, contraceptives, vitamin C deficiency, and menstruation [72].

Etiopathogenesis

Poor oral hygiene plays a major role in the development of periodontal disease. Gingivitis results when bacteria contained in plaque initiate an inflammatory response in the gingiva. Anaerobic and gram-negative bacteria have been found to have the strongest association with periodontal disease and include *Porphyromonas gingivalis*, *Actinobacillus*, *Tannerella forsythensis*, and *Treponema denticola* [72, 73]. Candida and other fungi are important causes in patients who are immunocompromised [74]. In response to invasion by bacteria and release of their toxins, immune cells including neutrophils, macrophages, plasma cells, and lymphocytes infiltrate the gingival connective tissue where they release cytokines. Inflammation results in increased vasodilation and vascular permeability leading to erythema and edema of the gingiva [75]. This stage of the disease is reversible with proper oral hygiene; however, if disease is allowed to progress to periodontitis, inflammation reaches alveolar bone resulting in bone resorption and, ultimately, tooth mobility and premature loss.

Clinical Manifestations

Clinical manifestations of gingivitis and periodontitis are mainly oral.

Oral Signs and Symptoms

Gingival discoloration and easy bleeding with or without halitosis are features of early gingivitis. Eversion of the gingival margin may also be seen, which encourages plaque formation and trauma from ingestion of food, leading to more inflammation [76] (Figs. 9.12 and 9.13). If allowed to progress, periodontitis results in tissue destruction, recession of gums, and tooth mobility. A serious complication of progressive disease is abscess formation, which can be seen in the canine, buccal, submandibular, or sublingual spaces.

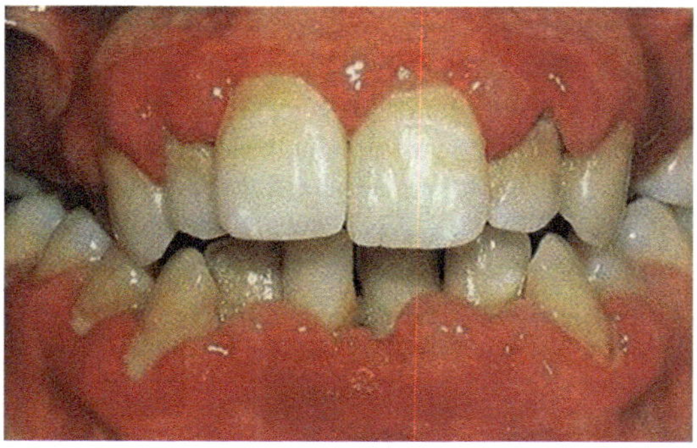

Fig. 9.12 Plaque-induced gingivitis. (Courtesy of Dr. Rochelle Torgerson)

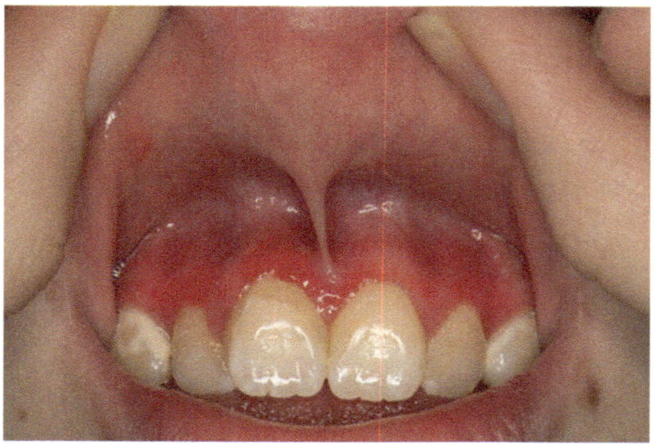

Fig. 9.13 Plaque-induced gingivitis. (Courtesy of Dr. Rochelle Torgerson)

Differential Diagnosis

Differential diagnoses include systemic diseases that have periodontal features. These include viral infections such as herpes, lichen planus, blistering disorders like pemphigus and pemphigoid, leukemia, lymphoma, tuberculosis, Wegener's granulomatosis, oral cancer, and metastatic cancer [72]. Medications like phenytoin, calcium channel blockers, and cyclosporin A may be associated with gingival enlargement [77].

The diagnosis of periodontal disease is based on clinical and radiographic features. The space between the gingiva and teeth should be 1–3 mm but will deepen as the disease progresses with increased loss of connective tissue and bone [78].

Treatment Recommendations

Periodontal disease is preventable by adhering to meticulous oral hygiene with both brushing and flossing, and periodic debulking of plaque by in-office cleanings. Minimizing risk factors such as smoking cessation and diabetes control are also effective. For cases of acute gingivitis, antibiotic therapy may be used but is only useful in combination with improvement in oral hygiene [73]. Selected antibiotics which have been recommended include metronidazole, clindamycin, tetracyclines, fluoroquinolones, and azithromycin [73]. Antibiotics are not effective for chronic gingivitis or periodontitis. Tooth destruction and premature loss are permanent consequences of chronic disease. Surgical reconstruction is the only means of repairing gingival contours and tooth loss.

Granuloma Inguinale

Epidemiology

Granuloma inguinale is caused by *Klebsiella granulomatis* and is also called donovanosis or granuloma venereum. It is a relatively rare tropical disease endemic to India, Papua New Guinea, South America, South Africa, the Caribbean, and

Australia [79, 80]. Incidence is higher in African Americans and those in lower socioeconomic communities.

Etiopathogenesis

The disease is caused by gram-negative coccobacilli that reside intracellularly within macrophages referred to as Donovan bodies. Transmission of the disease is not entirely understood. While some consider it to be a sexually transmitted infection, the occurrence in children and nonsexually active adults continues to puzzle experts [81]. The bacteria are not highly infectious, and it generally takes multiple contacts with an infected person for the disease to spread [1]. Should a person become infected, however, the bacteria invade genital and mucosal tissue where an ulcer is formed.

Clinical Manifestations

Initially, a painless granulomatous ulcer forms on the genitalia, which may bleed easily. There are four classifications of ulcers: ulcerogranulomatous, hypertrophic, necrotic, and sclerotic/cicatricial [82]. Genital and anal lesions are most common, but extragenital lesions and disseminated donovanosis occur as well. Disseminated disease is accompanied by systemic symptoms including fever, malaise, weight loss, and night sweats [80].

Infection with *K. granulomatis* increases the risk of acquiring HIV. Furthermore, coinfection with HIV makes the disease more difficult to treat resulting in persistent ulcers [80, 81].

Oral Signs and Symptoms

Oral donovanosis is well documented. The clinical appearance of the ulcers may vary making diagnosis difficult for examiners who do not encounter the disease frequently. Lesions may be purely ulcerative, granular, or cicatricial [83]. Lesions cause swelling and bleeding of the gingiva and palate and can invade underlying bone causing instability of the teeth [84–86]. Ulcers of the lips may extend into the oral cavity and cause enlargement of submental lymph nodes [87, 88]. Progression of ulcers in the posterior oropharynx can cause fistulas that extend into the neck or jaw [89].

Differential Diagnosis

Differential diagnoses should include other causes of granulomatous ulcers including cat scratch disease, tularemia, histoplasmosis, blastomycosis, and tuberculosis [90]. A case of oral donovanosis resembling actinomycosis has been reported [89]. If genital ulcers are present in addition to oral ulcers, one should consider the possibility of other sexually transmitted diseases, complex aphthosis, or Behcet disease.

Definitive diagnosis can be made by identification of Donovan bodies from a sample of the lesion fixed with Giemsa, Wright's, Leishman, or silver stain [81, 82]. Histological examination shows a dense inflammatory infiltrate with marked pseudoepitheliomatous hyperplasia [81].

Treatment Recommendations

There are several antibiotics that are effective in the treatment of donovanosis. Azithromycin and doxycycline are most commonly used; however, ciprofloxacin and trimethoprim/sulfamethoxazole have also been used, while erythromycin can be used in pregnancy. For persistent disease, an aminoglycoside can be added [79, 91].

Tularemia

Epidemiology

Tularemia is a zoonotic disease caused by *Francisella tularensis*, a gram-negative bacteria spread by animals including squirrels, rabbits, hares, muskrats, and other rodents or via bite from an arthropod [92–94]. It is found exclusively in the northern hemisphere with cases concentrated in Scandinavia, North America, Japan, Russia, Turkey, and Switzerland [92, 95–98]. Although rare, the disease is highly infectious and potentially life-threatening. Due to this fact and its ability to be aerosolized, the bacterium has been used as a weapon of bioterrorism in the past. The CDC reports that between 2001 and 2010, there were 1208 cases of tularemia in the USA with an average annual incidence of 0.041 per 100,000 persons [99]. In the USA, infection tends to be more common among whites (86%), children, and elderly males [99].

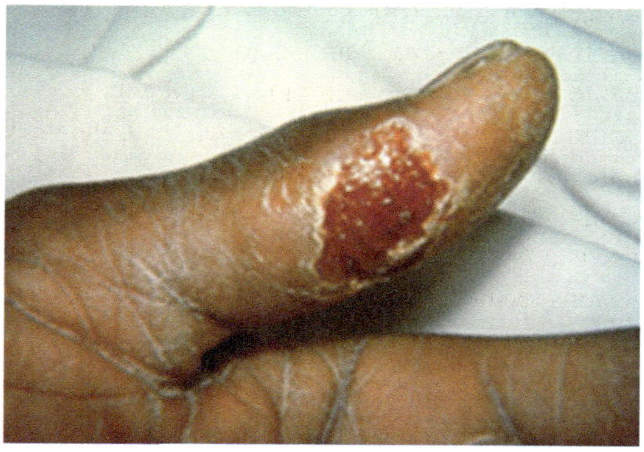

Fig. 9.14 Tularemia. Cutaneous ulcer. (Image courtesy of Centers for Disease Control and Prevention https://phil.cdc.gov/)

Etiopathogenesis

Infection by *F. tularensis* can occur through the skin, mucous membranes, gastrointestinal tract, or lungs. After entry, the incubation period is generally 3–5 days. During this time, bacteria invade macrophages and other cells where they multiply. In response, the body initiates an inflammatory response causing suppurative necrosis with polymorphonuclear cells, macrophages, and lymphocytes. Subsequently, an erythematous papule forms at the site of inoculation, which evolves into an ulcer with a necrotic base. Bacteria disseminate into the blood where they can reach the lymph nodes, spleen, liver, and lungs [1]. Granuloma formation follows once the bacteria reach the lymph nodes [46].

Clinical Manifestations

Clinical manifestations of tularemia are varied and depend upon the route of entry. The ulceroglandular form arises from the bite of an arthropod or from handling infected meat [94]. This form produces flu-like symptoms followed by a cutaneous ulcer and associated painful lymphadenopathy [94, 99] (Fig. 9.14). Glandular disease is similar but there are no cutaneous lesions. Typhoidal tularemia is difficult to diagnose, and its only manifestation is fever of unknown origin [1]. The most serious form of tularemia results from inhalation of bacteria. It produces a bronchopneumonia with dry cough, pleuritic pain, and dyspnea [1]. Infection via contaminated food or water can produce oropharyngeal or gastrointestinal symptoms. Tularemia of the eye has also been reported probably via self-inoculation from the hands. This oculoglandular form produces ulcers of the conjunctiva and can spread to surrounding lymph nodes [94]. Dermatologic signs of tularemia include erythema multiforme, urticaria, erythema nodosum, and cellulitis [100].

Oral Signs and Symptoms

Oral manifestations of tularemia occur due to consumption of contaminated water or food that has come in contact with urine or excrement from infected animals [97]. Signs of oropharyngeal tularemia include exudative tonsillopharyngitis, pharyngeal ulcers, and retropharyngeal lymphadenopathy. However, atypical cases of oropharyngeal tularemia have been reported. Uncommon presentations may appear as nonspecific pharyngitis without ulcers along with fever of unknown origin and persistent cervical lymphadenitis [101, 102]. Parapharyngeal abscess formation is another unusual presentation and may be confused with other diagnoses leading to a delay in proper treatment [103].

Differential Diagnosis

The features of oropharyngeal tularemia, mainly tonsillopharyngitis and cervical lymphadenitis, can appear similar to streptococcal and staphylococcal infections, mycobacterial infection, infectious mononucleosis, adenoviral infection, and diphtheria [55, 103]. Additionally, other causes of zoonotic infection should be considered including cat scratch disease and toxoplasmosis [104].

Definitive diagnosis of tularemia is by culturing *F. tularensis* on cysteine-enriched sheep blood agar. If culturing is unavailable, there are direct fluorescent antibody and PCR methods for identifying the bacterium.

Treatment Recommendations

Aminoglycosides (streptomycin or gentamicin) are first-line treatment for patients with severe tularemia. For mild to moderate disease, fluoroquinolones (ciprofloxacin or levofloxacin) are preferred [105]. Tetracyclines can be used for patients older than 8 years, but these are considered second-line therapy with a higher incidence of relapse [105]. Beta-lactams and macrolides are not effective against tularemia.

Cat Scratch Disease

Epidemiology

Cat scratch disease (CSD) is a zoonotic infection of cats caused by the *Bartonella* species, most commonly *Bartonella henselae*. Humans become infected after exposure to an infected cat either by scratch or bite. Fleas appear to be a vector, transferring infection between cats. In one study performed using a national database, the annual incidence of CSD in the USA was approximately 9.3 cases per 100,000 (22,000 cases) [106]. Peak incidence occurs in the fall, and winter seasons and infection seem to be more common in whites and males [106]. While CSD is one of the most common causes of chronic lymphadenopathy in children, overall infection occurs more often in adults.

Etiopathogenesis

Following inoculation, bacteria cause a local infection by disseminating to regional lymph nodes. The bacteria invade endothelial cells, thus initiating an inflammatory response marked by release of pro-inflammatory cytokines [107]. Subsequently, a granulomatous infiltrate develops in the lymph nodes. The immune system is generally able to control infection and bacterial isolation is rare [1]. Despite bacterial clearance within 1–2 weeks of infection, CSD causes a chronic but self-limited lymphadenitis. Occasionally, the bacteria may become blood-borne leading to visceral organ involvement and neuroretinitis.

Clinical Manifestations

In the immunocompetent patient, CSD first appears as a round, non-tender papule 3–10 days after the scratch. Systemic symptoms are not characteristic of the disease. Regional lymph nodes draining the area become enlarged and tender approximately 1–2 weeks after infection. Axillary and epitrochlear nodes are most commonly affected, with decreasing frequency in the head/neck and groin regions [108]. Although usually a self-limited process, chronic regional lymphadenitis may develop and can last for 12–24 months.

Visceral organ involvement is not uncommon and includes necrotizing granulomas of the liver or spleen [109]. Infection may also appear as fever of unknown origin. An analysis of 146 children by Jacobs and Schutze (1998) found that *B. henselae* was the third most common infectious cause of fever of unknown origin [110].

Atypical manifestations of CSD include hypercalcemia, encephalitis, pulmonary disease, thrombocytopenia, erythema nodosum, neuritis, neuroretinitis, and osteomyelitis [106, 108]. Parinaud's oculoglandular syndrome is the most common manifestation of ocular CSD and appears as a necrotic granuloma with ulceration of the conjunctiva. Patients complain of increased tear production and a foreign body sensation [111]. Immunodeficient patients are at risk of developing bacillary angiomatosis.

Oral Signs and Symptoms

Primary CSD of the mouth and mucous membranes has been reported and appears as an oral ulcer [112, 113]. Perioral areas should be inspected as well. Case reports have identified patients presenting with submandibular, submental, and parotid masses associated with CSD [114, 115]. Facial nerve palsy has been reported as a complication of CSD-induced parotid swelling [116].

Differential Diagnosis

The differential diagnosis of oral CSD should include other zoonotic infections including tularemia and toxoplasmosis. A diagnosis of CSD is based on clinical features and can be confirmed by serology. Serology via indirect immunofluorescent antibody assay can be used to establish a diagnosis. However, these serologic tests are not always sensitive enough to detect *B. henselae* antibodies [117]. On histopathology of a lymph node biopsy, CSD is characterized by microabscesses with reticulohistiocytic cells [118]. The presence of pleomorphic rod-shaped bacilli when stained with Warthin-Starry silver stain will confirm the diagnosis.

Treatment Recommendations

Most antibiotics have been proven ineffective in the treatment of CSD; therefore, mild cases can be managed without treatment. In fact, most cases of lymphadenopathy will resolve spontaneously in 2–4 months. For the immunocompetent patient with severe disease, however, azithromycin, rifampin, ciprofloxacin, or trimethoprim-sulfamethoxazole can be tried for 5–14 days [117]. Disease in the immunocompromised patient can be treated with macrolides, fluoroquinolones, rifampin, or gentamicin [119].

References

1. Goldman L, Schafter AI, editors. Cecil medicine: expert consult – online. Philadelphia: Elsevier Health Sciences; 2011.
2. Goldman L, Schafter AI, editors. Goldman's Cecil medicine. 24th ed. Philadelphia: Elsevier Saunders; 2012.
3. James WD, Berger T, Elston D. Andrew's diseases of the skin: clinical dermatology. Philadelphia: Elsevier Health Sciences; 2011.
4. Mandell GL, Bennett JE, Dolin R. Mandell, Douglas, and Bennett's principles and practice of infectious diseases. Philadelphia: Churchill Livingstone/Elsevier; 2010.
5. Bolognia JL, Jorizzo JL, Schaffer JV. Dermatology. UK: Elsevier Health Sciences; 2012.
6. Andreoli TE, et al. Andreoli and Carpenter's Cecil essentials of medicine. Philadelphia: Elsevier Health Sciences; 2010.
7. Schwarzenberger K, Werchniak AE, Ko CJ, editors. General dermatology. Edinburgh: Elsevier Limited; 2009.
8. Goering RV, Mims CA. Mims' medical microbiology. Philadelphia: Mosby Elsevier; 2008.
9. Leuci S, Martina S, Adamo D, Ruoppo E, Santarelli A, Sorrentino R, et al. Oral syphilis: a retrospective analysis of 12 cases and a review of the literature. Oral Dis. 2013;19(8):738–46. https://doi.org/10.1111/odi.12058.
10. Kent ME, Romanelli F. Reexamining syphilis: an update on epidemiology, clinical manifestations, and management. Ann Pharmacother. 2008;42(2):226–36. https://doi.org/10.1345/aph.1K086.
11. Drago F, Ciccarese G, Cogorno L, Tomasini CF, Cozzani EC, Riva SF, et al. Primary syphilis of the oropharynx: unusual location of a chancre. Int J STD AIDS. 2014; https://doi.org/10.1177/0956462414551235.
12. Hertel M, Matter D, Schmidt-Westhausen AM, Bornstein MM. Oral syphilis: a series of 5 cases. J Oral Maxillofac Surg. 2014;72(2):338–45. https://doi.org/10.1016/j.joms.2013.07.015.
13. Ficarra G, Carlos R. Syphilis: the renaissance of an old disease with oral implications. Head Neck Pathol. 2009;3(3):195–206. https://doi.org/10.1007/s12105-009-0127-0.
14. Captline AM, White NS, Merkow LP, Snyder SP. Atrophic luetic glossitis. Report of a case. Oral Surg Oral Med Oral Pathol. 1970;30(2):192–5. https://doi.org/10.1016/0030-4220(70)90360-9.
15. Centers for Disease Control and Prevention. Sexually transmitted diseases treatment guidelines. MMWR Morb Mortal Wkly Rep. 2010;59(RR-12):1–110.

16. Bolognia JL, Jorizzo JL, Schaffer JV, editors. Dermatology. 3rd ed. London: Elsevier Limited; 2012.
17. Skerlev M, Culav-Koscak I. Gonorrhea: new challenges. Clin Dermatol. 2014;32(2):275–81. https://doi.org/10.1016/j.clindermatol.2013.08.010.
18. Randle HW. Treatment of oral ulcers. Dermatol Clin. 1993;11(4):801–8.
19. Bruce AJ, Rogers RS 3rd. Oral manifestations of sexually transmitted diseases. Clin Dermatol. 2004;22(6):520–7. https://doi.org/10.1016/j.clindermatol.2004.07.005.
20. Centers for Disease Control and Prevention (CDC). Update to CDC's sexually transmitted diseases treatment guidelines, 2010: oral cephalosporins no longer a recommended treatment for gonococcal infections. MMWR Morb Mortal Wkly Rep. 2012;61(31):590–4.
21. Bignell C, Fitzgerald M. UK national guideline for the management of gonorrhoea in adults, 2011. Int J STD AIDS. 2011;22(10):541–7. https://doi.org/10.1258/ijsa.2011.011267.
22. Centers for Disease Control and Prevention (CDC). Tuberculosis outbreak associated with a homeless shelter – Kane County, Illinois, 2007–2011. MMWR Morb Mortal Wkly Rep. 2012;61(11):186–9.
23. Centers for Disease Control and Prevention (CDC). Notes from the field: tuberculosis cluster associated with homelessness – Duval County, Florida, 2004–2012. MMWR Morb Mortal Wkly Rep. 2012;61(28):539–40.
24. Kaplan JE, Benson C, Holmes KK, Brooks JT, Pau A, Masur H, et al. Guidelines for prevention and treatment of opportunistic infections in HIV-infected adults and adolescents: recommendations from CDC, the National Institutes of Health, and the HIV Medicine Association of the Infectious Diseases Society of America. MMWR Recomm Rep. 2009;58(Rr-4):1–207.. quiz CE1-4
25. Toossi Z, Mayanja-Kizza H, Hirsch CS, Edmonds KL, Spahlinger T, Hom DL, et al. Impact of tuberculosis (TB) on HIV-1 activity in dually infected patients. Clin Exp Immunol. 2001;123(2):233–8. https://doi.org/10.1046/j.1365-2249.2001.01401.x.
26. Brighenti S, Andersson J. Local immune responses in human tuberculosis: learning from the site of infection. J Infect Dis. 2012;205(Suppl 2):S316–24. https://doi.org/10.1093/infdis/jis043.
27. Mignogna MD, Muzio LL, Favia G, Ruoppo E, Sammartino G, Zarrelli C, et al. Oral tuberculosis: a clinical evaluation of 42 cases. Oral Dis. 2000;6(1):25–30.
28. Verma S, Prakash R, Mohan S, Singh U, Agarwal N. Primary oral tuberculosis. BMJ Case Rep. 2013; https://doi.org/10.1136/bcr-2013-010276.
29. Ishikawa H, Hyo Y, Ono T. Tuberculous submandibular lymphadenitis. J Oral Maxillofac Surg. 1982;40(5):302–5. https://doi.org/10.1016/0278-2391(82)90224-5.
30. Popowich L, Heydt S. Tuberculous cervical lymphadenitis. J Oral Maxillofac Surg. 1982;40(8):522–4. https://doi.org/10.1016/0278-2391(82)90017-9.
31. Garg RK, Singhal P. Primary tuberculosis of the tongue: a case report. J Contemp Dent Pract. 2007;8(4):74–80. https://doi.org/10.1016/S0278-2391(89)80019-9.
32. Centers for Disease Control and Prevention (CDC). Recommendations for use of an isoniazid-rifapentine regimen with direct observation to treat latent Mycobacterium tuberculosis infection. MMWR Morb Mortal Wkly Rep. 2011;60(48):1650–3.
33. American Thoracic Society, CDC, Infectious Diseases Society of America. Treatment of tuberculosis. MMWR Recomm Rep. 2003;52(Rr-11):1–77.
34. Melnick SL, Roseman JM, Engel D, Cogen RB. Epidemiology of acute necrotizing ulcerative gingivitis. Epidemiol Rev. 1988;10:191–211.
35. Wade DN, Kerns DG. Acute necrotizing ulcerative gingivitis-periodontitis: a literature review. Mil Med. 1998;163(5):337–42.
36. Osuji OO. Necrotizing ulcerative gingivitis and cancrum oris (noma) in Ibadan. Niger J Periodontol. 1990;61(12):769–72. https://doi.org/10.1902/jop.1990.61.12.769.
37. Listgarten MA. Electron microscopic observations on the bacterial flora of acute necrotizing ulcerative gingivitis. J Periodontol. 1965;36:328–39. https://doi.org/10.1902/jop.1965.36.4.328.
38. Turnbull RS. Periodontal disease part IV: periodontal infections. Can Fam Physician. 1988;34:1399–400.
39. Cogen RB, Stevens AW Jr, Cohen-Cole S, Kirk K, Freeman A. Leukocyte function in the etiology of acute necrotizing ulcerative gingivitis. J Periodontol. 1983;54(7):402–7. https://doi.org/10.1902/jop.1983.54.7.402.
40. Claffey N, Russell R, Shanley D. Peripheral blood phagocyte function in acute necrotizing ulcerative gingivitis. J Periodontal Res. 1986;21(3):288–97. https://doi.org/10.1111/j.1600-0765.1986.tb01461.x.
41. Horning GM, Cohen ME. Necrotizing ulcerative gingivitis, periodontitis, and stomatitis: clinical staging and predisposing factors. J Periodontol. 1995;66(11):990–8. https://doi.org/10.1902/jop.1995.66.11.990.
42. Zitelli BJ, McIntire SC, Nowalk AJ. Zitelli and Davis' atlas of pediatric physical diagnosis: expert consult – online. Philadelphia: Elsevier Health Sciences; 2012.
43. Pindborg JJ, Bhat M, Roed-Petersen B. Oral changes in South Indian children with severe protein deficiency. J Periodontol. 1967;38(3):218–21.
44. Uohara GI, Knapp MJ. Oral fusospirochetosis and associated lesions. Oral Surg Oral Med Oral Pathol. 1967;24(1):113–23. https://doi.org/10.1016/0030-4220(67)90297-6.
45. Falkler WA Jr, Martin SA, Vincent JW, Tall BD, Nauman RK, Suzuki JB. A clinical, demographic and microbiologic study of ANUG patients in an urban dental school. J Clin Periodontol. 1987;14(6):307–14. https://doi.org/10.1111/j.1600-051X.1987.tb00976.x.
46. Kliegman R. Nelson textbook of pediatrics. Philadelphia: Elsevier/Saunders; 2011.

47. Habif TP. Clinical dermatology. Philadelphia: Elsevier Health Sciences; 2009.
48. Ferri FF. Ferri's color atlas and text of clinical medicine. Philadelphia: Saunders/Elsevier; 2009.
49. Baren JM, Rothrock S, Brennan J, Brown L. Pediatric emergency medicine. Philadelphia: Elsevier Health Sciences; 2007.
50. Murray PR, Rosenthal KS, Pfaller MA. Medical microbiology. Philadelphia: Elsevier Health Sciences; 2012.
51. Berk DR, Bayliss SJ. MRSA, staphylococcal scalded skin syndrome, and other cutaneous bacterial emergencies. Pediatr Ann. 2010;39(10):627–33. https://doi.org/10.3928/00904481-20100922-02.
52. Braunstein I, Wanat KA, Abuabara K, McGowan KL, Yan AC, Treat JR. Antibiotic sensitivity and resistance patterns in pediatric staphylococcal scalded skin syndrome. Pediatr Dermatol. 2014;31(3):305–8. https://doi.org/10.1111/pde.12195.
53. Marx J, Hockberger R, Walls R. Rosen's emergency medicine – concepts and clinical practice. Philadelphia: Elsevier Health Sciences; 2013.
54. Global leprosy update, 2013; reducing disease burden. Wkly Epidemiol Rec 2014;89(36): 389–400.
55. Cohen J, Opal SM, Powderly WG. Infectious diseases. Philadelphia: Elsevier – Health Sciences Division; 2010.
56. Rodrigues LC, Lockwood D. Leprosy now: epidemiology, progress, challenges, and research gaps. Lancet Infect Dis. 2011;11(6):464–70. https://doi.org/10.1016/S1473-3099(11)70006-8.
57. Motta AC, Komesu MC, Silva CH, Arruda D, Simão JC, Zenha EM, et al. Leprosy-specific oral lesions: a report of three cases. Med Oral Pathol Oral Cir Bucal. 2008;13(8):E479–82.
58. de Abreu MA, Michalany NS, Weckx LL, Neto Pimentel DR, Hirata CH, de Avelar Alchorne MM. The oral mucosa in leprosy: a clinical and histopathological study. Braz J Otorhinolaryngol. 2006;72(3):312–6.
59. Dhawan AK, Verma P, Sharma S. Oral lesions in leprosy revisited: a case report. Am J Dermatopathol. 2012;34(6):666–7. https://doi.org/10.1097/DAD.0b013e3182485bcc.
60. Girdhar BK, Desikan KV. A clinical study of the mouth in untreated lepromatous patients. Lepr Rev. 1979;50(1):25–35.
61. Bucci F Jr, Mesa M, Schwartz RA, McNeil G, Lambert WC. Oral lesions in lepromatous leprosy. J Oral Med. 1987;42(1):4–6.
62. Scheepers A, Lemmer J, Lownie JF. Oral manifestations of leprosy. Lepr Rev. 1993;64(1): 37–43.
63. Costa A, Nery J, Oliveira M, Cuzzi T, Silva M. Oral lesions in leprosy. Indian J Dermatol Venereol Leprol. 2003;69(6):381–5.
64. Swain JP, Soud A, Agarwal SK. Necrotic erythema nodosum leprosum with oral mucosal involvement. Indian J Lepr. 2008;80(2):175–8.
65. Scheepers A, Lemmer J. Erythema nodosum leprosum: a possible cause of oral destruction in leprosy. Int J Lepr Other Mycobact Dis. 1992;60(4):641–3.. doi: 1299716
66. Martinez TS, Figueira MM, Costa AV, Gonçalves MA, Goulart LR, Goulart IM. Oral mucosa as a source of Mycobacterium leprae infection and transmission, and implications of bacterial DNA detection and the immunological status. Clin Microbiol Infect. 2011;17(11):1653–8. https://doi.org/10.1111/j.1469-0691.2010.03453.x.
67. Chimenos Kustner E, Pascual Cruz M, Pinol Dansis C, Vinals Iglesias H, Rodríguez de Rivera Campillo ME, López López J. Lepromatous leprosy: a review and case report. Med Oral Patol Oral Cir Bucal. 2006;11(6):E474–9.
68. Ishii N, Barua S, Mori S, Nagaoka Y, Suzuki K. Report of the tenth meeting of the WHO Technical Advisory Group on Leprosy Control. Nihon Hansenbyo Gakkai Zasshi. 2010;79(1):37–42.
69. Chemotherapy of leprosy. Report of a WHO Study Group. World Health Organ Tech Rep Ser 1994;847:1–24.
70. Petersen PE, Bourgeois D, Ogawa H, Estupinan-Day S, Ndiaye C. The global burden of oral diseases and risks to oral health. Bull World Health Organ. 2005;83(9):661–9.
71. Tomar SL, Asma S. Smoking-attributable periodontitis in the United States: findings from NHANES III. National Health and Nutrition Examination Survey. J Periodontol. 2000;71(5):743–51. https://doi.org/10.1902/jop.2000.71.5.743.
72. Pihlstrom BL, Michalowicz BS, Johnson NW. Periodontal diseases. Lancet. 2005;366 (9499):1809–20. https://doi.org/10.1016/S0140-6736(05)67728-8.
73. Slots J. Systemic antibiotics in periodontics. J Periodontol. 2004;75(11):1553–65. https://doi.org/10.1902/jop.2004.75.11.1553.
74. Robinson PG. The significance and management of periodontal lesions in HIV infection. Oral Dis. 2002;8(Suppl 2):91–7. https://doi.org/10.1034/j.1601-0825.2002.00019.x.
75. Newman MG, et al. Carranza's clinical periodontology. Philadelphia: Elsevier – Health Sciences Division; 2014.
76. Quick CRG, et al. Essential surgery: problems, diagnosis, and management. Philadelphia: Elsevier – Health Sciences Division; 2013.
77. Marshall RI, Bartold PM. A clinical review of drug-induced gingival overgrowths. Aust Dent J. 1999;44(4):219–32. https://doi.org/10.1111/j.1834-7819.1999.tb00224.x.
78. Pihlstrom BL. Measurement of attachment level in clinical trials: probing methods. J Periodontol. 1992;63(12 Suppl):1072–7. https://doi.org/10.1902/jop.1992.63.12s.1072.
79. Markle W, Conti T, Kad M. Sexually transmitted diseases. Prim Care. 2013;40(3):557–87. https://doi.org/10.1016/j.pop.2013.05.001.

80. Velho PE, Souza EM, Belda JW. Donovanosis. Braz J Infect Dis. 2008;12(6):521–5. https://doi.org/10.1590/S1413-86702008000600015.
81. O'Farrell N. Donovanosis. Sex Transm Infect. 2002;78(6):452–7. https://doi.org/10.1136/sti.78.6.452.
82. O'Farrell N, Moi H. European guideline for the management of donovanosis, 2010. Int J STD AIDS. 2010;21(9):609–10. https://doi.org/10.1258/ijsa.2010.010245.
83. Rajendran R, Sivapathasundharam B. Shafer's textbook of oral pathology. Philadelphia: Elsevier/Reed Elsevier; 2012.
84. Hanna CB, Pratt-Thomas HR. Extragenital granuloma venereum; report of six cases of lip, oral and cutaneous involvement with review of literature. S Med J. 1948;41(9):776–82.
85. Doddridge M, Muirhead R. Donovanosis of the oral cavity. Case report. Aust Dent J. 1994;39(4):203–5. https://doi.org/10.1111/j.1834-7819.1994.tb04776.x.
86. Brain P. Granuloma inguinale with extensive oral involvement. S Afr Med J. 1951;25(33):581–2.
87. Veeranna S, Raghu TY. Oral donovanosis. Int J STD AIDS. 2002;13(12):855–6. https://doi.org/10.1258/095646202321020170.
88. Hart G. Donovanosis. Clin Infect Dis. 1997;25(1):24–30.. quiz 31-2
89. Coovadia YM, Steinberg JL, Kharsany A. Granuloma inguinale (donovanosis) of the oral cavity. A case report. S Afr Med J. 1985;68(11):815–7.
90. Wysocki GP, Brooke RI. Oral manifestations of chronic granulomatous disease. Oral Surg Oral Med Oral Pathol. 1978;46(6):815–9. https://doi.org/10.1016/0030-4220(78)90313-4.
91. Workowski KA, Berman S. Sexually transmitted diseases treatment guidelines, 2010. MMWR Recomm Rep. 2010;59(Rr-12):1–110.
92. Boyce JM. Recent trends in the epidemiology of tularemia in the United States. J Infect Dis. 1975;131(2):197–9.
93. Tarnvik A, Sandstrom G, Sjostedt A. Epidemiological analysis of tularemia in Sweden 1931–1993. FEMS Immunol Med Microbiol. 1996;13(3):201–4. https://doi.org/10.1111/j.1574-695X.1996.tb00237.x.
94. Ellis J, Oyston PC, Green M, Titball RW. Tularemia. Clin Microbiol Rev. 2002;15(4):631–46. https://doi.org/10.1128/CMR.15.4.631-646.2002.
95. Berdal BP, Mehl R, Meidell NK, Lorentzen-Styr AM, Scheel O. Field investigations of tularemia in Norway. FEMS Immunol Med Microbiol. 1996;13(3):191–5. https://doi.org/10.1111/j.1574-695X.1996.tb00235.x.
96. Ohara Y, Sato T, Fujita H, Ueno T, Homma M. Clinical manifestations of tularemia in Japan – analysis of 1,355 cases observed between 1924 and 1987. Infection. 1991;19(1):14–7. https://doi.org/10.1007/BF01643750.
97. Gurcan S. Epidemiology of tularemia. Balkan Med J. 2014;31(1):3–10. https://doi.org/10.5152/balkanmedj.2014.13117.
98. Pilo P, Johansson A, Frey J. Identification of Francisella tularensis cluster in central and western Europe. Emerg Infect Dis. 2009;15(12):2049–51. https://doi.org/10.3201/eid1512.080805.
99. Tularemia – United States, 2001–2010. MMWR Morb Mortal Wkly Rep 2013;62(47):963–6.
100. Senel E, Satilmis O, Acar B. Dermatologic manifestations of tularemia: a study of 151 cases in the mid-Anatolian region of Turkey. Int J Dermatol. 2014; https://doi.org/10.1111/ijd.12431.
101. Polat M, Kara SS, Tapısız A, Tezer H. Unusual presentation of oropharyngeal tularemia: a case report. Vector Borne Zoonotic Dis. 2013;13(5):337–9. https://doi.org/10.1089/vbz.2012.1184.
102. Dentan C, Pavese P, Pelloux I, Boisset S, Brion JP, Stahl JP, et al. Treatment of tularemia in pregnant woman. France Emerg Infect Dis. 2013;19(6):996–8. https://doi.org/10.3201/eid1906.130138.
103. Koc S, Gürbüzler L, Yaman H, Eyibilen A, Salman N, Ekici A. Tularaemia presenting as parapharyngeal abscess: case presentation. J Laryngol Otol. 2012;126(5):535–7. https://doi.org/10.1017/S0022215112000096.
104. Dlugaiczyk J, Harrer T, Zwerina J, Traxdorf M, Schwarz S, Splettstoesser W, et al. Oropharyngeal tularemia – a differential diagnosis of tonsillopharyngitis and cervical lymphadenitis. Wien Klin Wochenschr. 2010;122(3–4):110–4. https://doi.org/10.1007/s00508-009-1274-8.
105. Boisset S, Caspar Y, Sutera V, Maurin M. New therapeutic approaches for treatment of tularaemia: a review. Front Cell Infect Microbiol. 2014;4:40. https://doi.org/10.3389/fcimb.2014.00040.
106. Jackson LA, Perkins BA, Wenger JD. Cat scratch disease in the United States: an analysis of three national databases. Am J Public Health. 1993;83(12):1707–11.
107. Dehio C. Molecular and cellular basis of bartonella pathogenesis. Annu Rev Microbiol. 2004;58:365–90. https://doi.org/10.2105/AJPH.83.12.1707.
108. Cook GC, Zumla A. Manson's tropical diseases. Philadelphia: Saunders; 2009.
109. Arisoy ES, et al. Hepatosplenic cat-scratch disease in children: selected clinical features and treatment. Clin Infect Dis. 1999;28(4):778–84.. NO DOI
110. Jacobs RF, Schutze GE. Bartonella henselae as a cause of prolonged fever and fever of unknown origin in children. Clin Infect Dis. 1998;26(1):80–4.. NO DOI
111. Farrar J, et al. Manson's tropical diseases: expert consult – online. UK: Elsevier Health Sciences; 2013.
112. Margileth AM. Dermatologic manifestations and update of cat scratch disease. Pediatr Dermatol. 1988;5(1):1–9. https://doi.org/10.1111/j.1525-1470.1988.tb00876.x.
113. Moriarty RA, Margileth AM. Cat scratch disease. Infect Dis Clin N Am. 1987;1(3):575–90.

114. Steiner M, Gould A, Wilkie W, Porter K. Cat-scratch disease in the submandibular region: report of a case. J Oral Maxillofac Surg. 1994;52(6):614–8. https://doi.org/10.1016/0278-2391(94)90100-7.
115. Mintz SM, Anavi Y. Cat scratch fever presenting as a submental swelling. J Oral Maxillofac Surg. 1988;46(11):1015–8. https://doi.org/10.1016/0278-2391(88)90343-6.
116. Premachandra DJ, Milton CM. Cat scratch disease in the parotid gland presenting with facial paralysis. Br J Oral Maxillofac Surg. 1990;28(6):413–5. https://doi.org/10.1016/0266-4356(90)90042-J.
117. Margileth AM. Recent advances in diagnosis and treatment of cat scratch disease. Curr Infect Dis Rep. 2000;2(2):141–6. https://doi.org/10.1007/s11908-000-0026-8.
118. Brunetti E, Fabbi M, Ferraioli G, Prati P, Filice C, Sassera D, et al. Cat-scratch disease in Northern Italy: atypical clinical manifestations in humans and prevalence of Bartonella infection in cats. Eur J Clin Microbiol Infect Dis. 2013;32(4):531–4. https://doi.org/10.1007/s10096-012-1769-5.
119. Conrad DA. Treatment of cat-scratch disease. Curr Opin Pediatr. 2001;13(1):56–9.

10 Oral Signs of Tropical, Fungal, and Parasitic Diseases

Ricardo Pérez-Alfonzo, Silvio Alencar-Marques, Elda Giansante, and Antonio Guzmán-Fawcett

Introduction

The tropical or equatorial regions include those regions of the world between the two North 23° parallels, Tropic of Cancer, and 23° South, where the difference between seasons occurs as a function of the amount of rainfall, expressed as the dry season and rainy season.

The absence of the four independent seasons, as seen in the Northern and Southern hemispheres, combined with the environmental humidity alternating with extreme draught, defines a characteristic infectious pathology.

The tropics and subtropics comprise about 74% of the world population. A large part of the diseases seen in the world's tropical regions are related to poor public health conditions, originating from poverty. Infectious and parasitic diseases along with emergent diseases such as AIDS constitute the majority of tropical dermatoses. More prevalent dermatologic conditions are mycoses, parasitoses, mycobacterioses, and treponematoses. The present chapter focuses on tropical diseases, which have the greatest mucocutaneous compromise.

R. Pérez-Alfonzo (✉)
Dermatologic Program, "Jacinto Convit" Institute of Biomedicine, Central University of Venezuela, Caracas, Venezuela

S. Alencar-Marques
Department of Dermatology and Radiotherapy, Botucatu School of Medicine – São Paulo State University (UNESP), Botucatu, Brazil

E. Giansante
University Hospital Caracas, Central University of Venezuela, Caracas, Venezuela

A. Guzmán-Fawcett
Pierre Fauchard Faculty of Dentistry, Autonomous University of Paraguay, Asunción, Paraguay

Candidiasis

Candidiasis is caused by opportunistic yeasts from the genus *Candida*, most frequently, *C. albicans*. It typically affects the skin and oral and genital mucous membranes. In some extreme cases such as in immunosuppressed patients, it can lead to more widespread infection and invade deeper tissues, producing systemic candidiasis [1].

Under certain environmental conditions such as those prevalent in tropical areas, high humidity and heat, *Candida*, which is usually part of the normal human flora, can proliferate becoming pathogenic. In addition, antibiotic therapy, which alters the normal equilibrium of the bacterial flora and immunosuppressive agents such as corticosteroids, can lead to candida infection. Other risk factors include pregnancy, obesity, and diabetes [1, 2].

Etiopathogenesis

Candida is part of the normal flora of the gastrointestinal and genital mucous membranes.

N. Fazel (ed.), *Oral Signs of Systemic Disease*, https://doi.org/10.1007/978-3-030-10863-2_10

Table 10.1 Candidiasis: predisposing factors [3]

Physiologic factors	
Pregnancy	
Menopause	
Prematurity	
Drugs	*Diseases*
Antibiotics	Diabetes mellitus
Steroids	Acquired immune deficiency syndrome (AIDS)
Immunosuppressive drugs	Thyroid disease
Oral contraceptives	
Local factors	
pH changes in the oral and vaginal mucosa	
Poor oral hygiene	
Poor dentition	
Ill-fitting dentures or dental prostheses	
Colonization of dental prosthesis	
Xerostomia	
Direct contact with products high in sugars (i.e., bakers, fruit-packers)	
Finger sucking	
Fingernail biting	
Overzealous manicures and pedicures	
Factors specific for oral candidiasis	
Radiation therapy	
Vitamin deficiencies (B_2, B_3, B_6, B_{12}, C, and folic acid)	
Mineral deficiencies (Ca, Fe, Zn)	
Malnutrition	
Inflammatory bowel disease	
Leukemia, lymphoma, metastatic carcinomas	
Addison's disease	

Approximately 50% of healthy individual harbor the organism, more frequently found at the posterior dorsum of the tongue. It is also the primary opportunistic pathogenic yeast for humans and is highly prevalent in AIDS patients. The most important pathogenic species is *C. albicans*, even though there are many others. Multiple factors contribute to a shift from its saphrophitic form to opportunistic infection, most commonly affecting the oral and genital mucous membranes [1] (Table 10.1).

Epidemiology

Candida causes up to 25% of the superficial mycoses involving the nails, skin, and mucous membranes. The pseudomembranous form or oral thrush, easily recognized, affects 4–8% of newborns. *Candida* vulvovaginitis, a frequent gynecological infection, occurs more commonly between 20 and 30 years of age. Candidal balanitis occurs in adult and elderly men [4]. Deep and systemic forms of candida are uncommon, which may arise due to the use of intravenous catheters or in intravenous drug abusers. Oral candidiasis can occur in the pediatric population as well as adults and immunocompromised patients [1].

Clinical Manifestations

Candidiasis can occur in a variety of clinical pictures among which the most common are the localized mucocutaneous and cutaneous forms. Other less common forms are chronic mucocutaneous candidiasis and disseminated disease such as *Candida* septicemia. The course may be acute, subacute, or chronic. Mucosal candidiasis is classified as acute and chronic (Table 10.2).

One of the more frequent presentations is intertriginous candidiasis seen interdigitally in the hands, feet, or axillary, inguinal, inframammary, or intergluteal areas as a result of moisture accumulation. In the diaper area, it is usually secondary to a previous dermatitis such as an irritant dermatitis. Neonatal candidiasis presents as thrush or disseminated pustular or vesicular lesions. *Candida* can also affect the nails, typically with yellow, green, or black discoloration of the nail plate. Systemic candidiasis can affect any organ most commonly the esophagus and heart. *Candida* septicemia usually has an intestinal origin, while iatrogenic candidemia is associated with parenteral nutrition.

Table 10.2 Classification of oral candidiasis [2, 4]

Acute candidiasis
Pseudomembranous
Atrophic
Chronic candidiasis
Atrophic subtype
Angular cheilitis (*perlêche*)
Hyperplastic
Chronic Mucocutaneous candidiasis

Oral Signs and Symptoms

Pseudomembranous Candidiasis

One of the most frequent forms of candidiasis affecting the oral mucous membranes is thrush. It presents as creamy, fluffy plaques overlying an erythematous mucosal area, which can be removed with gauze (Fig. 10.1). The buccal and labial mucosa, dorsum of the tongue, and palate are frequently involved sites, which can cause symptoms of dysphagia. It is the most frequent form of candidiasis seen in newborns, infants, elders, and immunocompromised patients (Figs. 10.2 and 10.3). In patients undergoing antibiotic or steroid treatment, atrophic lesions can develop in the palate. Oral candidiasis can extend to involve the esophagus, especially in immunosuppressed patients, producing significant dysphagia and retrosternal pain.

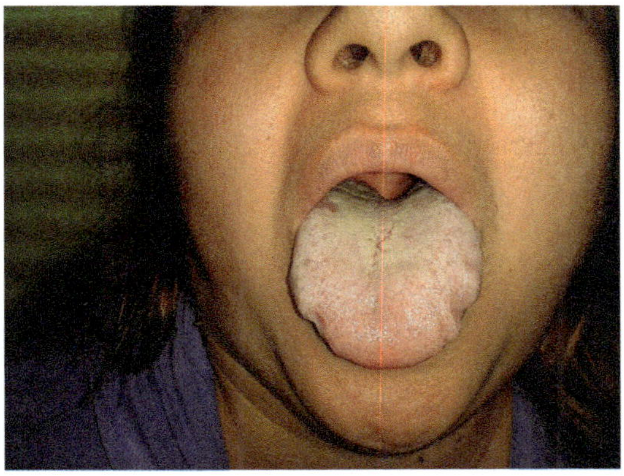

Fig. 10.1 Candidiasis: pseudomembranous form of the dorsal tongue

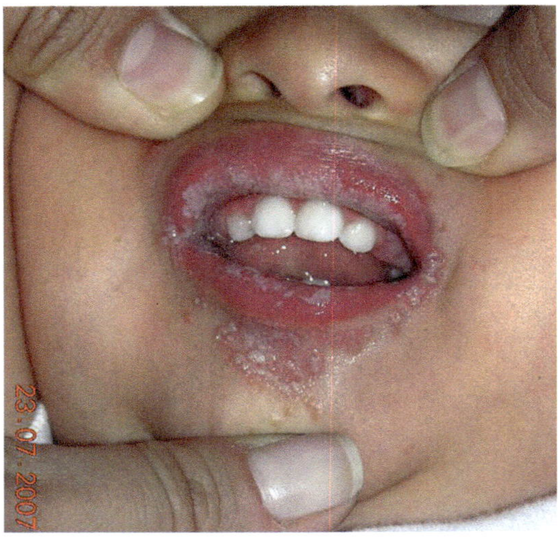

Fig. 10.2 Candidiasis: oral thrush in a young child

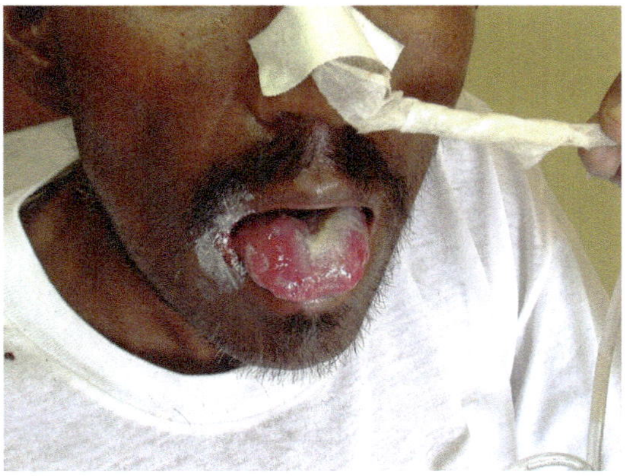

Fig. 10.3 Candidiasis in an HIV+ patient. (Courtesy of J. M. Ollague, Guayaquil, Ecuador)

Oral thrush in newborns typically occurs as a result of transmission from the mother during vaginal delivery and is rarely seen in cesarean births. In severe cases, the entire oral mucosa is affected, which can lead to compromise of the esophagus and airway causing difficulties with swallowing and breathing. Predisposing factors to oral thrush in newborns include salivary drooling, use of pacifiers, poor oral hygiene, and contamination with maternal saliva. In adults, thrush may have multiple associations and can be considered as an "illness of the ill" [2] (see Table 10.1).

Acute atrophic candidiasis is a frequent variant, which presents as red, atrophic, painful, patches (Figs. 10.4, 10.5, and 10.6). It is most frequently seen after oral antibiotic therapy.

Angular cheilitis is most commonly secondary to *Candida*. Angular cheilitis is characterized by fissuring and erythema at the labial commissures. It is a frequent finding in elderly patients, with accentuation of the marionette lines or loss of vertical dimension in poorly fitting dental prostheses [5] (Fig. 10.7). Predisposing factors for angular cheilitis are listed in Table 10.3.

In chronic *Candida* infections, the microorganism invades deeper into the mucosa and

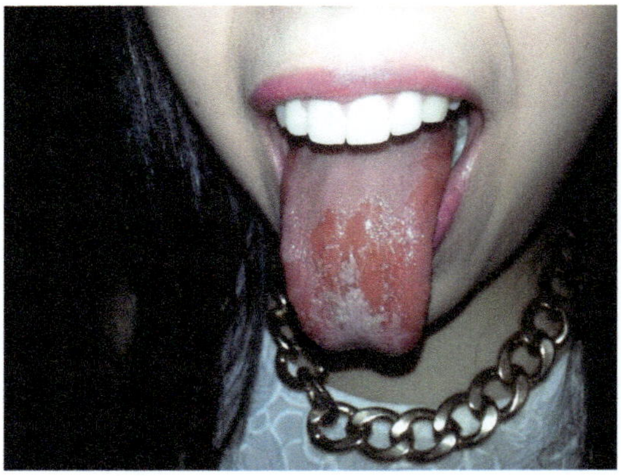

Fig. 10.4 Acute atrophic candidiasis: tongue

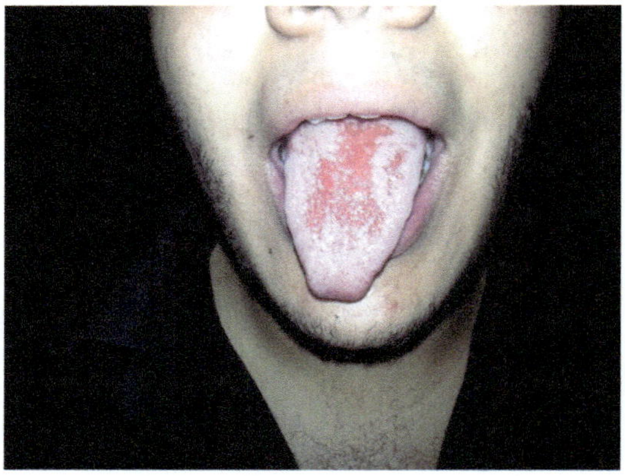

Fig. 10.5 Acute atrophic candidiasis: tongue

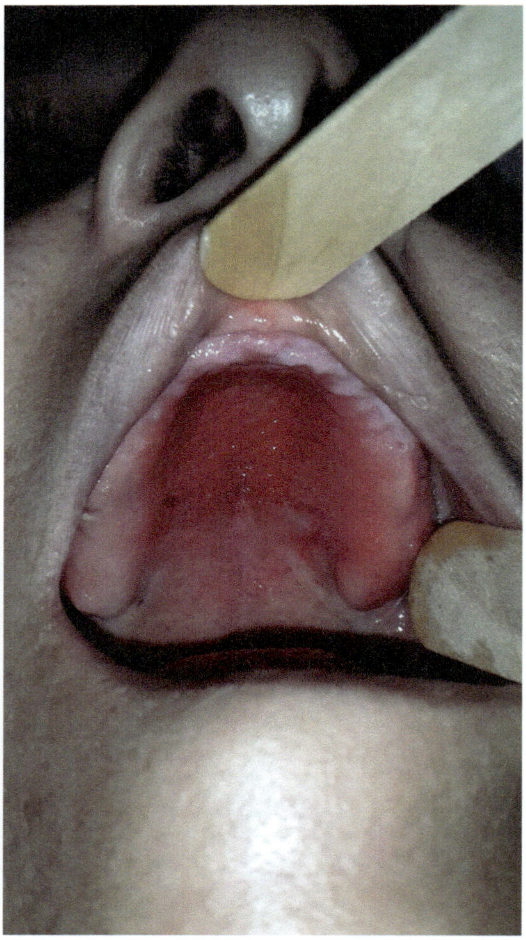

Fig. 10.6 Acute atrophic candidiasis: palate

induces a hyperplasic tissue reaction. The typical clinical presentation is a large whitish plaque similar to leukoplakia, which is strongly adherent to the mucosa, frequently seen in the commissural and retro-commissural areas, but also on the cheeks, palate, and tongue.

In all forms of leukoplakia, including precancerous lesions, secondary *Candida* infection is frequently seen. Median rhomboid glossitis is associated with *Candida* infection and can be considered a variant of chronic hyperplastic candidiasis.

Chronic atrophic forms are characterized by a solitary adherent erythematous or whitish plaque, which is frequently seen in patients with poorly fitting prostheses, especially in diabetic patients. The tongue may appear red and atrophic, similar to what is seen in the setting of vitamin deficiencies. *Candida* can colonize dental protheses

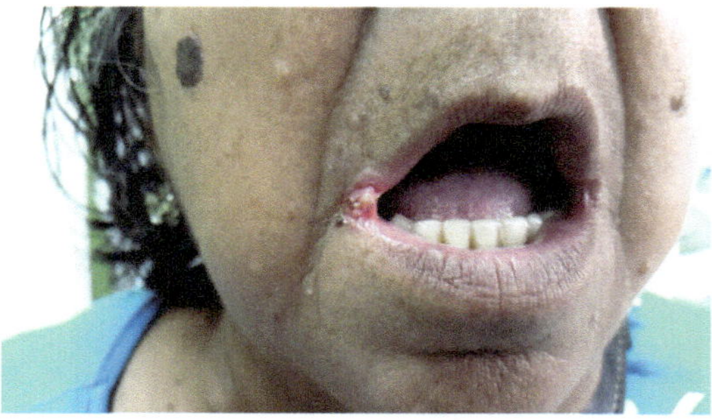

Fig. 10.7 Angular cheilitis

Table 10.3 Predisposing factors for angular cheilitis

Drooling
Fissures
Lip licking habit
Diabetes mellitus
Chronic mucocutaneous candidiasis
Accentuation of marionette lines secondary to aging

despite careful cleaning, becoming a reservoir for the microorganism.

The hyperplasic forms or black hairy tongue (*lingua villosa nigra*), common in AIDS patients, is frequently localized to the lateral borders of the tongue, being indistinguishable from the villous hyperplasia associated with the Epstein-Barr virus. These hyperplasic forms are rarely seen in smokers.

Chronic Mucocutaneous Candidiasis
Chronic mucocutaneous candidiasis is a rare condition that can affect the oral, genital, gastrointestinal mucosa or the lungs. It is seen in nursing infants or in early childhood and is related to thymus abnormalities, functional defects in lymphocytes and leukocytes, and endocrinopathies, and in rare cases, it is idiopathic. In adults, it can be associated with malignancy. Lesions appear on the skin, mucosa, and nails. Mucosal lesions are chronic affecting the face or scalp with a hyperkeratotic, vegetating, or granulomatous appearance. Involvement of all nails is often associated with paronychia and severe nail destruction.

Differential Diagnosis

Mucocutaneous candidiasis must be differentiated from entities such as coated tongue, geographic tongue, aphthous stomatitis, herpes simplex, and oral hairy leukoplakia due to the Epstein-Barr virus, among others.

The clinical suspicion should be corroborated by microscopic examination and/or culture of the sample. Oral candidiasis can be confirmed through microscopic examination of smears taken from the lesions or by culture. The sample taken from the lesions should be examined after the application of 10–20% KOH or with special stains such as Gram, Giemsa, PAS, Lugol, chlorazol black E, or methylene blue, in order to identify the hyphae or pseudohyphae.

Candida can be cultured via different media such as Sabouraud with whitish colonies appearing within 2–3 days. Other culture media such as Nickerson are more specific, allowing the distinction of yeast from fungi. The isolation of a *Candida* species in a culture medium should be correlated with the clinical presentation. Biopsies are not usually necessary, but when performed, the superficial forms show filaments and yeast within the thickened stratum corneum, which is more evident with PAS or the Gomori-Grocott stain. In the dermis, there is mild edema. Abscesses and a granulomatous reaction are noted with deeper involvement of the subcutis.

Treatment Recommendations

Treatment varies depending on the type of candidiasis and the degree of compromise of the patient such that in many instances topical therapy will suffice whereas in more serious cases systemic treatment is required.

Topical Therapy

A saturated sodium bicarbonate mouthwash is very useful in oral candidiasis associated with dental protheses. Angular cheilitis or *perleche* improves with ointments that preserve a dry environment and prevent contact with saliva. Also, the topical use of 1% gentian violet is effective but messy. Nystatin is an effective topical treatment for candidiasis in the form of creams, ointments, and ovules. Topical imidazoles have a wide range of action with similar efficacy including clotrimazole, econazole, miconazole, ketoconazole, and sertaconazole. Terbinafine and ciclopirox have comparable efficacy to that of imidazoles.

Systemic Therapy

Azoles are the treatment of choice in severe, chronic, topical treatment resistant cases of candidiasis. Ketoconazole, in most adult patients at a dose of 200–400 mg daily and in children at a 3 mg/kg daily dose, is very effective. Secondary hepatic and antiandrogenic effects with prolonged use must be kept in mind. Itraconazole has fewer side effects with a regimen of 100–200 mg daily for 3–5 days. Fluconazole as a single 150 mg dose can be used to treat adults without significant predisposing factors; the dose can be increased to

200–400 mg in severe cases. In children, the recommended dose is 3–6 mg/day; in children older than 6 years, a single 50 mg dose can be used. In mucocutaneous forms, itraconazole, 100 mg daily, is administrated until the signs and symptoms resolve.

Voriconazole is a second-generation wide spectrum triazole. It can be administered intravenously or orally and is particularly useful in cases of fluconazole-resistant candidiasis. It can also be used prophylactically in immunosuppressed or transplant patients. Posaconazole is also a second-generation broad spectrum antifungal that can be used in resistant cases of candidiasis. Amphotericin B, caspofungin, micafungin, and anidulafungin are indicated in deep and invasive forms, which do not respond to systemic azoles and in special cases such neutropenic and immunosuppressed patients.

In HIV/AIDS patients with recurrent oral candidiasis, topical therapies can be considered and if necessary, systemic therapies, preferably with itraconazole or fluconazole, reserving the triazolic derivatives as a last resort so as to avoid the generation of resistant strains [4].

Prophylactic systemic therapy should be considered in patients on prolonged oral antibiotic therapy and in immunosuppressed patients [6].

Actinomycosis

Actinomycosis is a rare chronic, suppurative, and granulomatous disease produced by anaerobic or microaerophilic bacteria, mainly *Actinomyces israelii.* Its clinical presentation is characterized by abscesses and multiple sinus tracts with extrusion of characteristic *grains*.

Etiopathogenesis

Despite its name, actinomycosis is a bacterial disease, mainly produced by *Actinomyces israelii*, an anaerobic, Gram-positive, slow-growing saprophytic microorganism of the oral cavity. It forms filamentous colonies, easily confused with fungal structures, which can become pathogenic.

Epidemiology

The source of infection is typically endogenous and localized to the neck and face, chest, or abdominal areas. These bacteria are considered part of the normal flora of the gastrointestinal tract, which can become pathogenic under special conditions. The disease is more frequent in individuals with poor oral hygiene, smokers, alcohol abusers, or following dental infections [7]. Individuals on immunosuppressive therapy and HIV/AIDS patients are at high risk, especially after dental procedures [8].

Clinical Manifestations

Cervicofacial actinomycosis is characterized by a diagnostic triad of induration, deformity, and fistulae that drain purulent material with grains [9]. It usually presents with multiple fistulae, but can be manifested by a single, chronic fistulous orifice, which must be differentiated from an odontogenic fistula.

The cervicofacial form is the most frequent subtype of actinomyces infection. It typically affects the mandible and, in some cases, can involve other areas of the face and the neck. Less often it can affect the maxilla with risk of spread to the paranasal sinuses and brain, and in rare cases, it can cause osteomyelitis [10].

Oral Signs and Symptoms

Oral actinomycosis can appear on the palate, tongue, tonsils, and gingiva as fistulous tracts [11] (Fig. 10.8).

Differential Diagnosis

In cases of cervicofacial actinomycosis, the differential diagnosis should include mycetoma, tuberculosis scrofula, lymphomas, osteomyelitis, dental fistulas, tularemia, and abscessed sebaceous cysts. Clinical suspicion for actinomycosis is confirmed by the presence of grains. Bacterial culture is also useful for corroborating the diagnosis and identifying the causative species.

The characteristic, but nonspecific, sulfur granules extruding from the fistulae can be visualized as tiny white-yellow clumps. They can also be seen on direct smears or in histological sections. They can measure up to 3 mm and are formed by compact microfilaments aggregates with thick spikes at the periphery (Figs. 10.9 and 10.10). When pressing them between two glass slides, a crunching noise is heard. It is important to differentiate them from *Nocardia* grains, which are alcohol-acid resistant as demonstrated with the Ziehl-Neelsen stain. Botryomycosis, actinomycetoma, and eumycetoma also have the characteristic of expelling grains, with different staining characteristics in each case.

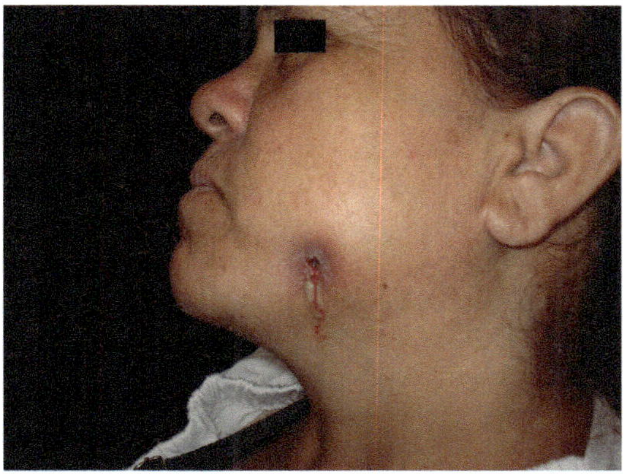

Fig. 10.8 Actinomycosis: Draining fistula of the mandibular area. (Courtesy of A. Bonifaz, México DF, Mexico)

Cultures are helpful in establishing a diagnosis; however, they need to be grown under anaerobic conditions. In general, yellowish filamentous colonies can be observed in about 3–6 days. They take various stains such as Gram, Giemsa, and Grocott and are Ziehl-Neelsen negative, a distinction from *Nocardia*. Histopathology demonstrates a necrotic, chronic granulomatous process with abundant polymorphonuclear cells, foreign body giant cells, and epithelioid cells, with yellowish sulfur granules and filamentous Gram-positive fungal-like pathogens. Nevertheless, the absence of granules does not exclude the diagnosis.

Treatment Recommendations

Cervicofacial actinomycosis, in general, has a good prognosis. Patients with actinomycosis require prolonged treatment with high-dose penicillin G (6–12 months). The treatment of choice is high-dose penicillin G, the duration of which

Fig. 10.9 Actinomycosis: microscopic examination of a grain showing microfilaments clumped together with thick spikes at the periphery

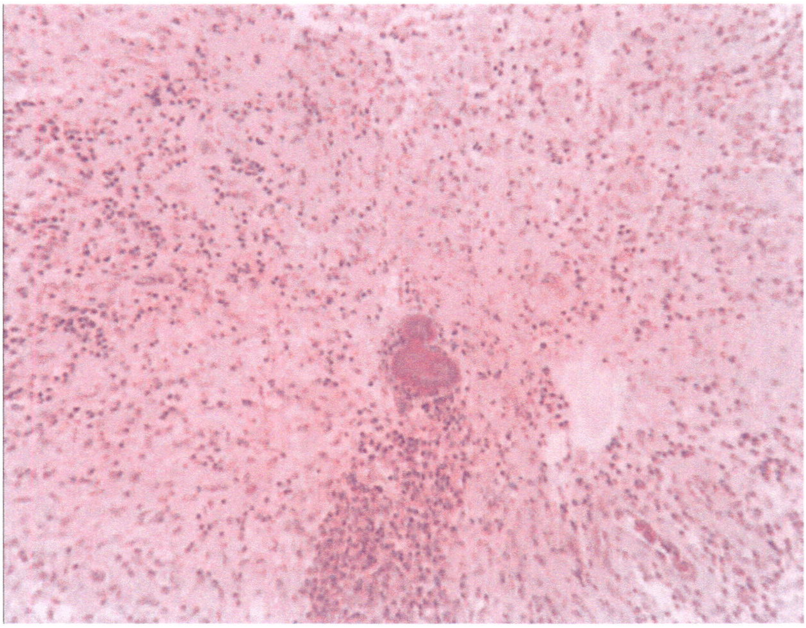

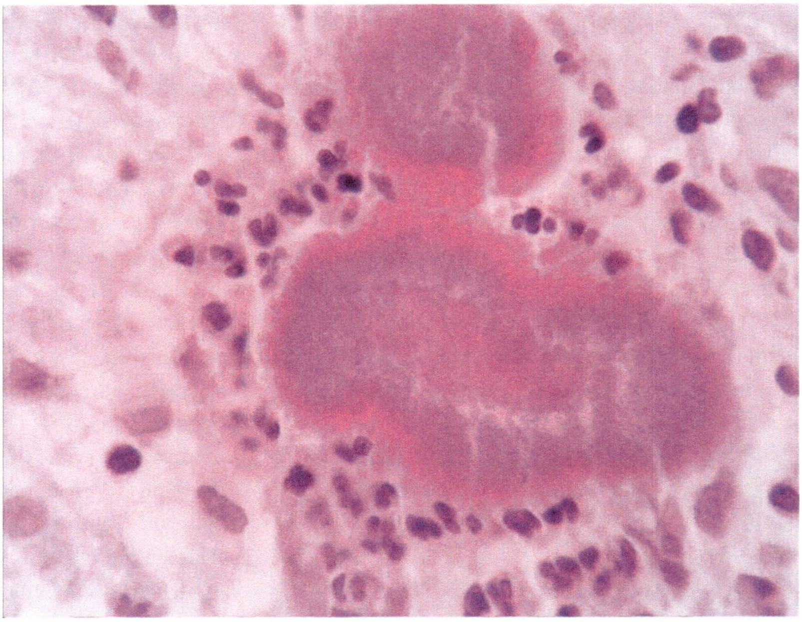

Fig. 10.10 Actinomycosis: basophilic grains in a hematoxylin-eosin stain, high magnification

is determined by the clinical response. In cases of allergy, resistance or intolerance to penicillin treatment with amoxicillin/clavulanate or trimethoprim/sulfamethoxazole can be considered. Debridement and surgical draining of the lesions are recommended.

Histoplasmosis

Etiopathogenesis

Histoplasmosis is a deep systemic mycosis produced by *Histoplasma capsulatum* within the *Ascomycota* phylum, which enters through respiratory pathways followed by possible oral, pharyngeal involvement or potential spread to other organs [2].

Epidemiology

Histoplasmosis constitutes the most frequent pulmonary mycosis worldwide. It is an opportunistic infection more commonly seen in HIV and immunosuppressed patients.

It is prevalent in tropical climates particularly in South America, Central and Southern Africa, and in Asia. In the USA, it has a high incidence in the Ohio and Mississippi River valleys. It can also be acquired when visiting caves, mines, and abandoned buildings, where bats and bat droppings are frequent. The feces of different birds such as hens, turkeys, gooses, doves, and starlings can also carry this pathogen.

Clinical Manifestations

Histoplasmosis characteristically arises from the inhalation of spores. In highly immunosuppressed patients, cutaneous infection is possible, but very rare. In most immunocompetent individuals, the infection is asymptomatic; however, it can cause mild respiratory symptoms. In isolated cases, it can present with symptoms and radiological imaging findings similar to pulmonary tuberculosis later evolving into a disseminated infection. However, in 1% of patients, the infection runs a severe course with remarkable pulmonary or extrapulmonary manifestations. Histoplasmosis is an AIDS-defining opportunistic disease; therefore, the diagnostic work-up should include a complete laboratory investigation including serologies to exclude HIV infection. HIV-infected patients are particularly susceptible to histoplasmosis such that oro-cutaneous lesions constitute a marker for HIV infection in endemic areas [12, 13].

Other groups of patients such as those who are undergoing prolonged steroid treatment and individuals with hematological diseases such as leukemia and lymphomas also have a higher risk of infection. In immunosuppressed patients with disseminated histoplasmosis, the cutaneous lesions can have varying morphologies such as erythematous macules, papules, nodules, pustules, herpetic, acneiform, erythema multiforme-like, molluscum contagiosum-like, vasculitic, and exfoliative eruptions [14] (Figs. 10.11, 10.12, and 10.13).

In some cases of disseminated cutaneous histoplasmosis occurring in HIV+ patients with AIDS, the clinical and histopathological features can be highly unusual, including atypical mucocutaneous lesions, which can present a diagnostic challenge (Fig. 10.14). These patients displayed unusual histopathological features, including a lichenoid, nodular pseudomyxoid, pyogenic granuloma-like, perifollicular, and deep perivascular dermatitis. Other more commonly encountered histopathological presentations include a histiocytic lobular panniculitis and focal nodular dermatitis [15].

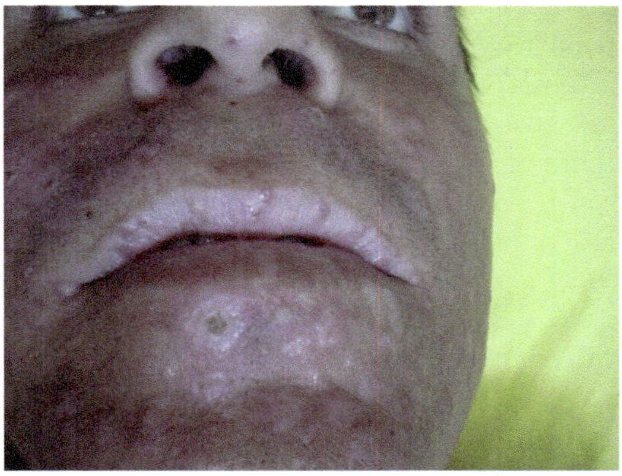

Fig. 10.11 Disseminated histoplasmosis in a young girl with myelodysplastic syndrome. (Courtesy of F. Gomez Daza,Valencia, Venezuela)

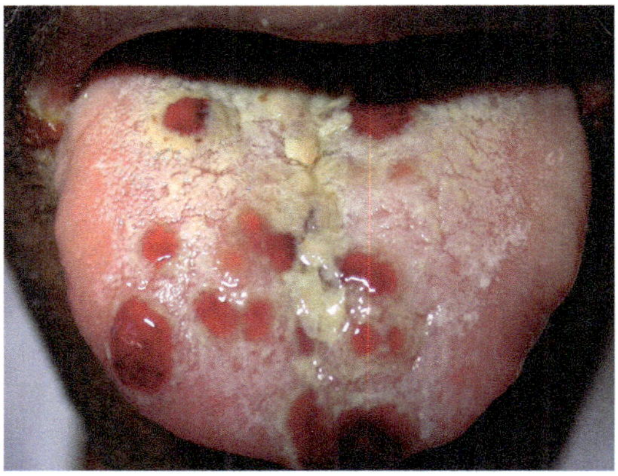

Fig. 10.12 HIV+ patient with disseminated histoplasmosis affecting the tongue. (Courtesy of F. Gomez Daza, Valencia, Venezuela)

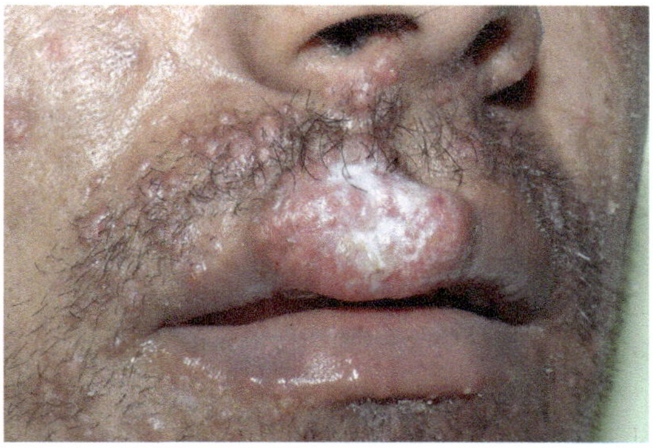

Fig. 10.13 Histoplasmosis presenting as molluscum contagiousum-like lesions. (Courtesy of P. Chang, Ciudad de Guatemala, Guatemala)

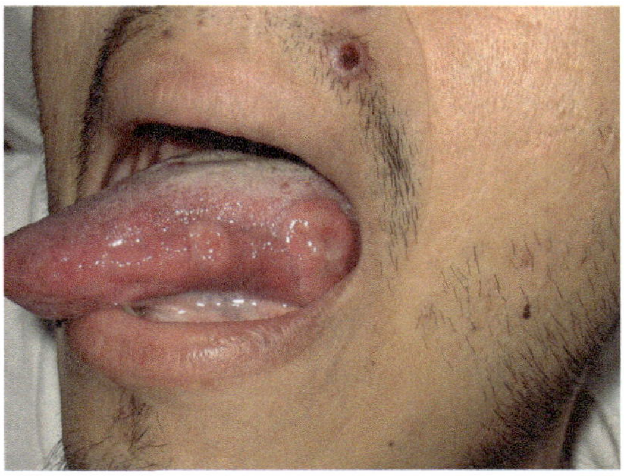

Fig. 10.14 Histoplasmosis: oral (tongue) and cutaneous in an HIV/AIDS patient. (Courtesy of J. M. Ollague, Guayaquil, Ecuador)

Oral Signs and Symptoms

Oral lesions of histoplasmosis are usually associated with other extrapulmonary manifestations

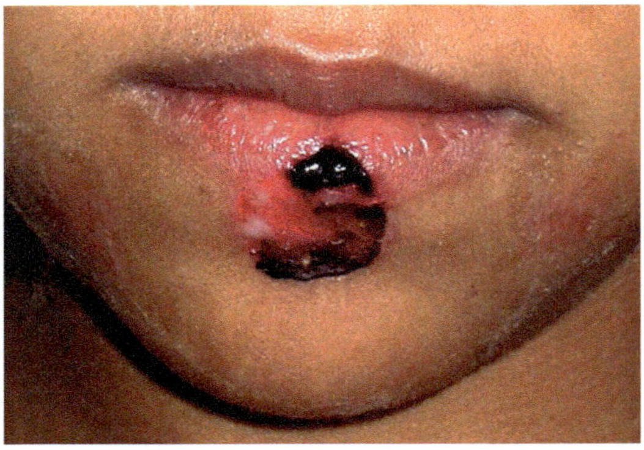

Fig. 10.15 Histoplasmosis: chronic non-healing ulceration in an HIV+ patient

and very seldom occur as the sole manifestation of the disease. Oral lesions are usually a manifestation of the disseminated form of the disease and are most frequently observed in severely immunocompromised patients. Isolated cases of primary histoplasmosis localized to the oral mucous membranes have been described in HIV-negative patients. The clinical presentation of the oral lesions is nonspecific and, in some cases, can be difficult to distinguish from oral squamous cell carcinoma. Histoplasmosis is an unusual and rare cause of chronic non-healing ulcerations in the oral cavity [16, 17] (Fig. 10.15).

Differential Diagnosis

Definitive diagnosis is established via culture, detection of the organism in tissues, the presence of antibodies on serology, and molecular identification of specific antigens. The differential diagnosis includes squamous cell carcinoma and paracoccidioidomycosis.

Treatment Recommendations

Itraconazole and amphotericin B (liposomal and deoxycholate) are effective therapies for histoplasmosis. For chronic pulmonary involvement and mild-to-moderate disease itraconazole, 200 mg three times daily for 3 days followed by itraconazole 200 mg once or twice daily for at least 1 year is recommended. In progressive disseminated histoplasmosis or moderate to severe disease, liposomal amphotericin B, 3.0 mg/kg per day for 1–2 weeks, is the drug of choice. Alternatively, itraconazole 200 mg three times daily for 3 days then 200 mg once or twice daily for at least 1 year can be considered. Amphotericin B desoxycholate, 0.75–1.0 mg/kg per day, is the treatment of choice [18].

Lifelong suppressive therapy with itraconazole, 200 mg daily, may be required in immunosuppressed patients and in patients who relapse despite receiving appropriate therapy. The Wheat's guidelines include a full range of recommendations for special situations such as histoplasmosis in children, pregnant women, CNS histoplasmosis, and moderate-to-severe acute pulmonary histoplasmosis.

Posaconazole, 800 mg per day for 6–34 weeks, has been used as *salvage treatment* in severe forms of histoplasmosis. Patients are eligible for *salvage therapy*, if standard therapy is not tolerated or in instances of refractory disease [19].

Mucormycosis

Etiopathogenesis

Mucormycosis is an uncommon severe opportunistic infection caused by fungi of the order *Mucorales*, mainly *Rhizopus*, *Absidia*, *Mucor*, and *Rhizomucor* [20]. It occurs in patients with diabetes mellitus (DM) in ketoacidosis, neutropenia, malignancy, or immunosuppressed transplant patients [21] (Fig. 10.16). Local trauma due to probes or other procedures in the nasal area can increase the risk of entry of the fungus in susceptible patients.

Epidemiology

The incidence of mucormycosis is expected to increase worldwide given the higher prevalence of predisposing factors. The mortality rate of mucormycosis has been cited as 40% despite aggressive surgical and antifungal therapy.

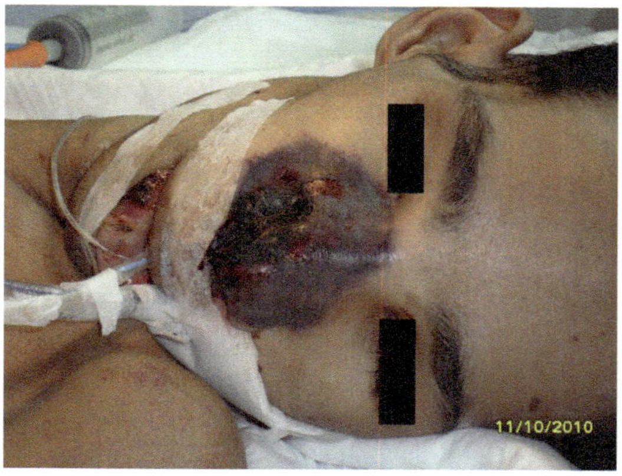

Fig. 10.16 Mucormycosis: Patient with Non-Hodgkin's lymphoma on immunosuppressive therapy. (Courtesy of E. Cavallera, Z. Rivera, A.M. Pulido, Caracas, Venezuela)

Patients with malignancies and hematopoietic stem cell transplant patients have mortality rates up to 65% and 90%, respectively [22–24].

Clinical Manifestations

The infection usually compromises the nasal cavity and can by contiguity affect the paranasal sinuses, palate, and buccal mucosa (Fig. 10.17). It has two clinical forms: primary and secondary cutaneous zygomycosis. The primary form has an overall good prognosis characteristically appearing as necrotic lesions after a traumatic injury. By contrast, the secondary form has a poor prognosis and starts as a fistula with necrotic tissue, generally as an extension of rhinocerebral involvement [25].

The possible clinical manifestations of mucormycosis include rhinocerebral invasion and pulmonary, cutaneous, and gastric disseminated disease [20, 21]. The original clinical description of the rhinocerebral type of mucormycosis is of oral/palatal necrosis. Bonifaz et al. presented 21 mucormycosis cases with palatal involvement (18.75%), from a total of 112 cases screened. All but one were associated with diabetic ketoacidosis (5 patients had type 1 DM and 15 had type 2 DM). The rhinocerebral clinical presentation was observed in 19 cases (90%), while in 2 cases there was disseminated disease. Nasal mucosal involvement occurred as the initial manifestation in most cases ($n = 16$). In three cases, the initial lesion presented as a palatal ulcer. All patients received amphotericin B desoxycholate combined with itraconazole in four cases and fluconazole in four other cases. Four cases were also subjected to surgical intervention. Clinical and mycological cure was achieved in only four cases (19%) [22].

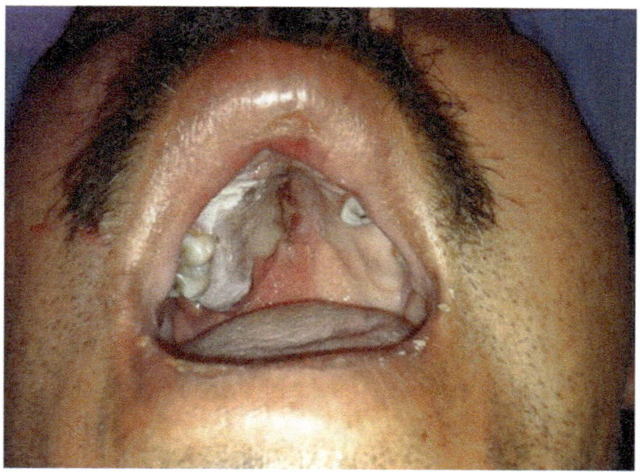

Fig. 10.17 Mucormycosis affecting the palate. (Courtesy of A. Bonifaz, Mexico DF, Mexico)

In children, the rhinocerebral form is the main clinical presentation, followed by the primary cutaneous and the pulmonary types. Predisposing factors such as DM and hematologic disease are similar to those seen in adults [26].

Differential Diagnosis

The diagnosis of mucormycosis is established based on clinical presentation and histopathological features showing vascular invasion by hyphae leading to thrombosis and tissue necrosis as the hallmark of the disease better demonstrated with the silver stain. The inflammatory response is sparse, and edema and necrosis are conspicuous. Samples must be sent for culture in order to identify the species and confirm the clinical diagnosis. Radiological imaging is important in cases with facial involvement in order to evaluate the extent of the disease and possible intracranial involvement [27]. Early clinical recognition and prompt therapy are crucial to preventing fatal outcomes.

Treatment Recommendations

A frequent tragic outcome in mucormycosis is unfortunately, the rule. In order to overcome this reality, the treatment strategy for mucormycosis is based on four factors: early diagnosis; correction of underlying predisposing risk factors when possible; prompt surgical debridement, if applicable; and timely initiation of antifungal therapy. Antifungal therapy with high doses of liposomal amphotericin B (5–7.5 mg/kg per day) or amphotericin B desoxycholate (1 mg/kg per day) is the treatment of choice [2].

Salvage therapy with deferasirox, a new iron chelator, proven to be fungicidal for clinical isolates of *Mucorales* in vitro, can be used [28]. Deferasirox should be administered for only 2–4 weeks because its toxicity increases after 4 weeks of therapy. Posaconazole is an option for patients refractory to or unable to tolerate amphotericin B therapy. The total duration of antifungal therapy for mucormycosis must be maintained until resolution of the clinical signs and symptoms of infection, resolution or stabilization of radiographic signs of activity, and reversal of underlying predisposing factors [20].

Paracoccidioidomycosis

Etiopathogenesis

Paracoccidioidomycosis is a systemic mycosis caused by a thermo-dimorphic fungus belonging to the *Paracoccidioides brasiliensis* complex. The *Paracoccidioides* genus is part of the *Ascomycota* phylum, Euromycetes class, Oxygenales order, and *Ajellomycetaceae* (Onygenaceae) family, similar to *Histoplasma capsulatum*, *Blastomyces dermatitidis*, *Coccidioides immites*, and *Coccidioides posadasii*. They all share thermo-dimorphism, the mycelium as the infective form, as well as a restricted geographic habitat [29]. In 2006, three novel *Paracoccidioides* species were suggested based on molecular studies, and in 2009, a new species, *Paracoccidioides lutzii*, was formally proposed. More recently, new species have been reported including *P.americana*, *P.restrepiensis*, and *P.venezuelensis* [30–34].

Subsequent to a pulmonary infection, most individuals develop a clinically silent chronic carrier state due to host-parasite equilibrium. The silent phase can be as long as 60 years. Evolution to overt disease is a consequence of disruption in the balance of the host-parasite relationship. Paracoccidioidomycosis is usually associated with high alcohol consumption, poor nutrition, tobacco use, and acquired or iatrogenic immunosuppression. These associated conditions contribute to an impaired immune response that favors fungal replication and dissemination [35].

Epidemiology

Paracoccidioidomycosis is endemic in continental Latin America from north of Argentina (34.5° south latitude) to south of Mexico (20° north latitude). Most cases are observed in Brazil, Colombia, Venezuela, Argentina, and Paraguay. However, sporadic cases have been reported throughout the world. It is seen more often in men and in rural areas and is contracted by inhalation of conidia produced by the saprophytic phase of the fungus [34].

Clinical Manifestations

The clinical manifestations of paracoccidioidomycosis vary. In 1987, Franco et al. proposed that paracoccidioidomycosis is best classified as a continuous spectrum [36]. The two poles of the disease consist of the acute-subacute form and the chronic form. In the acute-subacute clinical form (juvenile type), patients are usually young, either male or female, and present a clinical history of short duration. The clinical presentation of the juvenile type of the disease can include lymphadenopathy and hepatosplenomegaly as the main manifestations; however, involvement of the bone, joints, and skin does occur. The lungs are merely the portal of entry and usually show little or no damage. The mucous membranes are involved in less than 5% of acute-subacute cases [37].

The chronic clinical form is the classic presentation and accounts for 85–90% of all cases [37]. Most of these patients are men, over 30 years old, who present with a prolonged clinical course. Pulmonary with mucosal or cutaneous involvement are the hallmark of this clinical form. Moreover, every organ system can be involved, including the adrenals, lymph nodes, as well as the gastrointestinal and central nervous system [38].

Oral Signs and Symptoms

In a review of 152 dermatologic patients, cutaneous lesions were observed in 61.2% of chronic cases, while mucosal lesions were detected in 58.5% of patients, mostly affecting the oral mucosa [37]. The soft palate, gingiva, lower lip, buccal mucosa, and tongue are the most commonly affected sites. The classic clinical presentation of mucosal lesions is a superficial ulcer with a granular appearance and hemorrhagic points conferring a mulberry-like morphology [38] (Figs. 10.18, 10.19, 10.20, 10.21, 10.22, and 10.23). When the lips are involved, tissue infiltration resulting in macrocheilitis is also observed. Oral lesions observed in young patients are quite similar to those observed in adults. It is generally agreed that the mucosal or cutaneous lesions are a consequence of hematologic dissemination of the fungus and not the product of direct inoculation.

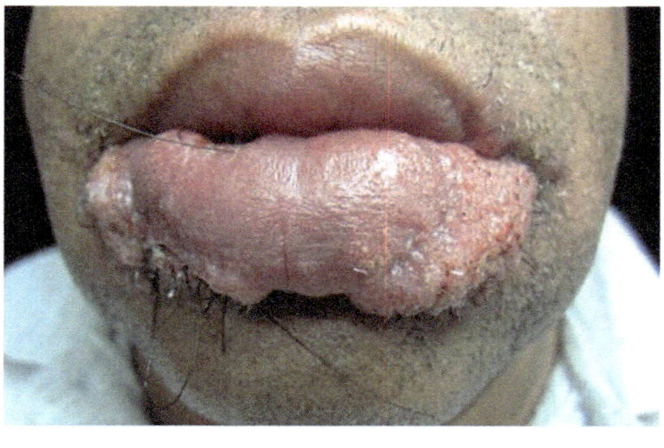

Fig. 10.18 Paracoccidiodomycosis: lip involvement. (Courtesy of E. Cavallera, E. Villasmil, Caracas, Venezuela)

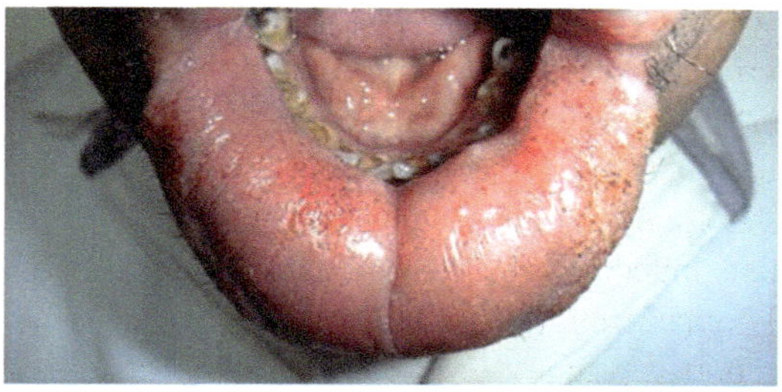

Fig. 10.19 Paracoccidiodomycosis: lip involvement. (Courtesy of E. Cavallera, E. Villasmil, Caracas, Venezuela)

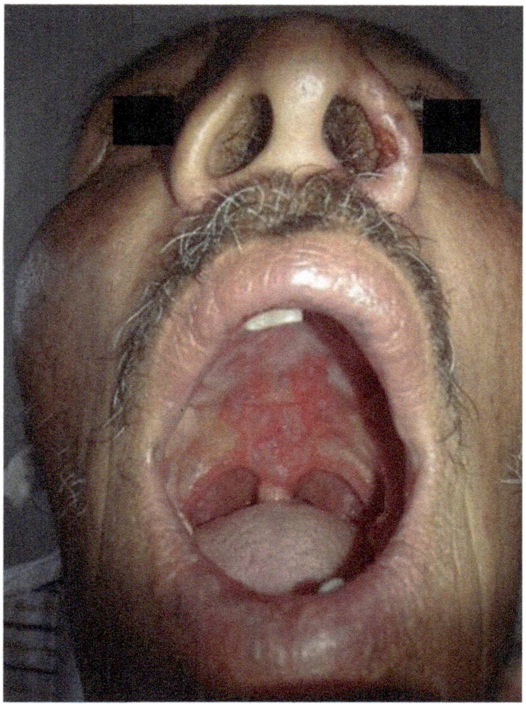

Fig. 10.20 Paracoccidioidomycosis: irregular shallow ulcer on palate. (Courtesy of M. Isernia, D. Bellorín, L. Crespo, E. Cavallera, Caracas, Venezuela)

Differential Diagnosis

Squamous cell carcinoma is the main differential diagnosis. Leishmaniasis and histoplasmosis must also be considered. The diagnosis of paracoccidioidomycosis depends on visualization and

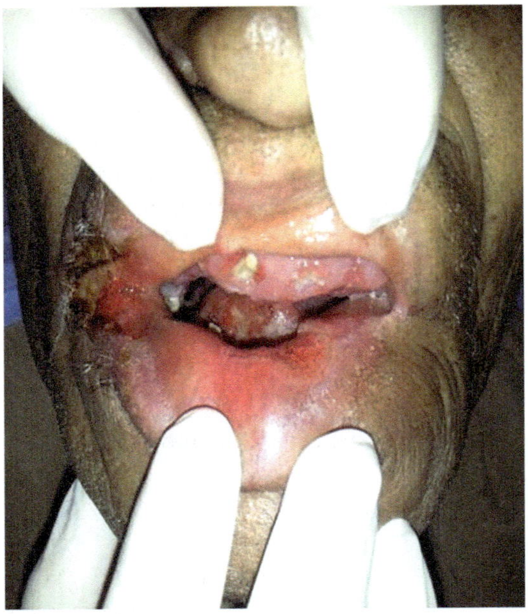

Fig. 10.21 Paracoccidioidomycosis: lip and buccal mucosa. (Courtesy of A. De La Torre, E. Cavallera, Caracas, Venezuela)

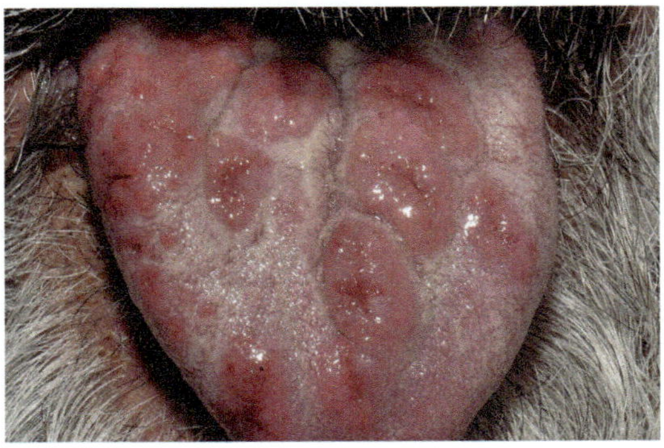

Fig. 10.22 Paracoccidioidomycosis: tongue

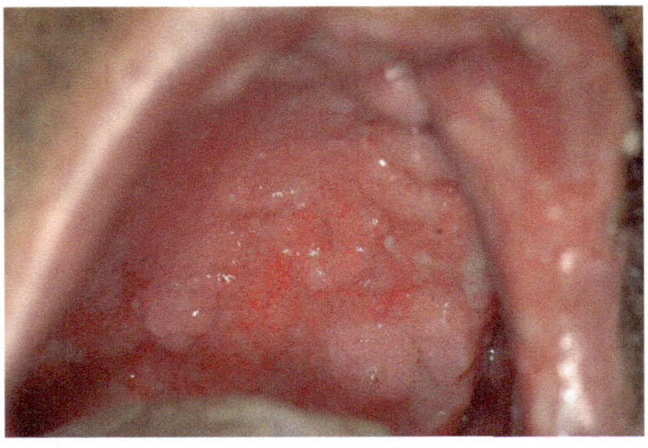

Fig. 10.23 Paracoccidioidomycosis: shallow ulcer on the palate with petechial hemorrhage

identification of the etiologic agent through direct examination via cytology, histopathology, or culture (Fig. 10.24). In practical terms, a biopsy for histopathological examination is the diagnostic procedure of choice. The classic presentation is an epithelioid granuloma mixed with polymorphonuclear leukocytes and mononuclear cells surrounding the fungus (Fig. 10.25). Serological testing is an adjunct to diagnosis of the disease and is a useful guide for monitoring the treatment response.

Treatment Recommendations

Treatment of paracoccidioidomycosis depends on the severity of disease. Itraconazole 200 mg per day for a duration of 6–9 months in mild cases and 12–16 months in moderate cases can be considered. For children who weigh less than 30 kg, itraconazole, 5–10 mg/kg/d, is recommended.

Treatment with trimethoprim-sulfamethoxazole for 12 months is indicated in mild disease, while moderate disease requires 18 months of treatment. In children, the recommended trimethoprim-sulfamethoxazole dose is 8–10 mg/kg twice a day for the same duration as in adults. Voriconazole is also as an option for treating mild and moderate disease. It is well-tolerated and as effective as itraconazole for long-term treatment [21, 39].

Amphotericin B desoxycholate is the drug of choice for severe cases starting at a dose of 10 mg daily, increasing by 10 mg with each successive dose until reaching 0.50 mg/kg per day or every other day. A maximum of 50 mg of amphotericin B desoxycholate in each infusion for adults and 25 mg/infusion for children is recommended. When dealing with life-threatening paracoccidioidomycosis, an initial dose of 30 mg per day, increasing by 20 mg with each successive dose and daily doses as high as 1.0–1.5 mg/kg, can be considered. Amphotericin B desoxycholate has well-known immediate and late side effects, which require careful monitoring. The most important of the late onset side effects is nephrotoxicity, which is characterized by decreased renal clearance, progressive hypokale-

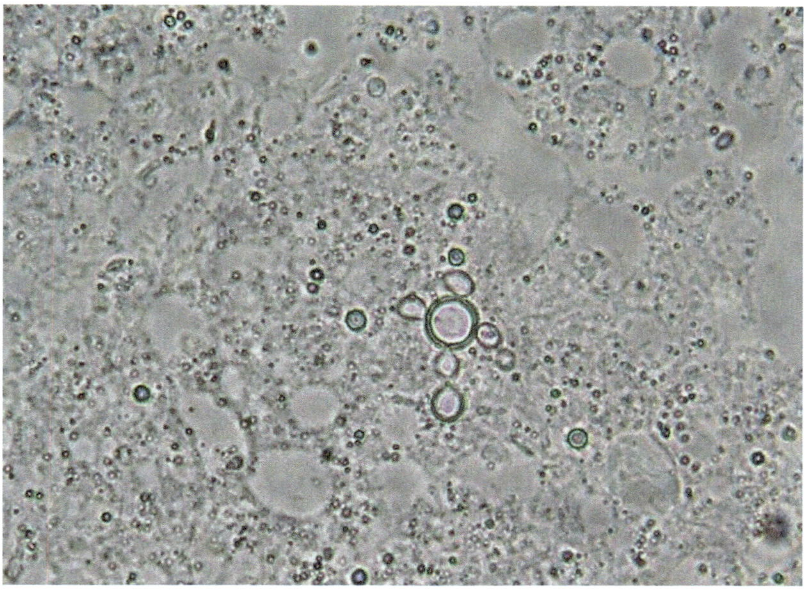

Fig. 10.24 Paracoccidioidomycosis: microscopic examination with KOH showing multiple buds attached to a mother cell

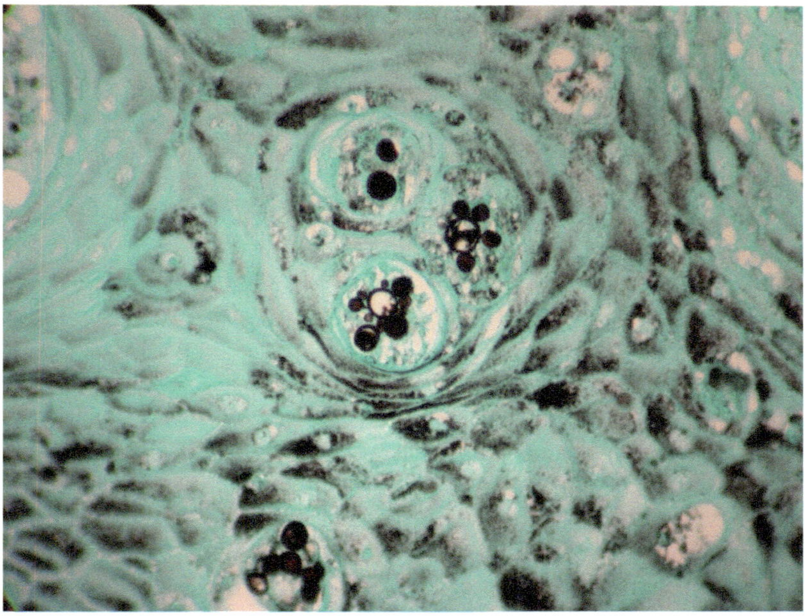

Fig. 10.25 Paracoccidioidomycosis: histopathology with Grocott silver stain

mia, hypomagnesemia, and renal tubular acidosis [40]. Amphotericin lipid complex 3.0–4.0 mg/kg/day for 15 days followed by itraconazole 200–400 mg/day can be an option for severe cases [21]. Fluconazole 800 mg per day is an alternative treatment regimen for patients with neurological involvement [21].

The clinical prognosis in paracoccidioidomycosis depends on the severity of the disease, presence of comorbidities, as well as treatment. Usually, there is a marked clinical improvement after 1 or 2 months of treatment with healing of mucosal and cutaneous lesions. Nevertheless, patients must be advised that healing of mucosal or cutaneous lesions is not an indicator of complete irradication of the disease. Complete cure is recognized when there are no more clinical signs of the disease, radiologic examination shows stabilization of pulmonary disease, and serological testing remains negative [41].

Blastomycosis

Subacute or chronic mycosis is caused by a dimorphic fungus called *Blastomyces dermatitidis* (*B. dermatitidis*). It is characterized by granulomatous suppurative lesions affecting the lungs, skin, and bones.

Etiopathogenesis

The *B. dermatitidis* spores or conidia penetrate the organism through inhalation into the respiratory pathways. Primary infection in most cases is asymptomatic. After inhalation of the conidia, there is a suppurative inflammatory reaction similar to caseation that can involve the lungs or affect other organs such as the skin and bones via hematogenous spread. In rare occasions, cutaneous inoculation can occur, forming a primary complex similar to that of sporotrichosis [2].

Epidemiology

The most important endemic focus of blastomycosis is found in the USA and Canada, located in the areas bordering the Great Lakes, St. Lawrence River, and the Ohio and Mississippi river valleys. Small foci have also been found in Mexico, Central America, and Africa. *B. dermatitidis* has been isolated in damp soil and can affect animals such as horses, beavers, and especially dogs. Men are affected more often than women and children because they are more likely to participate in activities that put them at risk for exposure to the organism [2].

Clinical Manifestations

Blastomycosis can affect the pulmonary, genitourinary, cutaneous, musculoskeletal, and central nervous system in addition to disseminated disease. Cutaneous blastomycosis is the main extrapulmonary form; it can occur in 40% of cases and is divided in primary and secondary cutaneous forms. The primary cutaneous form arises from inoculation of the fungus through skin trauma causing a chancre or nodular lesions with lymphangitis or adenitis similar to sporotrichosis. The secondary form arises from hematogenous and lymphatic dissemination. Localization to the face, particularly the nose, is very characteristic. The initial papular and nodular lesions eventually form abscesses, ulcers, and verrucous lesions [42].

Oral Signs and Symptoms

In general, mucosal involvement is very rare, in contrast to its counterpart, South American blastomycosis or paracoccidioidomycosis. Nevertheless, when it occurs, it can mimic the features of a squamous cell carcinoma. The larynx is the most commonly reported site of infection, followed by the oral cavity, neck, ears, nasal cavities/paranasal sinuses, and skull base/orbit [43, 44].

Differential Diagnosis

Blastomycosis is one of the great mimickers in medicine: verrucous cutaneous blastomycosis resembles malignancy and mass-like lung opacities due to *B. dermatitidis* are often confused with cancer. Blastomycosis may be clinically indistinguishable from tuberculosis and paracoccidioidomycosis.

The diagnosis of blastomycosis is frequently delayed due to its clinical presentation, which can be similar to more common clinical entities, most notably squamous cell carcinoma. A substantial portion of cases (42%) present without clinical or radiological evidence of pulmonary infection [42]. Sputum, pus, or wound exudates can be examined with potassium hydroxide, which reveals the mono-gemmating blastoconidia, with thick birefringent walls. Gemmation is very useful for differentiating the disease from the South American blastomycosis, since it presents with a single gemmation of the same size as the mother cell in contrast to multiple gemmations of various sizes in paracoccidioidomycosis. Culture reveals white, filamentous colonies with the presence of aerial hyphae. Biopsies are very useful for diagnostic purposes, especially with cutaneous involvement, which show the typical mono-gemmating cells after staining with hematoxylin-eosin, PAS, or Grocott. Typically, pseudoepitheliomatous hyperplasia with granulomas and multinucleated giant cells is noted on histopathology. PCR analysis is one of the most efficient and reliable diagnostic tests for the identification of *B. dermatitidis* [2].

Treatment Recommendations

Liposomal amphotericin B at a dose of 3–6 mg/kg/day is usually curative. If the lipid formulation is unavailable, amphotericin B deoxycholate at 0.5–1.0 mg/kg/day can be considered as an alternative. Itraconazole as monotherapy, 200 mg for 6–12 months, is also highly effective and is the mainstay of therapy for most patients with primary cutaneous blastomycosis. Voriconazole can be useful in cases refractory to other therapies.

Aspergillosis

Aspergillosis encompasses a group of diseases produced by pathogenic and opportunistic species belonging to the *Aspergillus* genus.

Etiopathogenesis

Aspergillus is an *Ascomycetes* (*Enascomycetes*) fungus, which includes *Aspergillus fumigatus*, *Aspergillus niger*, and *Aspergillus flavus*. It is ubiquitous in the environment with inoculation most frequently occurring through the respiratory tract. The external ear and nail can also be affected.

Epidemiology

Aspergillosis has been reported worldwide with a higher prevalence seen in workers who are exposed to grains (i.e., corn, wheat, and animal feed). It is associated with factors such as malnutrition, alcoholism, tuberculosis, lung cancer, immunosuppressive therapy, HIV disease, and lymphoproliferative disorders such as leukemia [2].

Clinical Manifestations

The most frequent types of aspergillosis are pulmonary, disseminated, cutaneous, otic, and ophthalmologic. The organism can be inhaled causing a delayed hypersensitivity reaction. It can occupy residual cavitary spaces in tuberculosis, histoplasmosis, and carcinomas and originate as the so-called fungus ball, composed of masses of mycelium mixed with mucus in the absence of alveolar invasion. In some cases, it invades the pulmonary parenchyma with risk of subsequent hematogenous spread to various organs such as the liver, spleen, heart, intestines, or brain.

The fungal rhinosinusitis seen in immunocompetent patients, which tends to have a nonspecific clinical presentation, is usually detected in imaging studies. Diagnosis is often delayed because the associated symptoms of headache, cough and facial pain, are similar to those of chronic bacterial sinusitis. It is caused by various filamentous fungi, especially belonging to the *Asperguillus fumigatus* and *Aspergillus flavus* species producing "*fungus balls*" in the paranasal sinuses [45, 46]. Cranio-cerebral involvement, seen more frequently in immunosuppressed patients, occurs through hematogenous spread or contiguous spread from the paranasal sinuses.

Oral Signs and Symptoms

Invasive *Aspergillus* granulomas can arise in immunocompetent individuals presenting as a palpable mass in the buccal mucosa following removal of an impacted mandibular third molar [47].

Differential Diagnosis

The differential diagnosis of aspergillosis cutaneous ulcers includes primary cutaneous mucormycosis, non-tuberculous mycobacterial infections, factitial dermatitis, and loxoscelism. Microscopic examination of cutaneous ulcer exudate or histopathological examination of tissue sections will reveal thin, septate, and hyaline hyphae. *Aspergillius* conidial heads are typical of pulmonary aspergillosis, and can be seen in its invasive form. Cultures should be done in culture media without cycloheximide since it inhibits growth of the fungus and repeated to exclude contamination from the environment. Biopsy for histopathologic examination is very useful in the setting of cutaneous ulcers, showing a granulomatous infiltrate with necrotic areas and abundant septate hyphae.

Immunological tests are useful above all in invasive pulmonary aspergillosis. Serological testing (i.e., gel immunodiffusion, complement fixation, RIA, and ELISA) is nonspecific. *Aspergillus* exo-antigens in the circulation at the moment of infection can be identified in various body fluids (such as blood serum, urine, cerebrospinal fluid, pericardial or pulmonary fluid, and bronchial lavage), which is a very useful test for the diagnosis of aspergillosis [2]. PCR analysis is the most useful test since it is highly specific and efficient and can be performed utilizing serum or paraffin-embedded tissue.

Treatment Recommendations

Amphotericin B can be effective in the treatment of aspergillosis; however, the potential toxic side effects require careful consideration. The azoles including ketoconazole, itraconazole, voriconazole, and posaconazole have been used successfully with fewer side effects. Voriconazole is the treatment of choice in invasive forms of the disease and can be administrated intravenously or orally. Caspofungin and micafungin, equinocandin derivatives that act on the fungal cell wall, do not have cross-resistance with azoles and have a limited number of drug interactions. They can be used in combination with Amphotericin B or azoles.

Cryptococcosis

Etiopathogenesis

Cryptococcosis is a systemic mycosis caused by the encapsulated fungus *Cryptococcus neoformans* or *Cryptococcus gattii*. The former is found worldwide as a microorganism in decaying wood, fruits, or bird droppings. *Cryptococcus gattii* has a more restricted geographic distribution being isolated from decomposing wood in tropical and subtropical areas as well as in temperate regions from the eucalyptus tree [48].

The fungus, *C. neoformans* or *C. gattii*, usually causes infection through inhalation or rarely, following injury to the skin or mucous membrane. Although the lungs are the focus of primary infection, its clinical presentation is mild, and the fungus remains silent in the lungs. Overt disease of the lung or other organ systems will occur when the host defense-fungus equilibrium is disrupted. Infection of the brain and meninges is the most common clinical manifestation and the most common cause of death from cryptococcosis emphasizing the tropism of the fungus for the CNS. Pulmonary disease results from primary lung infection or as a result of reactivation of latent foci of viable fungus. Cutaneous, bone, joint, and ocular involvement is a consequence of hematogenous spread of the fungus, particularly in immunosuppressed individuals [49].

Epidemiology

Cryptococcosis is a common opportunistic infection that affects immunosuppressed individuals, classically, HIV-infected and transplant patients. The introduction of highly active antiretroviral therapy (HAART) in the treatment of HIV-infected patients changed the epidemiology of cryptococcosis in developing countries with a clear reduction in number of cases and associated mortality. However, the overall incidence and mortality due to cryptococcosis remains high in underdeveloped regions where the incidence of HIV infection is still prevalent and access to HAART and healthcare resources is limited [49].

The clinical manifestations in the immunosuppressed individual are more commonly related to central nervous system (CNS) involvement.

Clinical Manifestations

Headache, nausea, dizziness, and irritability are the initial manifestations of cryptococcal meningoencephalitis. Decrease in cognitive function, impaired memory, and progressive ataxia followed by lassitude, blurred vision, or abrupt coma are strong indications of CNS involvement [50]. The shorter the duration of symptoms, the worse the prognosis. Pulmonary cryptococcosis is usually indolent with manifestations limited to dry cough, chest pain, and low fever with subsequent dissemination to the CNS or other organ systems [49]. Cutaneous cryptococcosis is usually secondary to hematogenous spread. Before the era of HAART, cutaneous cryptococcosis had been reported to occur in 15% of cases and was considered a sentinel sign of severe and disseminated disease [51, 52]. Molluscum-like papules and nodules more frequently affecting the head and upper trunk are the main clinical manifestation of cutaneous *Cryptococcus* [51, 52]. Primary cutaneous cryptococcosis has been reported more frequently in the last decade, both in immunosuppressed and non-immunosuppressed patients [53]. A diagnosis of primary disease is based on the presence of skin lesions either solitary or multiple in a limited area with a positive culture for *Cryptococcus* spp. in the absence of systemic disease [53]. Some authors include criteria such as involvement of an exposed area and prior history of exposure to trauma or a contaminated source [54–56]. Ulcerative or necrotic lesions usually affecting the forearm or hand are the most common presentation of primary cutaneous cryptococcosis (Fig. 10.26).

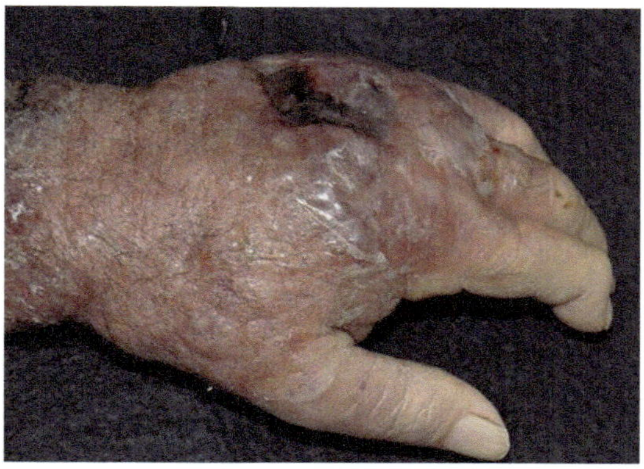

Fig. 10.26 Primary cutaneous *Cryptococcus* in an immunocompetent patient affecting the hand

Oral Signs and Symptoms

Oral mucosal lesions of cryptococcosis are extremely rare with very few cases reported in the literature. Review of the Medline databases from 2005 to 2017 has found only six cases of oral cryptococcosis published in the English literature [57–61]. Three cases occurred on the tongue producing, one case at the junction of the hard and soft palate presenting as an uncharacteristic shallow ulcer with discrete fibrin exudation. Other cases include a verrucous lesion in the retromolar space mimicking a squamous cell carcinoma and another affecting the gingiva in a leukemic patient. All of the cases except two were in HIV+ patients with concomitant skin lesions in three of them, suggesting disseminated disease [57–61]. An additional case of cryptococcosis restricted to the parotid gland in a patient wearing dentures has been reported [62]. Laryngeal cryptococcosis is also rare and often mimics laryngeal malignancy [63].

Differential Diagnosis

The differential diagnosis of cutaneous and oral cryptococcosis includes other opportunistic infections such as histoplasmosis, penicilliosis, paracoccidioidomycosis, and leishmaniasis.

The diagnosis of cryptococcosis of the CNS is based on examination of the cerebrospinal fluid (CSF), positive culture, or serologies. Magnetic resonance imaging (MRI) and computed tomography (CT) are useful tools to assess disease severity. MRI is preferred over CT for the evaluation of AIDS-associated cerebral cryptococcosis [57]. Pulmonary cryptococcosis does not have pathognomonic findings on imaging studies requiring biopsy of pulmonary tissue to establish the diagnosis.

Cutaneous or mucosal lesions can be diagnosed by histopathological examination, which is enhanced by stains such as mucicarmine, PAS, or alcian blue. Sabouraud's dextrose agar or other enriched media containing antibacterial antibiotics without cycloheximide are preferred media. The culture should be incubated at 30 °C with growth observed within 2–7 days. After an isolate has been established as *Cryptococcus*, the distinction between *C. neoformans* and *C.gattii* can be made using canavanine-glycine-bromothymol-blue (CGB) agar [53, 64]. After 1–5 days, the *C. gattii* turns the CGB medium from yellow green to blue, and the *C. neoformans* does not [53, 64]. This is a very sensitive and specific method to identify the *Cryptococcus* species. Nevertheless, molecular methods can be used with similar sensitivity and specificity. The serodiagnosis uses a latex agglutination kit devised to detect the polysaccharide capsule antigen with a sensitivity above 90% [64].

Treatment Recommendations

The strategies to treat the various clinical subtypes of cryptococcosis are beyond the scope of this chapter and are very well presented and discussed in the *Clinical Practice Guidelines for the Management of Cryptococcal Disease*, which is periodically updated [49]. For those patients with localized skin or mucosal disease for whom CNS, pulmonary, or disseminated disease has been ruled out, treatment options are fluconazole 400 mg per day or itraconazole 200 mg per day for 6–12 months [49].

Coccidioidomycosis

Etiopathogenesis

Coccidioidomycosis is a systemic mycosis caused by the dimorphic fungus *Coccidioides immitis* or *Coccidioides posadasii* [65, 66]. Similar to other systemic endemic mycoses, primary coccidioidomycosis is a consequence of inhaling the fungus [65–67]. Clinical pulmonary manifestations following infection will vary depending on the extent of infection and the immune status of the host. Overt disease can involve almost every organ system; however, pulmonary disease is the most common clinical manifestation [65–67].

The infection is a consequence of inhalation of arthroconidia, which results in asymptomatic, mild, or severe febrile respiratory illness [68]. The *Coccidioides* spp. is considered one of the most virulent among the etiologic agents of systemic mycosis. Inhalation of a few conidia can lead to infection in a normal healthy host. Accidental inhalation of conidia from *Coccidioides* culture is also a risk to laboratory workers and students [67]. There is no racial, sex, or age difference in susceptibility to primary pulmonary infection; however, a study in Kern County, California, done in 1995–1996 observed that independent risk factors for severe pulmonary disease included DM, recent history of cigarette smoking, low income, and older age [69]. Independent risk factors for disseminated disease include black race, low income, and pregnancy as well as immunocompromised patients [69, 70]. Other studies have reported that African Americans, Hispanics, Asians, and American Indians have a higher rate of extrapulmonary disease than Caucasians [71].

Epidemiology

Coccidioidomycosis is endemic in specific areas of the USA, Mexico, and Central and South America with a geographical distribution in semiarid or desert-like regions [65–67]. In the USA, the southwestern region of the country is the most important endemic area particularly the San Joaquin Valley and Southern California, Arizona, Nevada, Utah, and New Mexico [65, 67]. The incidence of coccidioidomycosis is growing in all endemic areas. In the USA, the incidence of coccidioidomycosis infection in endemic areas has considerably increased from 5.3 cases in 1998 to 42.6 cases per 100,000 population in 2011. Primary coccidioidal pneumonia accounts for 15–29% of all cases among patients with community-acquired pneumonia in Arizona [72]. Coccidioidomycosis can be considered an occupational hazard particularly in individuals who do agricultural work and construction, which has a higher risk of infection [65].

Clinical Manifestations

The majority of those exposed to the disease experience asymptomatic pulmonary infection. Typically, prior exposure does not lead to residual scarring in the lungs. In these instances, a positive coccidioidin skin test can confirm previous infection. Symptomatic pulmonary disease manifests 1–4 weeks following exposure. Most patients are febrile, and while chest pain is common, cough is less often observed as compared to other pulmonary infections [68]. Other possible symptoms are anorexia, malaise, myalgia, and backaches. Erythema nodosum and erythema multiforme are common cutaneous manifestations associated with pulmonary primary infection [68, 71]. The symptoms of pulmonary infection usually subside after 2 or 3 weeks but can progress to the development of cavitary disease, *coccidioidomas*, or progressive pulmonary disease. Disseminated disease occurring within the 1st weeks of primary disease is a predictor of a poor outcome. Single organ involvement is not infrequent in which case lesions affecting the eyes, bones, urogenital tract, or skin may be the only manifestation of the disease. Oral lesions tend to be extremely rare and most often occur in immunosuppressed patients with disseminated disease or occasionally as a solitary lesion affecting the tongue [73–75].

Differential Diagnosis

In endemic areas, primary pulmonary coccidioidomycosis is an important consideration in the setting of community-acquired pulmonary infection. Chronic pulmonary disease must be differentiated from tuberculosis, malignancy, and other systemic mycoses. Imaging studies such as CT or MRI do not have specific pathognomonic findings. Therefore, establishing a diagnosis will require a culture or biopsy. On histopathological examination, a purulent or granulomatous reaction is observed. Spherules with endospores in different stages of development and released endospores are frequently found in the cytoplasm of histiocytes, giant cells, or free in the tissue. Visual inspection of gross clinical specimens can be of great diagnostic value, as mature spherules are large and easily observed. Fresh tissue cultures can be performed using routine laboratory media at room temperature. However, because of risk of contamination, precautionary measures need to be taken in handling *Coccidioides* [67].

Treatment Recommendations

Amphotericin B in its different forms, itraconazole, and fluconazole are the most useful and frequently used treatments. Posaconazole and voriconazole can be administered as salvage therapy. Immunosuppressed patients, pregnant women, and elderly patients will require special attention [67, 76].

Parasitic Diseases

Leishmaniasis

Leishmaniasis is found worldwide; it is one of the most frequent tropical diseases constituting a significant public health problem in more than 88 countries. Leishmaniasis found in Central and South America has a more aggressive behavior and can affect the mucous membranes leading to a clinical form referred to as mucocutaneous leishmaniasis (MCL). Depending on the parasite species and the cell-mediated immune response of the patient, it can appear in four different clinical forms: localized cutaneous, disseminated cutaneous, mucocutaneous, and the visceral form (aka *Kala Azar*). Typically, an indolent ulcerated erythematous nodule arises after an insect bite, more frequently affecting the lower limbs or the head and neck [77].

Etiopathogenesis

It is caused by parasites of the *Leishmania* genus and transmitted to man by the bite of infected vectors belonging to the *Lutzomyia* and *Phlebotomus* genus. There are 20 different *Leishmania* species capable of producing the disease. The intrusion of man into environments where vectors proliferate, human migration, and more prevalent immunosuppression, especially that associated with HIV disease have gradually increased its incidence.

Leishmania are parasites belonging to the kinetoplastid order, protozoa which have their DNA in the form of a kinetoplast. The various species are grouped into two large complexes (*Leishmania brasiliensis and Leishmania mexicana)* causing different immunological responses in the host. The host's immunological response and nutritional status are very important in the development of the different clinical forms, as well as the number and location of the bites.

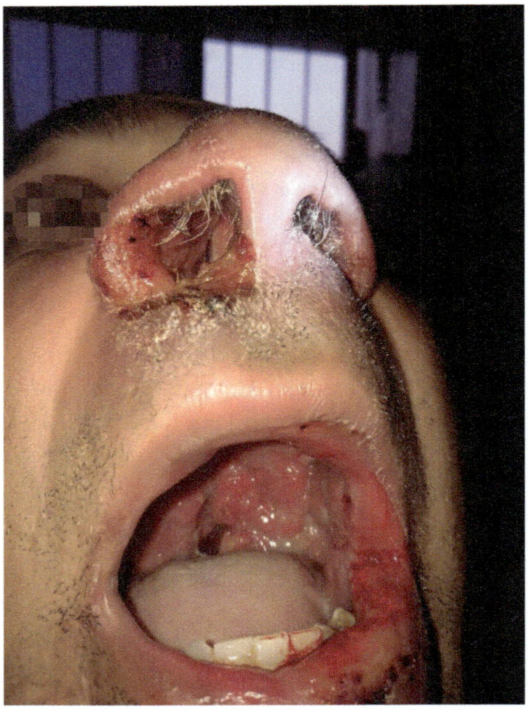

Fig. 10.27 Mucocutaneous Leishmaniasis: severe nasal-labial edema with nasal mucous membrane, lip and palatal involvement

Epidemiology

Cutaneous leishmaniasis (CL) is primarily a disease of the Near East (*Oriental Sore*) and the Mediterranean area. In Central and South America and Africa, it is frequent to find both cutaneous and mucocutaneous forms of the disease. In developed countries, its increased frequency is associated with leisure travel to endemic areas, immunosuppressive therapy, and the HIV/AIDS population.

Clinical Manifestations

Subsequent to the bite of an infected vector, a nodule or an erythematous plaque with variable degrees of induration with subsequent ulceration develops at the site.

Cutaneous leishmaniasis produced by *Leishmania tropica*, characteristic of the so-called *Old World Leishmaniasis*, tends to be limited. Mucocutaneous leishmaniasis can compromise the nasal and labial mucosa (Fig. 10.27). These forms have a variable presentation with nasal-labial edema in some cases, which can later affect the nasal septum and palate leading to perforation and disfiguring lesions of the centrofacial region (Figs. 10.28, 10.29, and 10.30). Mucous membrane involvement usually occurs due to hematogenous or lymphatic spread or via proximity with a localized cutaneous lesion.

Oral Signs and Symptoms

Mucosal involvement varies between 1% and 7% of cutaneous leishmaniasis cases primarily due to infection with the *Leishmania (Viannia) brazilensis complex.* Mucosal involvement may occur months or years after the cutaneous lesion has healed, independent of whether or not it was treated or arise spontaneously.

Nasal mucosal lesions initially appear with symptoms of nasal obstruction, rhinorrhea often

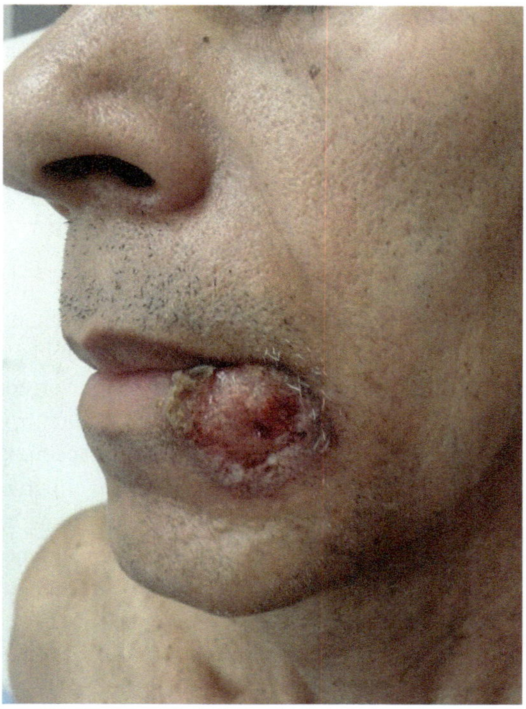

Fig. 10.28 Mucocutaneous leishmaniasis: lip. (Courtesy of A. Suarez, L. Camacaro, J. Guevara, O. Reyes, W. Vásquez, M.M. Hernández, Caracas, Venezuela)

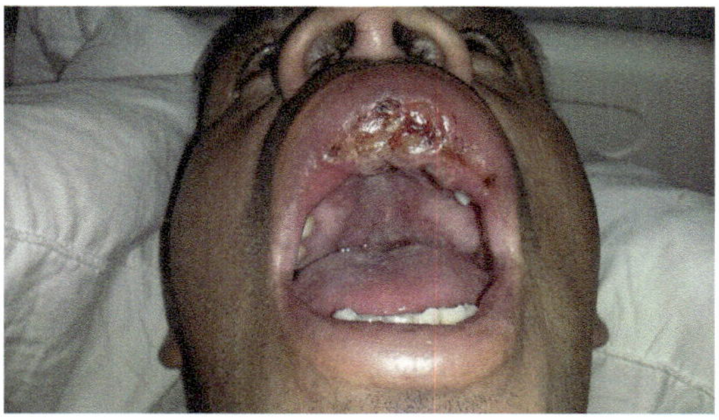

Fig. 10.29 Mucocutaneous leishmaniasis: lip and palatal ulceration

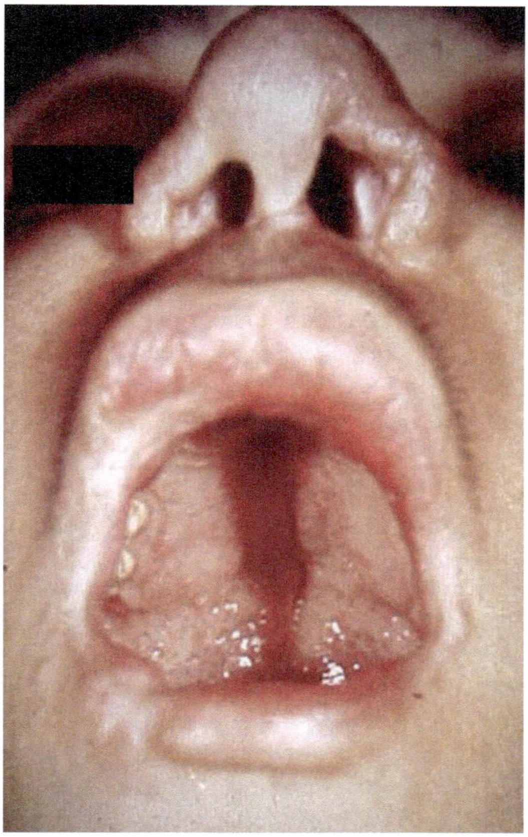

Fig. 10.30 Mucocutaneous leishmaniasis: nasal mucous membrane, lip and palatal involvement. (Courtesy of A.J. Rondón-Lugo, Caracas, Venezuela)

purulent due to bacterial infection, crusting, and epistaxis. Infiltration of the nasal mucosa by the *Leishmania* and the host's granulomatous response can lead to deformity and destruction of the nasal septum, producing a "tapir nose" appearance. If the destructive process progresses the posterior area of the nose, palate, pharynx, and larynx can also be affected.

Exclusive involvement of the oral mucosa is very rare. The nasal mucosa is mostfrequently affected. In general, the oral mucosa is affected due to the extension of cutaneous or nasal mucosal lesions, either due to contiguity or through hematogenous or lymphatic spread [78–80]. In general, mucosal manifestations of the disease can develop 1–5 years after the initial ulcerated cutaneous lesion has healed; nevertheless, in rare cases, the cutaneous and mucosal lesions can coincide. Epidemiological data show that in some countries approximately 5–7% of patients with cutaneous leishmaniasis will develop mucosal involvement.

Oral lesions in MCL are often confused with other oral diseases delaying diagnosis and treatment and increasing the likelihood of long-term sequelae. MCL most frequently affects the nose, followed by the mouth, pharynx, and larynx. Oral lesions have been reported in 37.9% of

MCL patients [81]. The presence of oral lesions was associated with involvement of the nasal, pharyngeal, and laryngeal mucous membranes, poor host response, and an indicator of treatment resistant disease [81]. Oral lesions affecting the labial mucosa, tongue, and hard and soft palate have been reported, which can present as labial or gingival hypertrophy, swelling or ulcerations of the tongue or palate with a cobblestone appearance, and vegetating tumors of the hard palate [79–84]. In immunocompromised patients, the oral mucosa is the second most frequently affected site of the head and neck region [82].

Differential Diagnosis

A definitive diagnosis is reached by visualization of the *Leishmania* amastigote parasite within tissue macrophages. The biopsy should be taken from the active border of the lesion, and, if possible, long-standing lesions should be avoided. Tissue biopsy or aspiration material should be used to prepare Giemsa stained slides for microscopic examination to confirm the presence of the amastigote parasite [85]. Tissue cultures can also facilitate diagnosis.

Species identification is critical in order to determine the expected clinical course, prognosis, and choice of treatment. PCR analysis can also be used to establish the diagnosis and determine the specific *Leishmania* species involved [77]. Other methods that can be used to confirm the diagnosis include immunohistochemistry using *Leishmania*-specific monoclonal antibodies, immunofluorescence, animal inoculation, and serologic assay. Montenegro's skin test can also be helpful; however, it cannot distinguish between past and active infection, which is important particularly in endemic areas [86].

The differential diagnosis of leishmaniasis includes paracoccidioidomycosis, cutaneous tuberculous, and histoplasmosis. Another important differential diagnosis is midline destructive disease such as Wegener's granulomatosis, vasculitis, and natural killer/T cell lymphoma (NKTCL) [87].

Treatment Recommendations

The role of therapy in cutaneous leishmaniasis is unclear since most cutaneous forms heal spontaneously with or without scarring. Various treatments have been used for the treatment of MCL [77] (Table 10.4). Antimonials, especially meglumine antimoniate, are the most effective treatment with a high cure rate. They can be administered intralesionally in localized cutaneous forms or intramuscularly at 20 mg/kg/d for 20 consecutive days in disseminated cutaneous forms, or patients at risk for mucosal involvement. Unfortunately, this drug has a high risk of untoward side effects such as myalgias, fever, headaches, and, less frequently, renal, hepatic, pancreatic, and hematologic toxicity. Serum sodium and potassium levels should be checked since hypokalemia can occur with increased risk of cardiac arrhythmias [88, 89].

Oral miltefosine 50 mg three times per daily for 28 days is effective in the treatment of visceral leishmaniasis caused by *L. donovani*. There are multiple reports of its effectiveness in cutaneous leishmaniasis, cases resistant to antimonial treatment, and in instances of intolerance to antimonials due to side effects. It has also been used successfully in the treatment of *Leishmania major*, *Leishmania donovani*, *Leishmania brasiliensis*, and *Leishmania mexicana*. However, gastrointestinal side effects may limit its use [84, 90, 91]. Some reports warn that although diffuse cutaneous leishmaniasis responds to miltefosine, relapse may occur with discontinuation

Table 10.4 Mucocutaneous leishmaniasis: treatment options

Antimonials	Amphotericin B	Miltefosine	Pentamidine
Rifampicin	Immunotherapy	Imiquimod	Ketoconazole
Terbinafine	Itraconazole	Thermotherapy	Cryotherapy
Trimethoropim/sulfamethoxazole			

[92]. Liposomal amphotericin B is an alternative therapy for MCL in South America particularly in cases due to *Leishmania braziliensis* and *Leishmania guyanensis*.

Immunotherapy with IFN, 5% imiquimod, or topical granulocyte-macrophage colony-stimulating factor as an adjunct to antimonial treatment was helpful in some series. Effective vaccination has been reported in patients with severe MCL and early diffuse CL by injecting killed *Leishmania braziliensis* promastigotes together with viable bacillus Calmette-Guerin [93, 94]. The potential of daylight-activated photodynamic therapy for treating localized forms of cutaneous leishmaniasis, in the setting of limited resources, could be a promising therapy [95].

Non-venereal Endemic Treponemal Infection: Yaws, Endemic Syphilis, and Pinta

The endemic treponemal diseases, yaws or frambesia, bejel or endemic syphilis, and pinta are a group of chronic relapsing non-venereal endemic treponemal infections closely related to syphilis, which are recognized by the WHO as neglected tropical diseases [96–100].

Etiopathogenesis

The genus *Treponema* contains both pathogenic and nonpathogenic species. Human pathogens cause four treponematoses: venereal syphilis (*T. pallidum* subsp. *pallidum*) and the endemic (non-venereal) treponematoses, yaws (*T. pallidum* subsp. *pertenue*), endemic syphilis (*T. pallidum* subsp. *endemicum*), and pinta (*T. carateum*) [98, 100]. Non-pathogenic treponemes can be part of the normal intestinal, oral, or genital flora.

Epidemiology

The endemic treponemal diseases are highly contagious. Transmission occurs through non-sexual human-to-human contact. Transmission of endemic syphilis, like that of yaws and pinta, is associated with poor hygiene. Despite extensive eradication campaigns, yaws remains widespread in the tropics predominantly affecting children living in certain tropical regions. It is endemic in parts of West Africa, Southeast Asia, and the Pacific. Pinta remains endemic in Central and South America, and endemic syphilis is present in certain regions of the Middle East [101–104]. With increasing worldwide travel, the diagnosis of the non-venereal treponematoses must be considered in appropriate clinical situations.

Clinical Manifestations

Treponemal infections are unique in that they are characterized by distinct clinical stages. Replication of the organism at the initial site of entry produces the primary stage. Dissemination of treponemes to other tissues results in the secondary stage. After a relatively prolonged period, in some cases up to 20–30 years later, the tertiary or late stage evolves. Oral treponemes have been associated with gingivitis and periodontal disease [100].

Yaws

Yaws is caused by *Treponema pallidum* ssp. *pertenue*, a gram-negative spirochete closely related to *Treponema pallidum* ssp. *pallidum*, the agent of venereal syphilis. The primary lesion is found at the site of cutaneous inoculation as an erythematous papule or group of papules or nodules known as *mother yaw or raspberry*. Lesions enlarge and ulcerate exuding a serous fluid rich in treponemes. These lesions heal spontaneously within one to several months, leaving an atrophic, depressed scar. Months after inoculation, the treponemes disseminate, a widespread rash develops, and secondary lesions quite similar to the mother yaw develop. Crops of lesions develop initially on the face and later spread to the trunk and arms. Lesions of the palms and soles are characteristic, as is the case with syphilis. Late yaws, sometimes called tertiary yaws, appears years later and is characterized by destructive lesions. It can affect the skin, mucous membranes, and bones. Oral lesions are uncommon. In the secondary stage, papillomas and intraoral plaques can be found on the lips and nose. As it progresses to the later stages, it can affect the nose with palatal perforation (*gangosa*) or lead to thickening of the nasal bones secondary to subperiosteal proliferation (*goundou*) [100–103].

Pinta

Pinta, caused by *T. carateum*, is endemic in the tropical areas of Central and South America. Most cases initially occur in children and adolescents. The primary lesions are flat, erythematous groups of papules that enlarge over the course of several months and produce scaly plaques. After a few months, the ulcerated lesions heal as hyperpigmented patches. Typically, the hands, feet, and scalp are affected. Late-stage pinta is characterized by hyperpigmented patches, which over time, become depigmented and hyperkeratotic due to scarring. The different stages of the disease are not clearly separated and commonly overlap [100].

Bejel (Endemic Syphilis)

Endemic syphilis, caused by *T. endemicum*, is still found in the Middle East and Central and South Africa. Clinical manifestations can be quite similar to those of syphilis and yaws. Primary lesions present as multiple papules affecting the mucous membranes of the eyes and mouth. The plaques of secondary bejel affect the mucous membranes and skin, becoming condylomatous in appearance, which usually heal spontaneously; it can also affect the muscles and bones. Clinical manifestations progress to a latency period that can last for several years. The late stage is characterized by deep skin *gummas* and destructive bone lesions with a predilection for the tibia [100].

Differential Diagnosis

The differential diagnosis of non-venereal treponemal infections includes syphilis and filiform warts. Diagnosis depends on epidemiological characteristics, clinical manifestations, demonstration of *Treponema* bacteria within exudate, and positive serological testing. In areas in which syphilis and yaws coexist, establishing a definitive diagnosis is unnecessary since both can be readily eradicated by penicillin. The two are virtually indistinguishable by morphology and serological testing [96]. Several minor genetic differences have been identified among the subspecies. Infection with yaws or syphilis results in reactive treponemal serology, and there is no widely available test to distinguish between these infections. Thus, migration of people from yaws-endemic areas to developed countries may present clinicians with diagnostic dilemmas.

Treatment Recommendations

T. pallidum pertenue, *T. pallidum endemicum*, and *T.carateum* are exquisitely sensitive to penicillin. As in syphilis, a single dose of penicillin G benzathine (1.2 million units) is curative. Azithromycin 30 mg/kg was shown to be equivalent to penicillin in patients with primary and secondary yaws, with a cure rate of 95% [105–107]. Treatment recommendations used for syphilis can be used to treat non-venereal endemic treponemal infections.

Atypical Mycobacteria

Epidemiology

Atypical mycobacteria produce infections in humans and animals. Better known as non-tuberculous mycobacteria (NTM) or mycobacteriosis, it is a mycobacterial species different from *M. leprae*, *M. tuberculosis, and M. bovis*. Atypical mycobacteria infections have been reported more often in the immunosuppressed, either HIV/AIDS associated or patients under therapeutic immunosuppression. In immunocompetent patients, the increasing prevalence of invasive cosmetic procedures has led to a dramatic increase in these infections. Therefore, NTM infections constitute an emergent infectious disease and a public health issue. The great majority of cases associated with cosmetic procedures are due to mesotherapy, use of fillers, liposuction, and breast implants [108, 109]. There are only a few studies reporting NTM infection of the oral cavity [110, 111].

Etiopathogenesis

NTM are saprophytic or opportunistic pathogens present in the environment including tap water or water processed for dialysis, which can contaminate medical equipment such as fiberscopes or liposuction cannulas due to improper sterilization. There is no evidence of transmission between people. The organism can survive in broad ranges of temperature, pH, salt concentration, and pO2. The high lipid cell wall favors *biofilm* formation, leading to a greater tendency for chronicity of infections and resistance to disinfectants and antibiotics.

In immunocompetent patients, invasive surgical and cosmetic procedures such as mesotherapy, fillers, prosthetic implants (such as breast, facial, gluteus, and testicular implants), cosmetic surgery (i.e., rhytidectomy, liposuction), tattoos, and body piercings have resulted in NTM infection, often causing outbreaks (Fig. 10.31). Cases have been reported secondary to acupuncture, oral surgery procedures, and non-sanitary pedicures and whirlpools. Surgical wound infections from NTM can arise from contaminated liposuction cannulas or gentian violet marking solution [112, 113]. Often improper disinfection procedures are the cause of infection.

Before highly active antiretroviral therapies (HAART) were available, disseminated Mycobacterium avium complex (MAC) infection was one of the most common opportunistic infections that affected AIDS patients. The clinical picture of MAC infections in patients treated with potent antiretroviral therapies has shifted from a disseminated disease with bacteremia to a localized infection, most often presenting with lymphadenopathy and osteomyelitis [12].

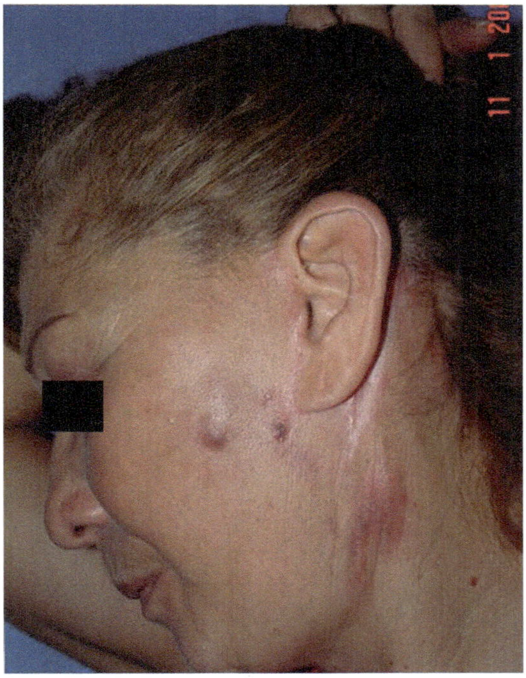

Fig. 10.31 Atypical mycobacteria: *M. abscessus* infection post facelift and liposuction of the neck

Clinical Manifestations

Cutaneous manifestations of NTM infections occurring after cosmetic procedures are nonspecific often presenting as nodules, cold abscesses, fistulae, and solitary or multiple ulcers. These manifestations depend on the species involved, the time of evolution of the infection, and the immunological profile of the patient [108].

Oral Signs and Symptoms

Oral ulcerations affecting the hard palate have been described in HIV as well as non-HIV patients with MAC infection [114, 115]. In AIDS patients, they arise in the later stages of the disease [111]. NTM infections in children commonly occur in the cervicofacial region, often

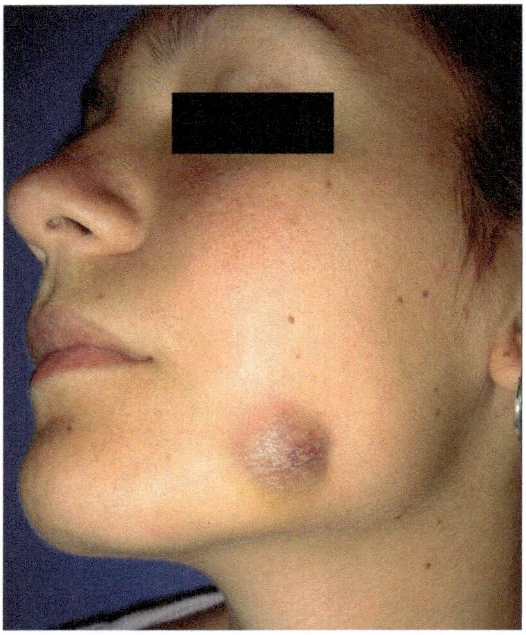

Fig. 10.32 Atypical mycobacteria: *M. fortuitum* infection after dental surgery

presenting as salivary gland masses. Thus, fine-needle aspiration cytology is useful in the investigation of these infections [116–118]. Also, in elderly immunocompetent patients, parotid gland infections have been described [119].

M. fortuitum infection can arise in surgical wounds of dental surgery such as molar extractions or in the setting of odontogenic abscesses, presenting as recurrent mandibular cutaneous abscesses responsive to treatment with intravenous amikacin and ciproflaxin as observed by Perez-Alfonzo (Figs. 10.32 and 10.33). Odontogenic infection has also been reported in the USA, in nine children who developed presumptive or confirmed *M. abscessus* infection after undergoing dental pulpotomy [110].

Differential Diagnosis

NTM infections should be differentiated from tuberculosis, sarcoidosis, and filler-induced foreign body granulomas, among others [120, 121]. Isolation of mycobacteria in culture can be used to establish a definitive diagnosis allowing

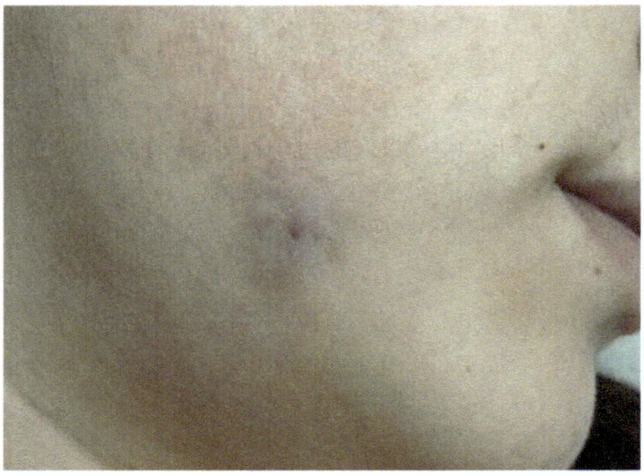

Fig. 10.33 Atypical mycobacteria: maxillary abscess produced by *M. fortuitum* infection after dental surgery

for species identification, which is critical for directing antibiotic therapy. NTM are classified according to their rate of growth in Lowenstein-Jensen culture: fast-growing *Mycobacteria* (visible growth <7 days); examples are *M. fortuitum*, *M. chelonae*, and *M. abscessus*. Examples of slow-growing *Mycobacteria* (>7 days) are *M. avium*, *M. kansasii*, *M. simiae*, *M. szulgai*, *M. scrofulaceum*, *M. haemophilum*, *M. ulcerans*, *M. marinum*, and *M. gordonae*.

The capacity for producing pigment in culture can also be a useful tool in identification of the mycobacteria subtype. For example, pigment-producing *Mycobacteria* include *M. marinum* and *M. kansasii.* Non-pigment-producing *Mycobacteria* include the fast growers such as *M. fortuitum*, *M. chelonae*, and *M. abscessus*. Other tests, which can be used for species identification, are biochemical tests, chromatographic techniques, and, above all, molecular identification, specifically, PCR analysis for the gene hsp65 (PRA), followed by restriction fragment analysis. The analysis is done by comparing fragment patterns with published patterns found in the Parasite database [108]. Determination of the antibiotic susceptibility of each identified species is highly recommended.

The most frequent mycobacteria, found after complications of cosmetic procedures, are *M. abscessus (30–40%)* followed by *M. fortuitum* and *M. chelonae*. *M. abscessus* can be differentiated into two genotypes based on gene hsp65 polymorphism: Type 1, which includes *M.*

abscessus subsp. *abscessus*, and Type 2, which includes *M. abscessus* subsp. *bolletii* and *M. abscessus* subsp. *massiliense*. Differentiation between these subspecies is important for the detection of inducible clarithromycin-resistant species in the *M. abscessus* group, a core drug for the treatment of NTM infections.

Treatment Recommendations

Treatment is based upon an initial 14–21-day treatment phase with two drugs and a 3–12-month maintenance phase. *M. abscessus* is generally sensitive to amikacin and clarithromycin (PRA type 1). *M. fortuitum* infections typically respond to amikacin, cefoxitin, ciprofloxacin, gatifloxacin, imipenem, levofloxacin, linezolid, and trimethoprim-sulfamethoxazole. *M. chelonea* is sensitive to amikacin, clarithromycin, gatifloxacin, linezolid, and tobramycin.

Acknowledgment The authors would like to acknowledge the valuable suggestions made by Lic. María Eugenia Gallinoto (Instituto de Biomedicina "Dr. Jacinto Convit," Universidad Central de Venezuela) and Dr. Jacobus H. de Waard (Microbiologist Tuberculosis Department, Instituto de Biomedicina "Dr. Jacinto Convit," Universidad Central de Venezuela).

References

1. Arenas R, Estrada R. Tropical dermatology, Vademècum. Georgetown: Landes Biosciences; 2001. ISBN1-57059-493-7.
2. Bonifaz A. Micología Médica Básica cuarta Edición. New York: McGraw Hill; 2012.
3. Martins N, Ferreira IC, Barros L, Silva S, Henriques M. Candidiasis: predisposing factors, preventions, diagnosis and alternative treatment. Mycopathologia. 2014;177:223–40.
4. Bork K, Hoede N, Korting G, Burgdorf W, Young S. Diseases of the oral mucosa and the lips. 2nd ed. Philadelphia: WB Saunders; 1996.
5. Sakaguchi H. Treatment and prevention of oral candidiasis in elderly patients. Med Mycol J. 2017;58: J43–9.
6. Hani U, Shivakumar HG, Vaghela R, Osmani RAM, Shrivastava A. Candidiasis: a fungal infection- current challenges and progress in prevention and treatment. Infect Disord – Drug Targets. 2015;15: 42–52.
7. Moghimi M, Salentijn E, Debets-Ossenkop Y, Karagozoglu KH, Forounzanfar T. Treatment of cervicofacial actinomycosis: a report of 19 cases and review of literature. Med Oral Patol Oral Cir Bucal. 2013;18:e627–32.
8. Kolm I, Aceto L, Hombach M, Kamarshev J, Hafner J, Urosevic-Maiwald M. Cervicofacial actinomycosis: a long forgotten infectious complication of immunosuppression – report of a case and review of the literature. Dermatol Online J. 2014;20:22640.
9. Valour F, Sénéchal A, Dupieux C, Karsenty J, Lustig S, Breton P, et al. Actinomycosis: etiology, clinical features, diagnosis, treatment, and management. Infect Drug Resist. 2014;7:183–97.
10. Fadda GL, Gisolo M, Crosetti E, Fulcheri A, Succo G. Intracranial complication of rhinosinusitis from actinomycosis of the paranasal sinuses: a rare case of abducens nerve palsy. Case Rep Otolaryngol. 2014;2014:601671.
11. Cohen PR, Tschen JA. Tonsillar actinomycosis mimicking a tonsillolith: colonization of the palantine tonsil presenting as a foul-smelling, removable, unilateral, giant tonsillar concretion. Int J Dermatol. 2010;49:1165–8.
12. Eidbo J, Sanchez RL, Tschen JA, Ellner KM. Cutaneous manifestations of histoplasmosis in the acquired immune deficiency syndrome. Am J Surg Pathol. 1993;17:110–6.
13. Marques SA, Silvares MR, Camargo RM, Marques ME. Cutaneous histoplasmosis disclosing an HIV-infection. An Bras Dermatol. 2013;88:420–3.
14. Corti M, Villafañe MF, Palmieri O, Negroni R. Rupioid histoplasmosis: first case reported in an AIDS patient in Argentina. Rev Inst Med Trop Sao Paulo. 2010;52:279–80.
15. Ollague Sierra JEI, Ollague Torres JM. New clinical and histological pattern of acute disseminated histoplasmosis in human immunodeficiency virus positive patients with acquired immunodeficiency syndrome. Am J Dermatophatol. 2013;35:203–12.
16. Ge L, Zhou C, Song Z, Zhang Y, Wang L, Zhong B, Hao F. Primary localized histoplasmosis with lesions restricted to the mouth in a Chinese HIV negative patient. Int J Infect Dis. 2010;14(Suppl 3): e325–8.
17. Iqbal FL, Schifter M, Coleman HG. Oral presentation of histoplasmosis in an immunocompetent patient: a diagnostic challenge. Aust Dent J. 2014;59:386–8.
18. Wheat J, Freifeld AG, Kleiman MB, Baddley JW, McKinsey DS, Loyd JE, Kauffman CA, Infectious Diseases Society of America. Clinical practice guidelines for the management of patients with histoplasmosis: 2007 update by the Infectious Diseases Society of America. Clin Infect Dis. 2007;45:807–25.
19. Restrepo A, Tobon A, Clark B, Graham DR, Corcoran G, Bradsher RW, et al. Salvage treatment of histoplasmosis with posaconazole. J Inf Secur. 2007;54:319–27.
20. Spellberg B, Walsh TJ, Kontoyiannis DP, Edwards J Jr, Ibrahim AS. Recent advances in the management

of mucormycosis: from bench to bedside. Clin Infect Dis. 2009;48:1743–51.
21. Marques SA. Fungal infections of the mucous membrane. Dermatol Ther. 2010;23:244–51.
22. Bonifaz A, Macias B, Paredes-Farreira F, Arias P, Ponce RM, Araiza J. Palatal zygomycosis: experience of 21 cases. Oral Dis. 2008;14:569–74.
23. Kontoyiannis DP, Wessel VC, Bodey GP, Rolston KV. Zygomycosis in the 1990s in a tertiary-care cancer center. Clin Infect Dis. 2000;30:851–6.
24. Marr KA, Carter RA, Crippa F, Wald A, Corey L. Epidemiology and outcome of mould infections in hematopoietic stem cell transplant recipients. Clin Infect Dis. 2002;34:909–17.
25. Bonifaz A, Vázquez-González D, Tirado-Sánchez A, Ponce-Olivera RM. Cutaneous zygomycosis. Clin Dermatol. 2012;30:413–9.
26. Bonifaz A, Tirado-Sánchez A, Calderón L, Romero-Cabello R, Kassack J, Ponce RM, et al. Mucormycosis in children: a study of 22 cases in a Mexican hospital. Mycoses. 2014;57(Suppl 3):79–84.
27. Ameen M, Arenas R, Martinez-Luna E, Reyes M, Zacarias R. The emergence of mucormycosis as an important opportunistic fungal infection: five cases presenting to a tertiary referral center for mycology. Int J Dermatol. 2007;46:380–4.
28. Reed G, Ibrahim A, Edwards J Jr. Deferasirox, an iron-chelating agent, as salvage therapy for rhinocerebral mucormycosis. Antimicrob Agents Chemother. 2006;50:3968–9.
29. Bagagli E, Theodoro RC, Bosco SM, McEwen JG. Paracoccidioidesbrasiliensis: phylogenetic and ecological aspects. Mycopathologia. 2008;165: 197–207.
30. Matute DR, McEwen JG, Puccia R, Montes BA, San-Blas G, Bagagli E, et al. Cryptic speciation and recombination in the fungus Paracoccidioidesbrasiliensis as revealed by gene genealogies. Mol Biol Evol. 2006;23:65–73.
31. Matute DR, Sepulveda VE, Quesada LM, Goldman GH, Taylor JW, Restrepo A, et al. Microsatellite analysis of three phylogenetic species of Paracoccidioidesbrasiliensis. J Clin Microbiol. 2006;44:2153–7.
32. Teixeira MM, Theodoro RC, de Carvalho MJ, Fernandes L, Paes HC, Hahn RC. Phylogenetic analysis reveals a high level of speciation in the Paracoccidioides genus. Mol Phylogenet Evol. 2009;52:273–83.
33. Theodoro RC, Teixeira Mde M, Felipe MS, Paduan Kdos S, Ribolla PM, San-Blas G, et al. Genus Paracoccidioides: species recognition and biogeographic aspects. PLoSOne. 2012;7:e37694.
34. Turissini DA, Gomez OM, Teixeira MM, McEwen JG, Matute DR. Species boundaries in the human pathogen *Paracoccidioides*. Fungal Genet Biol. 2017;106:9–25.
35. Bellissimo-Rodrigues F, Machado AA, Martinez R. Paracoccidioidomycosis epidemiological features of a 1,000-cases series from a hyperendemic area on the Southeast of Brazil. Am J Trop Med Hyg. 2011;85:546–50.
36. Marques SA. Paracoccidioidomycosis: epidemiological, clinical, diagnostic and treatment up-dating. An Bras Dermatol. 2013;88:700–11.
37. Franco M, Montenegro MR, Mendes RP, Marques SA, Dillon N, Mota NGS. Paracoccidioidomycosis: a recently proposed classification of its clinical forms. Rev Soc Bras Med Trop. 1987;20:129–32.
38. Marques SA, Cortez DB, Lastória JC, Camargo RMP, Marques MEA. Paracoccidioidomycosis: frequency, morphology and pathogenesis of tegumentary lesions. An Bras Dermatol. 2007;82:411–7.
39. Queiroz-Telles F, Goldani LZ, Schlamm HT, Goodrich JM, Espinel-Ingroff A, Shikanai-Yasuda MA. An open-label comparative pilot study of oral voriconazole and itraconazole for long-term treatment of paracoccidioidomycosis. Clin Infect Dis. 2007;45:1462–9.
40. Peçanha PM, Souza S, Falqueto A, Grão-Veloso TR, Lírio LV, Ferreira CUG Jr, et al. Amphotericin B lipid complex in the treatment of severe paracoccidioidomycosis: a case series. Int J Antimicrob Agents. 2016;48:428–30.
41. Shikanai-Yasuda MA, TellesFilho FQ, Mendes RP, Colombo AL, Moretti ML. Grupo de Consultores do Consenso em Paracoccidiodomicose. Consenso em paracoccidioidomicose. Rev Soc Bras Med Trop. 2006;39:297–310.
42. Saccente M, Woods GL. Clinical and laboratory update on blastomycosis. Clin Microbiol Rev. 2010;23:367–81.
43. Rucci J, Eisinger G, Miranda-Gomez G, Nguyen J. Blastomycosis of the head and neck. Am J Otolaryngol. 2014;35:390–5.
44. Kruse AL, Zwahlen RA, Bredell MG, Gengler C, Dannemann C, Grätz KW. Primary blastomycosis of oral cavity. J Craniofac Surg. 2010;21:121–3.
45. Fanucci E, Nezzo M, Neroni L, Montesani L Jr, Ottria L, Gargari M. Diagnosis and treatment of paranasal sinus fungus ball of odontogenic origin: case report. Oral Implantol (Rome). 2014;6(3):63–6.
46. Grosjean P, Weber R. Fungus balls of the paranasal sinuses: a review. Eur Arch Otorhinolaryngol. 2007;264:461–70.
47. Ganesh P, Nagarjuna M, Shetty S, Kumar P, Bhat V, Salins PC. Invasive aspergillosis presenting as swelling of the buccal mucosa in an immunocompetent individual. Oral Surg Oral Med Oral Pathol Oral Radiol. 2015;119:e60–4.
48. MacDougall L, Fyfe M, Romney M, Starr M, Galanis E. Risk factors for Cryptococcus gattii infection, British Columbia. Canada Emerg Infect Dis. 2011;17:193–9.
49. Perfect JR, Dismukes WE, Dromer F, Goldman DL, Graybill JR, Hamill RJ, et al. Clinical practice guidelines for the management of cryptococcal disease: 2010 update by the infectious diseases society of America. Clin Infect Dis. 2010;50: 291–322.

50. Viviani MA. Cryptococcal meningitis: diagnosis and treatment. Int J Antimicrob Agents. 1996;6: 169–73.
51. Thomas I, Schwartz RA. Cutaneous manifestations of systemic cryptococcosis in immunosuppressed patients. J Med. 2001;32:259–66.
52. Negroni R. Cryptococcosis. Clin Dermatol. 2012;30:599–609.
53. Marques SA, Bastazini I Jr, Martins AL, Barreto JÁ, Barbieri D'Elia MP, Lastória JC, et al. Primary cutaneous cryptococcosis in Brazil: report of 11 cases in immuno competent and immunosuppressed patients. Int J Dermatol. 2012;51:780–4.
54. Nascimento E, Bonifácio da Silva ME, Martinez R, Von ZeskaKress MR. Primary cutaneous cryptococcosis in an immunocompetent patient due to Cryptococcus gattii molecular type VGI in Brazil: a case report and review of the literature. Mycoses. 2014;57(7):442–7.
55. Patel P, Ramanathan J, Kayser M, Baran JJR. Primary cutaneous cryptococcosis of the nose in an immunocompetent woman. J Am Acad Dermatol. 2000;43:344–5.
56. Pau M, Lallai C, Aste N, Aste N, Atzori L. Primary cutaneous cryptococcosis in an immunocompetent host. Mycoses. 2010;53:256–8.
57. Iatta R, Napoli C, Borghi, Montagna MT. Rare mycosis of oral cavity: a literature epidemiological review. Oral Surg Oral Med Oral Pathol Oral Radiol Endod. 2009;108:647–55.
58. Faria PF, Vargas PA, Saldiva PH, Böhm GM, Mauad T, de Almeida OP. Tongue disease in advanced AIDS. Oral Dis. 2005;11:72–80.
59. Liew C, Barreto L, Mills C. Interesting case: an unusual case of oral ulceration. Br J Oral Maxillofac Surg. 2006;44:350.
60. Mohamad I, Abdullah B, Salim R, Rajet KA, Naik VR. Cryptococcosis: a rare fungal infection of the tongue. Southeast Asian J Trop Med Public Health. 2010;41:1188–91.
61. Patel S, Navas M, Batt C, Jump RLP. Oral cryptococcosis in a patient with chronic lymphocytic leukemia. Int J Infect Dis. 2016;50:18–20.
62. Kantarcioglu AS, Gulenc M, Yücel A, Uzun N, Taskin T, Sakiz D, Altas K. Cryptococcal parotid involvement: an uncommon localization of Cryptococcus neoformans. Med Mycol. 2006;44:279–83.
63. Wong DJY, Stanley P, Paddle P. Laryngeal cryptococcosis associated with inhaled corticosteroid use: case report and review of the literature. Front Surg. 2017;4:e63.
64. Kwon-Chung KJ, Bennett JE. Cryptococcosis. In: Kwon-Chung KJ, Bennett JE, editors. Medical mycology. Philadelphia: Lea & Febiger; 1992. p. 397–446.
65. Benedict K, Park BJ, Thompson GR 3rd. Coccidioidomycosis: epidemiology. Clin Epidemiol. 2013;5:185–97.
66. Welsh O, Vera-Cabreira L, Rendon A, Gonzalez G, Bonifaz A. Coccidioidomycosis. Clin Dermatol. 2012;30:573–91.
67. Kwon-Chung KJ, Bennett JE. Coccidioidomycosis. In: Kwon-Chung KJ, Bennett JE, editors. Medical mycology. Philadelphia: Lea & Febiger; 1992. p. 357–97.
68. Blair JE, Chang YH, Cheng MR, Vaszar LT, Vikram HR, Orenstein R, et al. Characteristics of patients with mild to moderate primary pulmonary coccidioidomycosis. Emerg Infect Dis. 2014;20:983–90.
69. Rosenstein NE, Emery KW, Werner SB, Kao A, Johnson R, Rogers D, et al. Risk factor for severe pulmonary and disseminated coccidioidomycosis: Kern County, California, 1995–1996. Clin Infect Dis. 2001;32:708–16.
70. Odio CD, Marciano BE, Galgiani JN, Holland SM. Risk factor for disseminated coccidioidomycosis, United States. Emerg Infect Dis. 2017;23: 308–11.
71. Galgiani JN, Ampel NM, Blair JE, Catanzaro A, Johnson RH, Stevens DA, Williams PL, Infectious Diseases Society of America. Coccidioidomycosis. Clin Infect Dis. 2005;41(9):1217–23.
72. Center of Disease Control and Prevention. Increase in reported coccidioidomycosis: United States 1998–2011. MMWR Morb Mortal Wkly Rep. 2013;62:217–21.
73. Rodriguez RA, Konia T. Coccidioidomycosis of the tongue. Arch Patol Lab Med. 2005;129:e4–6.
74. Stich A, Müller A, Tintelnot K. Coccidioidomycosis with manifestation on the tongue. Pathologe. 2013;34:548–51.
75. Mendez LA, Florez SA, Martinez R, Almeida OP. Ulcerated lesion of the tongue as manifestation of systemic coccidioidomycosis. Case Rep Med. 2017; https://doi.org/10.1155/2017/1489501.
76. Galgiani JN, Ampel NM, Blair JE. 2016 Infectious Diseases Society of America (IDSA) clinical practice guidelines for the treatment of Coccidioidomycosis. Clin Infect Dis. 2016;61:717–22.
77. Ameen M. Cutaneous leishmaniasis: advances in disease pathogenesis, diagnostics and therapeutics. Clin Exp Dernatol. 2010;35:699–705.
78. Ramos-e-Silva M. Diseases of the oral cavity caused by Protozoa. In: Lotti TM, Parish LC, Rogers IIIRS, editors. Oral diseases. Textbook and Atlas. Berlin: Springer-Verlag; 1999. p. 122–5.
79. Mignogna MD, Celentano A, Leuci S, Cascone M, Adamo D, Ruoppo E, Favia G. Mucosal leishmaniasis with primary oral involvement: a case series and a review of the literature. Oral Dis. 2015;21(1):e70–8.
80. García de Marcos JA, Dean Ferrer A, Alamillos Granados F, Ruiz Masera JJ, Cortés Rodríguez B, Vidal Jiménez A, et al. Localized Leishmaniasis of the oral mucosa. A report of three cases. Med Oral Patol Oral Cir Bucal. 2007;12(4):E281–6.
81. Da Costa DC, Palmeiro MR, Moreira JS, Martins AC, da Silva AF, Madeira Mde F, et al. Oral manifestations in the American tegumentary leishmaniasis. PLoS One. 2014;9:e109790.
82. Milián MA, Bagán JV, Jiménez Y, Pérez A, Scully C. Oral leishmaniasis in a HIV-positive patient.

Report of a case involving the palate. Report of a case involving the palate. Oral Dis. 2002;8:59–61.
83. Passi D, Sharma S, Dutta, S, Gupta C. Localized leishmaniasis of oral mucosa: Report of an unusual clinicopathological entity. Hindawi Publishing Corporation. Case Reports in Dentistry. 2014;753149. https://doi.org/10.1155/2014/753149.
84. Kassam K, Davidson R, Tadrous PJ, Kumar M. Lingual Leishmaniasis presenting to maxillofacial surgery in UK with successful treatment with miltefosine. Case Rep Med. 2013;2013:975131.
85. Daneshbod Y, Oryan A, Davarmanesh M, Shirian S, Negahban S, Aledavood A, et al. Clinical, histopathologic, and cytologic diagnosis of mucosal leishmaniasis and literature review. Arch Pathol Lab Med. 2011;135:478–82.
86. Almeida TF, da Silveira EM, Dos Santos CR, León JE, Mesquita AT. Exclusive primary lesion of oral leishmaniasis with Immunohistochemical diagnosis. Head Neck Pathol. 2016;10:533–7.
87. Crovetto-Martínez R, Aguirre-Urizar JM, Orte-Aldea C, Araluce-Iturbe I, Whyte-Orozco J, Crovetto-De la Torre MA. Mucocutaneous leishmaniasis must be included in the differential diagnosis of midline destructive disease: two case reports. Oral Surg Oral Med Oral Pathol Oral Radiol. 2015;119(1):e20–6.
88. Minodier P, Parola P. Cutaneous leishmaniasis treatment. Travel Med Infect Dis. 2007;5:150–8.
89. Amato VS, Tuon FF, Siqueira AM, Nicodemo AC, Neto VA. Treatment of mucosal leishmaniasis in Latin America: systematic review. Am J Trop Med Hyg. 2007;77:266–74.
90. Zerpa O, Blanco B, Kannee C, Ulrich M, Sindermann H, Engel J, Convit J. Treatment of diffuse cutaneous leishmaniasis with miltefosine: a case report. Int J Dermatol. 2006;45:751–3.
91. Vélez I, López L, Sánchez X, Mestra L, Rojas C, Rodriguez E. Efficacy of miltefosine for the treatment of American cutaneous leishmaniasis. Am J Trop Med Hyg. 2010;83:351–6.
92. Zerpa O, Ulrich M, Blanco B, Polegre M, Avila A, Matos N, et al. Diffuse cutaneous leishmaniasis responds to miltefosine but then relapses. Br J Dermatol. 2007;156:1328–35.
93. Convit J, Ulrich M, Zerpa O, Borges R, Aranzazu N, Valera M, et al. Immunotherapy of american cutaneous leishmaniasis in Venezuela during the period 1990–99. Trans R Soc Trop Med Hyg. 2003;97(4):469–72.
94. Convit J, Ulrich M, Polegre MA, Avila A, Rodríguez N, Mazzedo MI, et al. Therapy of Venezuelan patients with severe mucocutaneous or early lesions of diffuse cutaneous leishmaniasis with a vaccine containing pasteurized Leishmania promastigotes and bacillus Calmette-Guerin: preliminary report. Mem Inst Oswaldo Cruz. 2004;99:57–62.
95. Ameen M. The potential of daylight-activated photodynamic therapy for treating localized forms of cutaneous leishmaniasis in resource-limited settings. Br J Dermatol. 2015;172:1192–3.
96. Marks M, Solomon AW, Mabey DC. Endemic Treponemal disease. Trans R Soc Trop Med Hyg. 2014;108:601–7.
97. Koff AB, Rosen T. Non venereal treponematoses: yaws, endemic syphilis, and pinta. J Am Acad Dermatol. 1993;29:519–35.
98. Antal GM, Lukehart SA, Meheus AZ. The endemic treponematoses. Microbes Infect. 2002;4:83–94.
99. Giacani L, Lukehart SA. The endemic treponematoses. Clin Microbiol Rev. 2014;27:89–115.
100. Radolf JD. Treponema. In: Baron S, editor. Medical microbiology. 4th ed. Galveston: University of Texas Medical Branch at Galveston; 1996. Chapter 36.
101. Marks M, Mitjà O, Solomon AW, Asiedu KB, Mabey DC. Yaws. Br Med Bull. 2015;113:91–100.
102. Marks M, Lebari D, Solomon AW, Higgins SP. Yaws. Int J STD AIDS. 2015;26:696–703.
103. Mitjà O, Asiedu K, Mabey D. Yaws. Lancet. 2013;381:763–73.
104. Kazadi WM, Asiedu KB, Agana N, Mitjà O. Epidemiology of yaws: an update. Clin Epidemiol. 2014;6:119–28.
105. Mitjà O, Hays R, Ipai A, Penias M, Paru R, Fagaho D, et al. Single-dose azithromycin versus benzathine-benzylpenicillin for treatment of yaws in children in Papua New Guinea: an open-label, non-inferiority, randomised trial. Lancet. 2012;379:342–7.
106. Kwakye-Maclean C, Agana N, Gyapong J, Nortey P, Adu-Sarkodie Y, Aryee E, et al. A single dose oral azithromycin versus intramuscular benzathine penicillin for the treatment of yaws-a randomized non inferiority trial in Ghana. PLoS Negl Trop Dis. 2017;11(1):e0005154.
107. Fegan D, Glennon MJ, Kool J, Taleo F. Tropical leg ulcers in children: more than yaws. Trop Dr. 2016;46:90–3.
108. Rivera-Olivero IA, Guevara A, Escalona A, Oliver M, Pérez-Alfonzo R, Piquero J, et al. Soft-tissue infections due to non-tuberculous mycobacteria following mesotherapy. What is the price of beauty. Enferm Infecc Microbiol Clin. 2006;24:302–6.
109. Torres-Coy JA, Rodríguez-Castillo BA, Pérez-Alfonzo R, DE Waard JH. Source investigation of two outbreaks of skin and soft tissue infection by Mycobacterium abscessus subsp. abscessus in Venezuela. Epidemiol Infect. 2016;144:1117–20.
110. Peralta G, Tobin-D'Angelo M, Parham A, Edison L, Lorentzson L, Smith C, et al. Notes from the field: Mycobacterium abscessus infections among patients of a pediatric dentistry practice – Georgia, 2015. MMWR Morb Mortal Wkly Rep. 2016;65:355–6.
111. Lange CG, Woolley IJ, Brodt RH. Disseminated mycobacterium avium-intracellulare complex (MAC) infection in the era of effective antiretroviral therapy: is prophylaxis still indicated? Drugs. 2004;64:679–92.
112. Safraneck TJ, Jarvis WR, Carson LA, Cusick LB, Bland LA, Swenson JM, Silcox VA. Myobacterirum chelonae wound infections after plastic surgery

employing contaminated gentian violet skin-marking solution. N Engl J Med. 1987;317:197–201.
113. Murillo J, Torres J, Bofill L, Ríos-Fabra A, Irausquin E, Istúriz R, et al. Skin and wound infection by rapidly growing mycobacteria: an unexpected complication of liposuction and liposculpture. The Venezuelan Collaborative Infectious and Tropical Diseases Study Group. Arch Dermatol. 2000;136: 1347–52.
114. Robinson P, Farthing P, Scott GM, Bennett JH. Oral Mycobacterium avium complex infection in a patient with HIV-related disease. A case report. Oral Surg Oral Med Oral Pathol Oral Radiol Endod. 1996;81:177–9.
115. Alagarswamy RK, Halfpenny W, Thiruchelvam JK, Mohamid W. Rare presentation of Mycobacterium avium-intracellulare infection. Br J Oral Maxillofac Surg. 2007;45:670–2.
116. Cox HJ, Brightwell AP, Riordan T. Non-tuberculous mycobacterial infections presenting as salivary gland masses in children: investigation and conservative management. J Laryngol Otol. 1995;109:525–30.
117. Berkovic J, Vanchiere JA, Gungor A. Non tuberculous mycobacterial lesion of the parotid gland and facial skin in a 4 year old girl: a proposed treatment strategy. Am J Otolaryngol. 2016;37:89–94.
118. Bonali M, Mattioli F, Alicandri-Ciufelli M, Presutti L. Atypical mycobacteriosis involving parotid and para-retropharyngeal spaces. Eur Arch Otorhinolaryngol. 2016;273:4031–3.
119. Yamanaka T, Okamoto H, Hosoi H. Non-tuberculous mycobacterial infection of the parotid gland in an immunocompetent elderly patient. BMJ Case Rep. 2013;16:2013.
120. Motswaledi MH, Khammissa RA, Jadwat Y, Lemmer J, Feller L. Oral sarcoidosis: a case report and review of the literature. Aust Dent J. 2014;59:389–94.
121. Sharma P, Saxena S, Aggarwal P, Reddy V. Tuberculosis of odontogenic cyst. Indian J Tuberc. 2013;60:50–4.

11 Oral Signs of Genetic Disease

Julio C. Sartori-Valinotti and Jennifer L. Hand

Incontinentia Pigmenti (Bloch-Sulzberger Syndrome)

Epidemiology

Incontinentia pigmenti (IP) is an ectodermal dysplasia with an estimated prevalence of 0.7 cases per 100,000 births, almost exclusively affecting females [1].

Etiopathogenesis

IP is an X-linked disease caused by mutation in the IKK-gamma gene (inhibitor of nuclear factor kappa-B kinase subunit gamma), previously known as NEMO, located on chromosome Xq28. Disruption, usually by deletion, of the IKK-gamma gene is responsible for downstream activation of cellular apoptosis. Programmed cell death in different tissues such as the skin, teeth, nails, eyes, skeleton, and central nervous system (CNS) accounts for the clinical manifestations of the disease. The disease is lethal in males, usually prenatally.

J. C. Sartori-Valinotti · J. L. Hand (✉)
Department of Dermatology, Mayo Clinic and Foundation, Rochester, MN, USA
e-mail: hand.jennifer@mayo.edu

Clinical Manifestations

In affected females, the striking cutaneous findings evolve sequentially in four distinct, overlapping stages that follow developmental skin lines (Fig. 11.1):

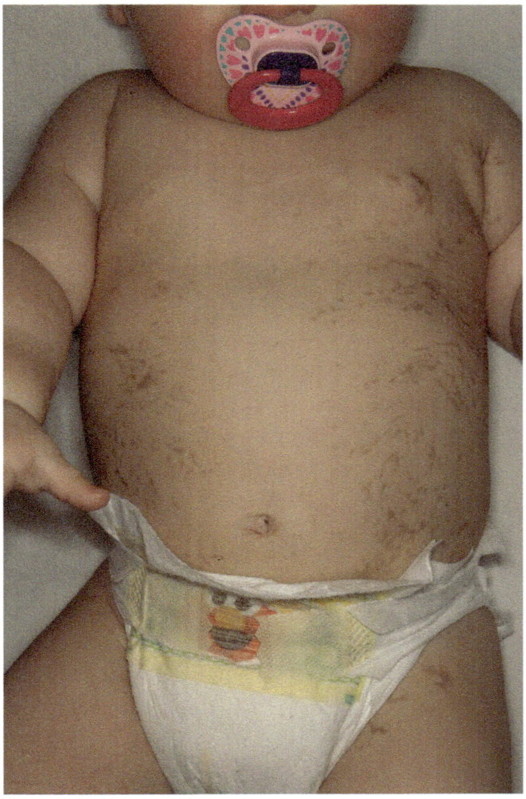

Fig. 11.1 Female infant with cutaneous hyperpigmentation along developmental skin (Blaschko's) lines, typical of incontinentia pigmenti

N. Fazel (ed.), *Oral Signs of Systemic Disease*, https://doi.org/10.1007/978-3-030-10863-2_11

inflammatory vesicles, verrucous phase, hyperpigmentation, and finally hypopigmented linear or reticular lesions. The latter is due to epidermal atrophy and dermal scarring [2]. Mild, patchy alopecia is a common feature. Anomalies of the eyebrows and eyelashes have also been reported [3]. Dystrophic nail changes may vary from mild to severe [2]. Retinal abnormalities (telangiectasias, hemorrhages, neovascularization, disorders of the retinal pigment epithelium, etc.) may unexpectedly cause blindness in early childhood, and non-retinal abnormalities (microphthalmia, vitreous and lens anomalies) may present in the neonatal period [3, 4]. CNS complications of IP, present in up to 30–46% of patients, include microcephaly, mental retardation, motor incoordination, and seizures [5, 6]. Unilateral breast and nipple hypoplasia as well as supernumerary nipples may be seen [2].

Oral Signs and Symptoms

The most comprehensive review of the oral and dental manifestations of IP included 1286 IP patients from 1993 to 2010. In this study, Minić and coworkers found that 54% of patients had dental and/or oral anomalies. Most recently, dental and/or oral changes have been regarded as the most important minor diagnostic criteria for IP. While dental changes are not appreciable until after tooth eruption, they are often the feature most concerning to parents, which brings the disorder to medical attention. Cleft and high-arched (gothic) palate present at birth and may aid in early diagnosis. Dental anomalies are, however, more common than oral anomalies in IP. In descending order of frequency, dental shape anomalies (coni- or peg-like teeth) (Fig. 11.2), hypodontia, and delayed dentition are the most common. Enamel and tooth strength are normal [7]. Other manifestations include extensive dental decay and early loss of dentition [8]. The mean number of missing permanent teeth is 5.9 [9]. In a small case series, salivary secretion was lower than normal in 43% of patients [10].

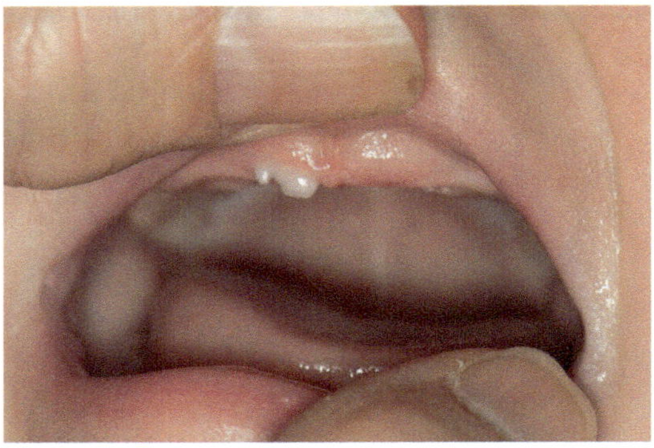

Fig. 11.2 Misshapen deciduous tooth in female infant with incontinentia pigmenti

Differential Diagnosis

Several skin disorders may present with cutaneous findings similar to IP. The differential diagnosis relies on the age/stage of the lesions. From an orodental perspective, abnormally-shaped teeth are seen in other forms of ectodermal dysplasias; extensive tooth loss and dental decay are seen in dyskeratosis congenita. Inflammatory periodontitis and premature loss of deciduous teeth are features of Papillon-Lefevre syndrome (PLS). The associated skin and oral (cleft and gothic palate) findings help distinguish IP from other genodermatoses.

Treatment Recommendations

Orthopedic and/or orthodontic repositioning of malpositioned teeth and bone expansion are recommended for subsequent prosthesis procedures [11, 12]. Early treatment is thought to improve self-esteem and nutrition. The National Foundation for Ectodermal Dysplasias (http://www.nfed.org) discusses strategies for affected families to obtain insurance coverage for necessary dental treatment.

Pachyonychia Congenita

Epidemiology

Pachyonychia congenital (PC) is a group of disorders unified by painful, plantar keratoderma [13] and characteristic, distinct nail changes with distal

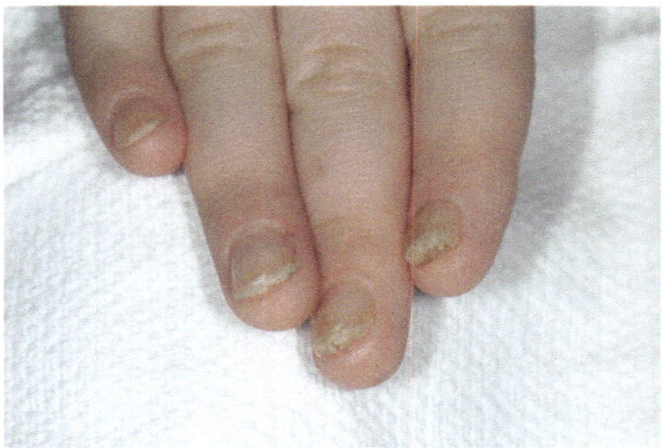

Fig. 11.3 Thickened nails with yellowish discoloration and transverse arching in a 6-year-old girl with pachyonychia congenita

onycholysis, subungual hyperkeratosis that causes transverse arching of the distal nail plate, and yellow-brown discoloration [14] (Fig. 11.3). There is a paucity of data regarding the incidence and prevalence of the disease, but approximately 1000 cases have been published in the literature [1].

Etiopathogenesis

PC is an autosomal dominant disorder. Keratins are structural proteins usually expressed in pairs [15]. The keratin pair K6b/K17 is expressed in nails and the palmoplantar surface. Mutations in either of these keratins cause PC type 2. Mutations in either K16 or K6a cause PC type 1 [15]. The genes for keratin 6a and 6b are on chromosome 12, and the genes for keratin 16 and 17 are on chromosome 17. A clinical genetic test is available.

Clinical Manifestations

In PC type 1 (aka Jadassohn-Lewandowsky syndrome), hyperkeratosis of the palms, soles, knees, and elbows, follicular hyperkeratosis (Fig. 11.4), and hyperhidrosis of the hands and feet are associated features. Oral leukokeratosis may be mild or absent in PC type 2 (aka Jackson-Lawler syndrome), which is associated with natal teeth, milder keratoderma, epidermal cysts, and steatocysts. Oral leukokeratosis may be found but is less marked than in PC type 1 [15].

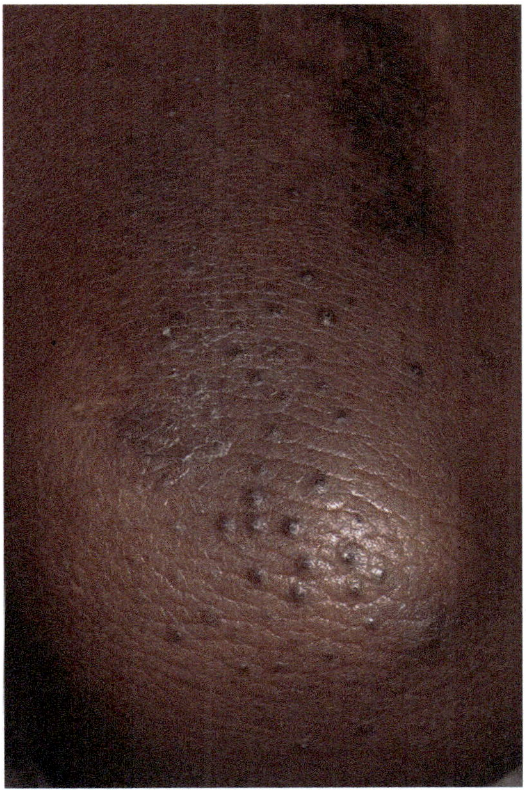

Fig. 11.4 Follicular hyperkeratosis over the extensor elbow in a young man with pachyonychia congenita

Oral Signs and Symptoms

Oral lesions of PC are white, opaque thickenings in small areas of the tongue or buccal mucosa (Fig. 11.5) or confluently covering the entire surface of the tongue, lips, and cheeks [14], with the tongue being the most common location [16]. Oral leukokeratosis is seen in 70% of patients with genetically confirmed PC [17]. Onset at birth has been reported in 54% of patients [17] and may represent the earliest manifestation of the disease. It can also be exacerbated by or interfere with breastfeeding [18]. The oral plaques can be painful as a result of trauma due to food intake or entirely painless [18–20]. Involvement of the oropharynx may create a hoarse voice. Histologic examination demonstrates acanthosis, marked hyperkeratosis, and absence of the granular layer. Malignant transformation of the leukokeratosis has not been reported [14].

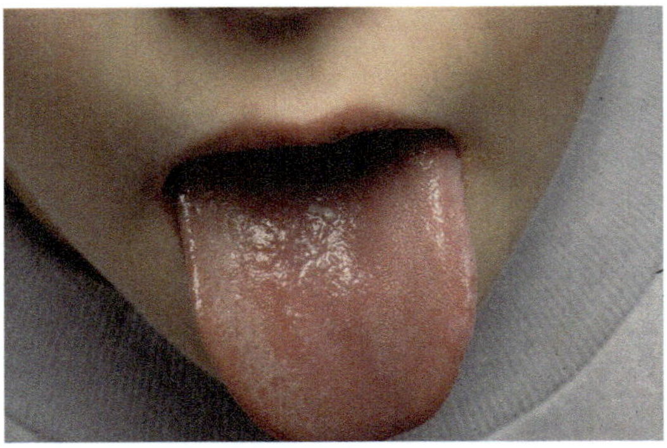

Fig. 11.5 Leukokeratosis over the lateral tongue in a young girl with pachyonychia congenita

Fifteen percent of patients with keratin 17 mutations have "natal teeth" compared to only 3% of patients with keratin 6a mutation and none with keratin 6b or 16 [17]. Natal teeth are either soft or crumbly and rapidly lost or normal appearing and persistent until permanent tooth eruption [16]. Angular cheilitis and median rhomboid glossitis have been described in patients with PC [18, 21].

Differential Diagnosis

Oral leukokeratosis in PC can be mistaken for white sponge nevus, oral leukoplakia, hairy tongue, and oral candidiasis [20]. Oral leukokeratosis is often misdiagnosed as thrush but does not improve with antifungal therapy. Interestingly, superinfection with *C. albicans* has been described [14, 22]. In a patient reported by Hannaford and Stapleton [22], lesions did not respond to anti-candidal treatment despite a positive culture.

Treatment Recommendations

Oral rehabilitation to eliminate the possibility of chronic trauma to the oral mucosa may be accomplished with the use of a well-designed prosthesis or intraoral devices [20]. Systemic retinoids may lead to improvement of oral leukoplakia [23]. However, the development of side effects limits its use in patients with PC [24].

Dyskeratosis Congenita

Epidemiology

Dyskeratosis congenita (DC) is a very rare genetic disease with a prevalence of 0.1/100,000 births [1].

Etiopathogenesis

All forms of the disease are caused by a disorder in telomere maintenance and feature short telomeres. Multiple genes with different mechanisms of inheritance have been described. The most common type, X-linked DC, is caused by a mutation in DKC1, which encodes dyskerin, on chromosome Xq28. Autosomal dominant DC is due to heterozygous mutations in either TERT or TERC. Autosomal recessive DC is caused by homozygous or compound heterozygous mutation in NOLA2, TCAB1, RTEL1, and TERT genes [25–27].

Clinical Manifestations

Typically, DC presents with a triad of reticulated hyperpigmentation of the skin (usually neck and chest), dystrophy of the nails, and oral leukoplakia. In addition, patients have a predisposition to hematologic abnormalities and bone marrow failure [28, 29]. Bone marrow failure is the chief cause of early death. New treatments are under development, but currently no treatments are found to be uniformly effective in all patients [28]. Patients with DC are also predisposed to pulmonary complications and malignancy.

Oral Signs and Symptoms

Oral leukoplakia is a diagnostic feature of this disorder and usually appears early in life in association with skin hyperpigmentation [29]. In a cohort of 17 patients with DC, oral leukoplakia was noted in 65% of patients. Other findings included decreased root/crown ratio and mild taurodontism [30]. Leukoplakia is generally

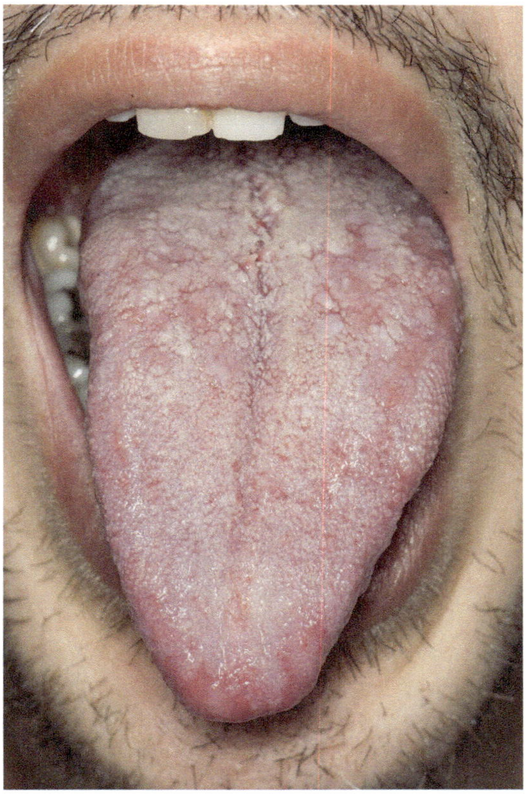

Fig. 11.6 Leukoplakia of the tongue in a man with dyskeratosis congenita

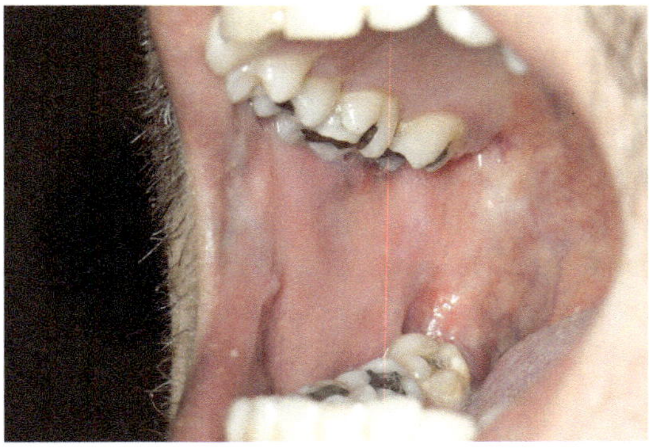

Fig. 11.7 Leukoplakia and telangiectasias on the buccal mucosa with evidence of prior dental caries in a man with dyskeratosis congenita

only seen in the mucous membranes of the mouth (Figs. 11.6 and 11.7) but may also be found in the esophagus and anogenital mucosa. The leukoplakia tends to progress with time and may undergo malignant transformation [29]. Extensive dental caries and loss of teeth are reported in 18% of patients with DC [28]. Anomalies in ectodermal structures coupled with neutropenia lead to a suboptimal host response and periodontal disease. Gingival inflammation, bleeding, recession, and alveolar bone loss trigger periodontitis [31, 32].

Differential Diagnosis

Oral leukoplakia in DC should be distinguished from that of PC. Periodontal disease may mimic changes of Papillon-Lefevre syndrome. As with many of the genodermatoses, the presence of accompanying cutaneous findings is a useful aid in establishing the correct diagnosis.

Treatment Recommendations

Appropriate dental and periodontal care are imperative in DC. In addition, due to the risk of malignant transformation, these patients should be followed closely. Most recently, the use of photodynamic therapy and CO2 laser therapy has emerged as effective and safe options for the treatment of oral premalignant lesions [33, 34].

Rothmund-Thomson Syndrome

Epidemiology

Rothmund-Thomson syndrome (RTS) is a rare autosomal recessive disorder with only 300 cases reported in the literature.

Etiopathogenesis

RTS is due to a compound heterozygous mutation in the DNA helicase gene RECQL4 on chromosome 8q24.3 [35]. The gene product plays a role in sister-chromatid cohesion that, when defective, leads to chromosomal instability with subsequent increased cancer susceptibility and cutaneous and skeletal abnormalities [36].

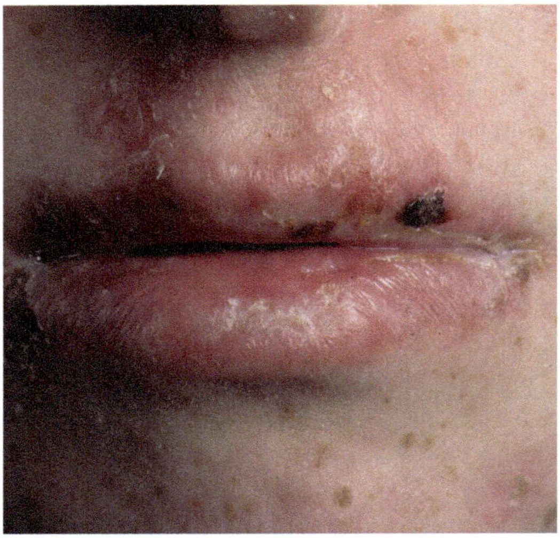

Fig. 11.8 Poikiloderma and atrophy of the skin and lips in an individual with Rothmund-Thomson syndrome V

Clinical Manifestations

The most salient cutaneous finding in RTS is the presence of poikiloderma (skin atrophy, telangiectasias, hyper-, and hypopigmentation) on the face (Fig. 11.8) and extensor extremities, hence the synonym poikiloderma congenitale. Afflicted patients have skeletal abnormalities (short stature, absent or hypoplastic thumbs, severe kyphoscoliosis, and hip dislocation), soft tissue contractures, juvenile cataracts, anemia, hypogonadism, and increased risk of malignancy (especially osteogenic sarcoma and lymphomas) [37–40].

Oral Signs and Symptoms

Numerous dental malformations of deciduous teeth, ectopic eruptions, and failed tooth eruption have been recognized in RTS [41]. In 1985, Starr and colleagues described hypodontia as one of the non-dermatologic complications of RTS [42]. Early periodontal disease has also been noted in this patient population [43] as well as microdontia, dystrophic teeth, and short root anomaly [44].

Differential Diagnosis

RAPADILINO syndrome is a rare disorder caused by RECQL4 mutation. Therefore, overlap with RTS exists. Hypoplastic radius and thumb are common features (RA in RAPADILINO stands for radial ray malformations). From a dental/oral perspective, patients with RAPADILINO syndrome may have a high-arched palate and micrognathia, but other dental or periodontal changes are usually not seen [45, 46]. In contrast, Papillon-Lefevre, Haim-Munk, and Ehlers-Danlos syndromes feature early periodontal disease and should be considered in the differential diagnosis of RTS.

Treatment Recommendations

Treatment should be individualized on a case-by-case basis. Periodontal care is of utmost importance to prevent or minimize tooth decay. For patients with tooth abnormalities (anodontia, microdontia, etc.), prosthetic devices are necessary to ensure proper masticatory function.

Hereditary Hemorrhagic Telangiectasia

Epidemiology

Hereditary hemorrhagic telangiectasia (HHT), aka Osler-Weber-Rendu syndrome, has an estimated prevalence of at least 1 in 5000 [47].

Etiopathogenesis

HHT is an autosomal dominant disorder. Four main genetic subtypes have been described. The disease-causing mutation in HHT1 is in the endoglin (ENG) gene on chromosome 9q34.1 (8162076). For HHT2, the mutation is in the activin receptor gene on chromosome 12q1 [48]. HHT3 and HHT4 are mapped to chromosome 5 and 7, respectively. The candidate genes have

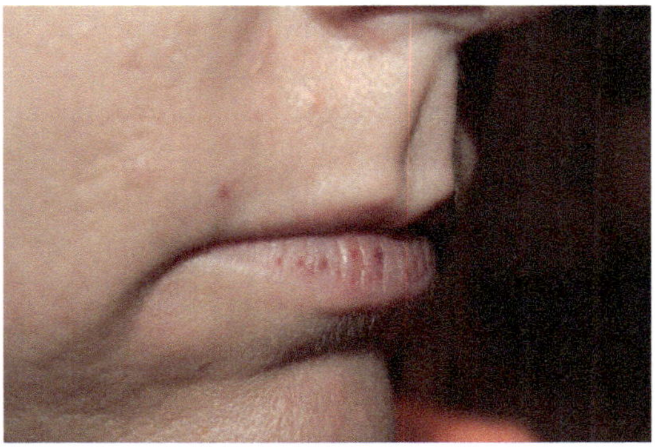

Fig. 11.9 Telangiectasias of the lip in a man with hereditary hemorrhagic telangiectasia

not been elucidated. HHT5 is caused by heterozygous mutation in the GDF2 gene (also known as BMP9) on chromosome 10q11 [49]. In addition, mutations in SMAD4 on chromosome 18q21 cause a form of HHT called juvenile polyposis/hereditary hemorrhagic telangiectasia syndrome [50].

Clinical Manifestations

HHT is characterized by multiple small and large arteriovenous malformations that become more prominent with age. The most common areas of involvement include the mucous membranes, skin (Fig. 11.9), gastrointestinal tract, liver, brain, and lung. Bleeding may cause sudden and devastating consequences. The earliest manifestation of the disease is epistaxis during childhood [47].

Oral Signs and Symptoms

Oral lesions may be punctate, spider-like, or nodular and can be found on the buccal mucosa, tongue, lips, palate, and gingivae [51]. Punctate telangiectasias on the tip of the tongue may be the first sign to present in childhood. More lesions usually develop after puberty. Color may vary from bright red to purple [4] but in the oral mucosa is usually cherry red [51]. Presentation of HHT as oral vascular malformations, hemorrhagic vesicles, and ulcers of the gingivae and oral mucosa has also been reported [52, 53]. Brain abscess formation following dental extractions and other dental procedures is a feared complication [54, 55]. Use of a very soft toothbrush may help prevent trauma from routine oral hygiene [53].

Differential Diagnosis

In the setting of mucosal telangiectasias in a patient with a history of epistaxis, multiple cutaneous telangiectasias, and a positive family history, the diagnosis should be straightforward. However, for atypical presentations, a high index of suspicion is needed. Patients with hereditary benign telangiectasia develop cutaneous plaque-like, arborizing, radiating, or punctate telangiectasias beginning in childhood. However, there are no mucosal or systemic vascular lesions [56].

Treatment Recommendations

Patients should be educated on the importance of avoiding oral trauma to prevent hemorrhage. Vascular malformations are amenable to treatment with sclerotherapy which obviates the need for more invasive surgical procedures and reduces the risk for postsurgical complications [52]. Nd:YAG laser has also been successfully used in the management of oral hemorrhage secondary to telangiectasias [57]. Some authors advocate the use of prophylactic antibiotics before oral procedures using the same guidelines as for patients at high risk of bacterial endocarditis [55].

Hermansky-Pudlak Syndrome

Epidemiology

Overall, the prevalence of Hermansky-Pudlak syndrome (HPS) is very low with approximately 0.15 cases per 100,000 births. However, in Puerto

Rico HPS likely represents the most frequent single-gene disorder. It is also prevalent in a village of canton Valais, Switzerland [58]. In Puerto Rico, the carrier frequency is estimated to be 1 in 21 [59].

Etiopathogenesis

HPS is an autosomal recessive condition. Nine subtypes have been identified, each of which is caused by homozygous or compound heterozygous mutations in several different genes. HPS1 is due to mutations in the HPS1 gene on chromosome 10q23 [60]. These genes encode components of the biogenesis of the lysosome-related organelles complexes (BLOC 1-3) or play a role in protein sorting to lysosomes (AP3B1). Dysfunction of cytoplasmic organelles related to lysosomes (melanosomes, platelet-dense granules, and lysosomes) accounts for the variety of symptoms seen in this disease [61].

Clinical Manifestations

As previously mentioned, clinical findings are a reflection of defective intracellular organelle trafficking/sorting and include pigmentary dilution of the skin, hair, and eyes, freckles in sun-exposed areas, pigmented nevi, nystagmus, reduced vision, epistaxis, bloody diarrhea, bleeding diathesis leading to prolonged bleeding time, and easy bruisability. Lysosomal ceroid storage results in interstitial pulmonary fibrosis, granulomatous colitis, renal failure, and cardiomyopathy [62].

Oral Signs and Symptoms

From an orodental viewpoint, the most important consideration in HPS patients is their bleeding tendency, which makes them prone to gingival hemorrhage. Indeed, fatal bleeding following tooth extraction has been documented [63]. Pediatric dentists should be aware of this possibility, especially when practicing in areas of high prevalence. Dental care practice recommendations including the use of protective UV glasses, as to avoid excessive glare from dental light, to administration of blood derivatives to assist with hemostasis are available [64].

Differential Diagnosis

Other disorders of hemostasis that may cause excessive gingival bleeding either with minor trauma or following dental procedures are Bernard-Soulier syndrome, Glanzmann thrombasthenia, gray platelet syndrome, and Chediak-Higashi syndrome [65].

Treatment Recommendations

For information regarding use of eyeglasses with UV filters, brushing techniques, antifibrinolytic agents, and local hemostatic measures during dental procedures, please refer to the article by Feliciano NZ and colleagues [64].

Lesch-Nyhan Syndrome

Epidemiology

The estimated prevalence of Lesch-Nyhan syndrome (LNS) at birth is about 0.34/100,000 [1].

Etiopathogenesis

LNS is an X-linked recessive disease caused by mutation in the HPRT gene, which encodes hypoxanthine guanine phosphoribosyltransferase. This enzyme catalyzes conversion of hypoxanthine to inosine monophosphate and guanine to guanosine monophosphate via transfer of the 5-phosphoribosyl group from 5-phosphoribosyl 1-pyrophosphate. Therefore, it has a pivotal role in the purine salvage pathway [66].

Clinical Manifestations

Clinical features are secondary to abnormal purine metabolism. Affected patients have short stature, growth and mental retardation (IQ 45–75), gout, nephrolithiasis, motor delay, hypotonia, extrapyramidal signs, choreoathetosis, spasticity, hyperreflexia, dysarthria, hyperuricemia, and hyperuricosuria [67].

Oral Signs and Symptoms

One of the most striking findings of the disease is the self-mutilating behavior with biting of the fingers and lips. The median age of onset is 2 years when eruption of the primary dentition is almost complete. The sites more frequently affected are the lower lip, inner cheeks, and tongue [67, 68].

Differential Diagnosis

Self-injury with involvement of the oral and perioral regions and the hands may be seen in a variety of neurological disorders (congenital, posttraumatic, and degenerative), congenital insensitivity pain with anhidrosis, and mental retardation [69, 70]. Limeres et al. proposed that the pattern of oral self-injury is not disease specific [68]. As such, the diagnosis relies on other condition-specific findings, which are usually apparent before self-mutilation ensues. Classic LNS features near complete absence of residual HPRT activity (less than 1.5%), whereas patients with Kelley-Seegmiller syndrome have a residual enzyme activity of at least 8%. The latter group of patients develops gout after puberty. Up to 25% of patients may have mild neurologic abnormalities but no self-injurious behavior [71].

Treatment Recommendations

According to Limeres and colleagues, intraoral devices alone (i.e., soft mouthguard or nonsurgical splint) or in combination with pharmacologic therapy offer the best management strategy for patients with oral self-injury of organic origin including LNS [68]. Psychologic therapy and uric acid reduction have not been shown to be of value in the treatment of self-mutilating behavior [68]. Extraction of primary and permanent teeth may be necessary [72].

Peutz-Jeghers Syndrome

Epidemiology

The reported prevalence of Peutz-Jeghers syndrome (PJS) is 2.2 cases per 100,000 births [1].

Etiopathogenesis

The disorder is due to mutations in the serine/threonine kinase, STK11, gene located at chromosomal locus 19p13 [73]. It is estimated that in 50% of cases, the condition is inherited from a parent, and in 50% of cases, the condition is the result of a new or de novo mutation [73]. A clinical genetic test is currently available for PJS.

Clinical Manifestations

PJS is a genetic condition characterized by gastrointestinal polyposis and tan to dark brown or blue macules on the skin and oral mucosa (Figs. 11.10 and 11.11) [74]. Diagnosis is based

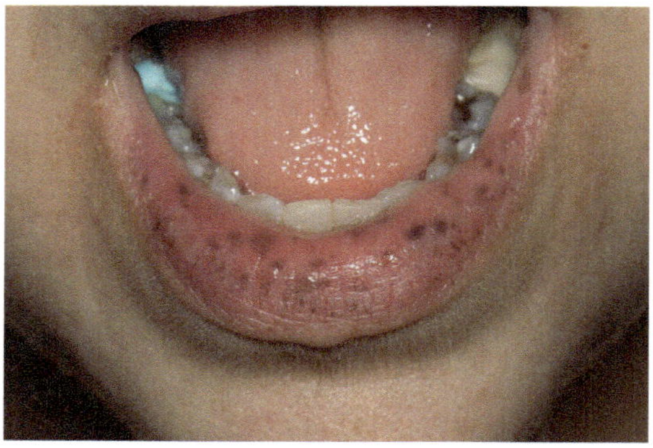

Fig. 11.10 Hyperpigmented macules affecting the lips in Peutz-Jeghers syndrome

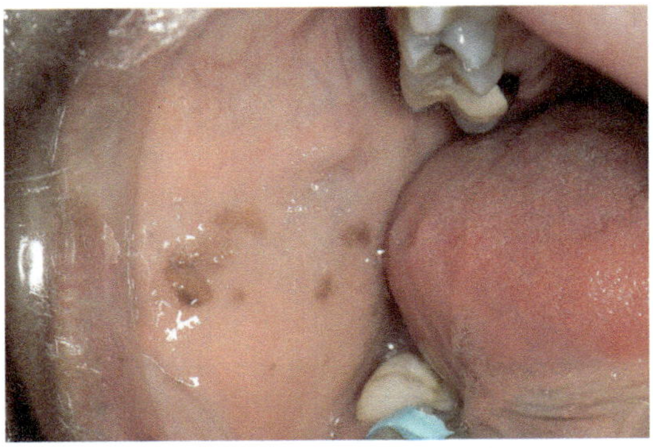

Fig. 11.11 Hyperpigmented macules over the buccal mucosa in a patient with Peutz-Jeghers syndrome

on these clinical findings. Polyps may cause intussusception or bowel obstruction. A study by Boardman et al. [75] determined that patients with Peutz-Jeghers syndrome had a 9.9 times relative risk for cancer. The incidence of gastrointestinal cancers and breast cancer is particularly increased [73, 75]. Therefore, cancer surveillance comprises an important part of management for these patients.

Oral Signs and Symptoms

The pigmented macules are usually present at birth or are first noted in early childhood [74]. The macules are usually found on the lips, buccal mucosa, and perioral skin. In the mouth, they may also be found on the palate and tongue. On the skin, distribution may include the face, dorsum of the hands, feet, fingers, eyes, umbilicus, and anus. Macules may be found in a periorificial distribution around the eyes in some patients. Skin macules are reported to fade with age, but the macules involving the oral mucosa tend to be persistent [74].

Differential Diagnosis

Lentigines with a distribution similar to that of PJS are found in Bandler syndrome and Laugier-Hunziker syndrome. Periorificial pigmented macules are seen in Carney Complex. Centrofacial lentiginosis and inherited patterned lentiginosis feature lentigines on the lips. Patients with Cronkhite-Canada syndrome develop lentigines on the buccal mucosa.

Treatment Recommendations

While lentigines in PJS are asymptomatic, they can be cosmetically distressful. Q-switched alexandrite laser is considered the treatment of choice for mucocutaneous melanosis associated with PJS [76, 77]. Q-switched ruby has also been used with satisfactory results [78]. Other treatment modalities such as dermabrasion, cryotherapy and CO2, or Argon laser may be associated with incomplete removal, scarring, or pigmentary changes [78].

Pseudoxanthoma Elasticum

Epidemiology

Pseudoxanthoma elasticum (PXE) occurs in 2.5 per 100,000 births [79].

Etiopathogenesis

PXE is an autosomal recessive condition due to mutations in the ATP-binding cassette, subfamily C, member 6 (*ABCC6*) gene. ABCC6 belongs to the multidrug resistance-associated protein (MRP) subfamily of ATP-binding cassette (ABC) transmembrane transporters [80].

Clinical Manifestations

The hallmark of the disease is the accumulation of fragmented and calcified elastic fibers in the skin, blood vessel walls, and Bruch's membrane in the eye resulting in soft, ivory-colored papules in a reticular pattern on the neck and intertriginous areas, as well as coronary artery occlusive disease, gastrointestinal hemorrhage, and retinal angioid streaks and choroidal neovascularizations [80]. Carriers of heterozygous mutations in ABCC6 gene may present with partial manifestations of the disease.

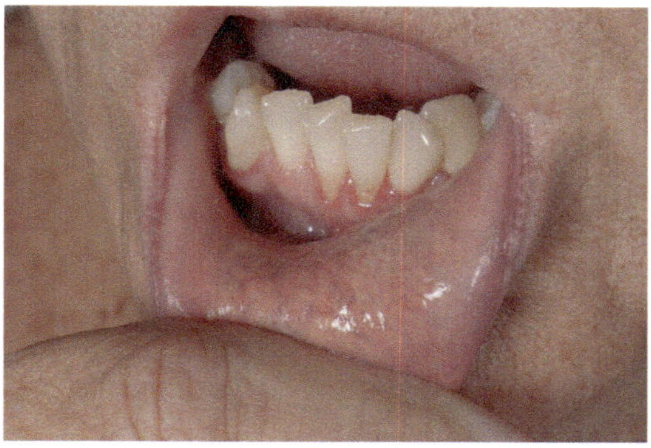

Fig. 11.12 Whitish papules on the inner lower lip caused by abnormal elastin in a patient with pseudoxanthoma elasticum

Oral Signs and Symptoms

Mucosal lesions of PXE are yellowish-to-white, macules and papules coalescing into reticulated patches or plaques. They appear on the inner aspect of the lower lip, cheeks, and palate [81] (Fig. 11.12). In patients without classic cutaneous findings, mucosal involvement of the lower lip may be the only clue to the diagnosis [82]. Oligodontia with agenesis of most of the permanent teeth has been reported [83]. More importantly, the presence of mucosal lesions may be a surrogate marker for potentially life-threatening cardiovascular disease [84].

Differential Diagnosis

Because of their location and color, the lesions may be misdiagnosed as Fordyce spots [85].

Treatment Recommendations

Oral lesions in PXE are asymptomatic, and no treatment is necessary. For rare cases with tooth abnormalities, treatment of the specific dental problem should be undertaken. Patients are vulnerable to early death from cardiovascular disease. Increasing evidence links poor oral health and vascular endothelial cell dysfunction. Therefore, meticulous oral hygiene may be especially important for affected individuals.

White Sponge Nevus

Epidemiology

The exact prevalence of white sponge nevus of Canon is unknown, but it is estimated to affect less than 1 in 200,000 individuals [86].

Etiopathogenesis

White sponge nevus (WSN) is a rare autosomal dominant condition due to heterozygous mutations in the keratin-4 gene on chromosome 12q13 or the keratin-13 gene on chromosome 17q21 [87, 88].

Clinical Manifestations

WSN is a disorder of non-keratinizing squamous epithelial differentiation that presents with leukokeratosis of the oral mucosa. However, the nose, esophagus, genitalia, and rectum may also be involved.

Oral Signs and Symptoms

The buccal mucosa is most commonly affected with white, bilateral, velvety, or "spongy" plaques (Fig. 11.13). The lesions are asymptom-

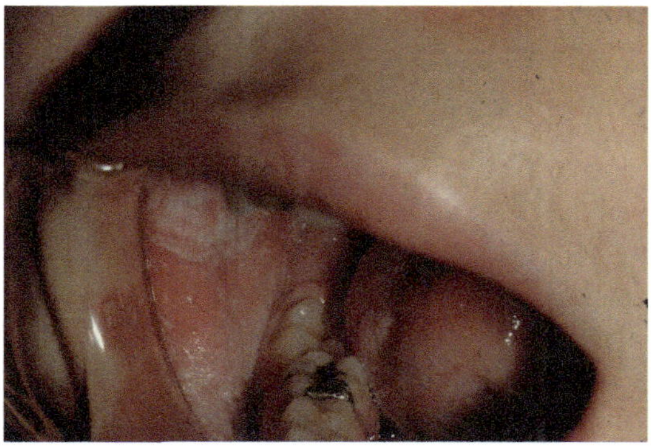

Fig. 11.13 Hyperkeratosis on the buccal mucosa in white sponge nevus

atic and first noted at birth or in early childhood. The labial and gingival mucosa, the floor of the mouth, or the entire oral cavity may be involved. While the lesions are painless, patients complain of an altered texture of the mucosa or that the lesions are cosmetically unappealing [89].

Differential Diagnosis

WSN should be differentiated from morsicatio buccarum (chronic cheek chewing), oral lichen planus, candidiasis, leukoedema, leukokeratosis nicotina palati (from smoking), dyskeratosis congenita, Darier's disease, benign intraepithelial dyskeratosis, and pachyonychia congenita. Early onset, bilateral involvement of the buccal mucosa, the lack of other systemic symptoms or signs, and a positive family history help distinguish WSN from the abovementioned conditions.

Treatment Recommendations

Most treatment recommendations are based on a handful of case reports/case series. Oral amoxicillin and tetracycline may afford some improvement, but prolonged treatment with a low maintenance dose is required [89]. Tetracycline mouth rinse and chlorhexidine have been used successfully [90–92]. Recurrence after CO2 laser therapy has been noted. Surgical excision may be curative [93].

Familial Adenomatous Polyposis (Gardner Syndrome)

Epidemiology

Familial adenomatous polyposis (FAP) occurs in 1 in 7500 births.

Etiopathogenesis

FAP is caused by heterozygous mutation in the adenomatous polyposis coli (APC) gene on chromosome 5q22.2. APC encodes a tumor suppression protein that antagonizes the WNT signaling pathway [94]. It is inherited in an autosomal dominant fashion.

Clinical Manifestations

The hallmark of FAP is the development of hundreds of adenomatous colorectal polyps, which have a 100% risk of malignant transformation, if prophylactic colectomy is not performed [95]. The polyps typically develop in the second or third decade of life. Extraintestinal manifestations include congenital hypertrophy of the retinal pigment epithelium which is found in up to 80% of patients and is usually present at birth allowing for early diagnosis [96], cutaneous lesions (epidermoid cysts, lipomas, fibromas, pilomatricomas, leiomyomas), desmoid tumors, as well as malignancies of the thyroid, pancreas, stomach, adrenals, and gallbladder [97].

Oral Signs and Symptoms

Supernumerary, impacted, and missing teeth have been reported in GS [98]. Supernumerary teeth are small and peg shaped [99]. The impacted teeth are usually canines [100]. Osteomas are the most common skeletal manifestation of the disease. They are present in 46–93% of patients and can arise in the skull, mandible, maxilla, and long bones. The largest are located at the angle of the mandible [101]. Osteomas of the mandibular condyle may be diagnostic; they are usually asymptomatic but can cause limited mandibular movement [102] or cause facial asymmetry [103]. In general, osteomas of the mandible and maxilla are common incidental findings on routine dental panoramic radiography. However, the presence of three or more should raise suspicion for the possibility of FAP [104].

Odontomas are also more frequent in FAP than in the general population [105]. They are well-defined, encapsulated, hard tissue growths with an odontogenic origin.

Differential Diagnosis

Full-blown FAP offers no diagnostic challenge. For early disease, the differential diagnosis is that of the individual lesions or findings. However, if two or more of the above listed cutaneous or maxillofacial findings coincide in the same patient, evaluation for colonic polyposis should be undertaken.

Treatment Recommendations

Osteomas are asymptomatic and usually removed for cosmetic reasons or when they restrict the oral aperture and/or mandibular movement [106]. Recurrence after surgical resection is rare [102].

Osteogenesis Imperfecta

Epidemiology

Osteogenesis imperfecta (OI) has an estimated prevalence of 1 in 12,000–15,000 children [107, 108].

Etiopathogenesis

OI is a genetically and phenotypically heterogeneous disorder with autosomal dominant and recessive inheritance. Autosomal dominant OI is due to mutations in COL1A1 gene on chromosome 17, COL1A2 on chromosome 7, or IFITM5 gene, encoding interferon-induced transmembrane protein-5, on chromosome 11p15. Genes responsible for autosomal recessive OI include SERPINF1, CRTAP, LEPRE1, PPIB, SERPINH1, FKBP10, BMP1 SP7, and WNT1 [109]. Mutations in COL1A1 and COL1A2 are responsible for about 90% of cases of OI [110].

Clinical Manifestations

OI is characterized by varying degrees of bone fragility and low bone mass leading to multiple bone fractures from minimal trauma. Wormian (intra sutural) bones of the skull, osteopenia, biconcave flattened vertebrae, femoral bowing, and joint hypermobility are among the most common skeletal abnormalities. Patients may present with blue sclera, thin skin, and easy bruisability. In addition, there are numerous extraskeletal manifestations such as progressive sensorineural and/or conductive hearing loss, otosclerosis, mitral valve prolapse, aortic root dilatation, basilar impression, macrocephaly, and hydrocephalus. The presence and severity of the aforementioned findings are highly variable owing to multiple genetic defects implicated in this condition [109, 111–113].

Oral Signs and Symptoms

Dentinogenesis imperfecta (DI) may be a feature of some forms of OI with an estimated prevalence of about 28% [114]. The teeth are typically yellow/brown or opalescent gray with significant attrition. Discoloration is due to dentin dysplasia. There is no correlation between the type of OI and the type/shade of discoloration [115]. Radiographically, the teeth have short roots and dentin hypertrophy leading to pulpal obliteration either before or just after eruption [116]. Individuals with OI types III and IV have more severe oral problems such as malocclusion (anterior and posterior cross bites and open bites), micrognathia, and delayed, accelerated, or ectopic tooth eruption [114].

Differential Diagnosis

DI types II and III are not associated with other inherited disorders. The main differential diagnosis is dentin dysplasia. The latter has an incidence of 1 in 100,000 [116].

Treatment Recommendations

Early institution of treatment will ensure good occlusion, adequate mandibular and maxillary growth, and preservation of the temporomandibular joints [117]. Initial management of the primary dentition includes placement of stainless steel crowns for the posterior teeth and acrylic crowns for the anterior teeth in conjunction with meticulous oral hygiene for prevention of dental caries and periodontal disease [118]. When eruption of the permanent dentition is complete, prosthetic restoration of the permanent teeth can be considered [119]. Nowadays, dental implants and ceramometal restoration (for posterior teeth) and glass-ceramic pressed veneers and crowns (for anterior teeth and premolars) offer a more functional and cosmetically appealing solution [120].

Basal Cell Nevus Syndrome

Epidemiology

The prevalence of basal cell nevus syndrome or Gorlin syndrome is between 1 in 31,000 [121] and 1 in 164,000 [122].

Etiopathogenesis

Basal cell nevus syndrome (BCNS) is caused by mutations in the PTCH1 gene on chromosome 9q22, the PTCH2 gene on 1p32, or the SUFU gene on 10q24-q25 [123]. PTCH1 encodes the receptor for Sonic hedgehog protein and accounts for most cases of BCNS [124]. The mechanism of inheritance is autosomal dominant.

Clinical Manifestations

Individuals with BCNS develop multiple basal cell carcinomas early in life, and the rate increases with age up to a frequency of about 97% in patients older than 40 years old, with the first tumor occurring at a mean age of 23 [125]. Other commonly observed features are frontal and biparietal bossing, broad nasal root, strabismus, iris coloboma, glaucoma [126], bifid ribs [127], calcification of the falx cerebri [128], medulloblastomas, ovarian fibromas/carcinomas, and palmoplantar pits [129].

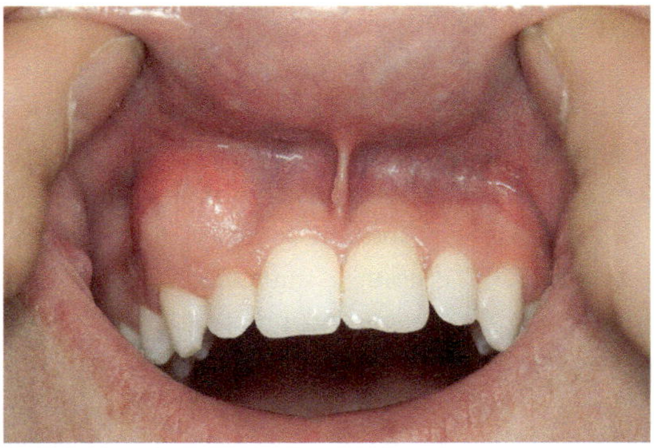

Fig. 11.14 Odontogenic keratocyst in the right upper jaw in a patient with basal cell nevus syndrome

Oral Signs and Symptoms

Keratocyst odontogenic tumors (KCOT), formerly odontogenic keratocysts, are benign cystic lesions reclassified as neoplasms due to their potential for slow growth and locally destructive behavior [130] (Fig. 11.14). KCOTs may be the presenting sign of NBCS [131]. Indeed, they are considered a major diagnostic criterion for this syndrome. The mandible: maxilla ratio is 2:1. The most common locations are the posterior mandible, near the third molars, and the ramus areas [132]. The most common complaint is jaw swelling (45%). Other symptoms include pain and altered taste. About 25% are asymptomatic and incidentally discovered on radiographs [133]. Seventy five percent of patients with BCNS develop KCOTs, 80% of them before the age of 20. They are usually multiple (median, 3; range, 1–28) [125]. Recurrence after surgical removal is common. Cleft lip and palate have also been documented in BCNS [134, 135]. An uncommon finding is bilateral hyperplasia of the mandibular coronoid processes [136].

Differential Diagnosis

BCNS has a limited number of oral manifestations. Nonetheless, because KCOTs are very common and arise early in this condition, the finding of a histologically proven KCOT should prompt further investigation to exclude BCNS.

Treatment Recommendations

Treatment of KCOTs is a matter of debate [137]. Conservative management (enucleation or marsupialization) may be attempted for small lesions [138, 139]. For more complex and large lesions, surgical removal via intraoral or endoscopic approaches is recommended [140]. BCNS patients are especially vulnerable to ionizing radiation which increases their risk of cutaneous basal cell skin cancers. Minimization of diagnostic X-rays is recommended. Because of the risk of odontogenic keratocysts, panoramic radiography is indicated every 12–18 months in those older than age 8 [141].

Tuberous Sclerosis Complex

Epidemiology

Tuberous sclerosis complex (TSC) affects about 2,000,000 people worldwide with an incidence of about 1 in 5000–10,000 live births [142–144].

Etiopathogenesis

TSC complex is inherited in an autosomal dominant manner and considered to be a heterogeneous disorder. About two-thirds of cases represent new mutations in patients with no family history of the disorder. The majority of cases are caused by a mutation of the TSC1 gene on chromosome 9q34 or the TSC2 gene on chromosome 16p13. In addition, TSC has a high rate of somatic mosaicism among affected individuals estimated to be 10–25% [144].

Clinical Manifestations

Tuberous sclerosis complex (TSC) has been described and studied for more than 160 years [145, 146]. As a result, diagnostic criteria have been well defined [147]. Abnormalities of the skin, central nervous system, kidney, and heart are prominent features of this disorder. TSC shows a great deal of variability in the degree of severity even among affected family members. Central nervous system abnormalities such as cognitive deficits and seizures affect long-term prognosis the most. Up to 14% of patients with TSC develop subependymal giant cell astrocytomas. Associated skin findings such as hypomelanotic macules, facial angiofibromas, and ungual fibromas have been reviewed in detail [147].

Oral Signs and Symptoms

Current diagnostic criteria include the oral finding of gingival fibromas (Fig. 11.15). These are described as small, fibrous nodules on the gingiva. Oral fibromas in TSC have also been described on the buccal mucosa and dorsum of the tongue [148]. Gingival fibromas are found in some patients with TSC and, therefore, are not essential to establishing a diagnosis. Also, gingival hyperplasia caused by antiseizure medication such as phenytoin may obscure gingival fibromas in these patients. A lack of oral hygiene has been associated with TSC, but this is thought to be due to mental deficiency rather than a growth or neoplastic change [145].

Multiple randomly distributed enamel pits provide another diagnostic feature of TSC. Enamel pitting may be seen by direct inspection and usually affects the labial sur-

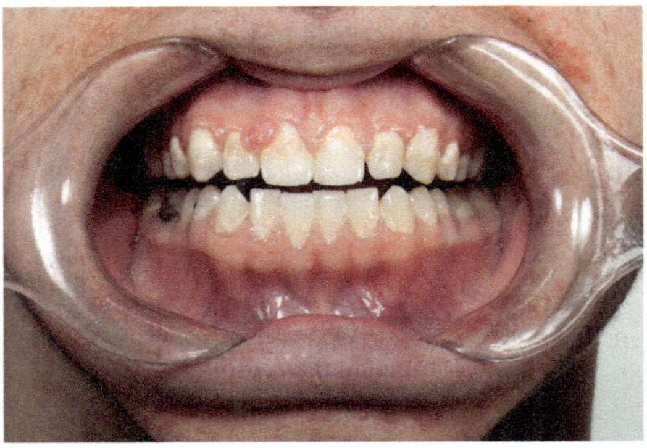

Fig. 11.15 Gingival hyperplasia in a patient with tuberous sclerosis

faces of the central and lateral incisors and canine teeth [145]. The prevalence of enamel pits in patients with TS is thought to range from 48% to 100% [145, 149]. Smaller pits can be better appreciated using dental plaque-disclosing stain on the surfaces of the teeth. Electron microscopy can also be used, once a tooth has been extracted. Enamel pits may be found on the teeth of otherwise healthy patients but are usually fewer and less obvious. A study by Flanagan et al. [149] found that the majority of patients with TSC had greater than 14 pits per person, whereas the majority of normal controls had less than 6 pits per person.

Differential Diagnosis

Oral fibromas can be misdiagnosed as fibrous hyperplasias, focal papillomas, hemangiomas, lymphangiomas, or lipomas [150].

Treatment Recommendations

Oral fibromas may interfere with oral hygiene. As such, education on oral hygiene and dietary habits, fluoride therapy, and frequent in-office cleanings are advisable [151]. Surgical resection of the most prominent ones could be considered on an individual basis.

Darier Disease

Epidemiology

Darier disease (DD) has an estimated prevalence of 1 in 55,000. Disease onset is usually before the third decade of life [152].

Etiopathogenesis

DD, an autosomal dominant disorder, results from a heterozygous mutation in the ATP2A2 gene, which encodes the sarcoplasmic reticulum Ca(2+)-ATPase-2 (SERCA2), on chromosome 12q23-q24.1. The SERCA2b pump specifically maintains low cytosolic Ca(2+) concentrations by actively transporting Ca(2+) from the cytosol into the sarco/endoplasmic reticulum lumen of keratinocytes [153, 154]. Gene penetrance may be complete by age 10, but expressivity is variable [155].

Clinical Manifestations

Disease onset is usually between the ages of 6 and 20 years. The characteristic skin findings are brown, warty, hyperkeratotic, 2–4 mm papules with predilection for the seborrheic areas (scalp, forehead, trunk, and intertriginous regions). Acral involvement is almost universal (96% of patients) with palmar keratotic plaques, palmoplantar pits, and acrokeratosis verruciformis-like lesions on the dorsal hands [156]. The hyperkeratotic plaques are often malodorous and moderately pruritic. Nail changes include longitudinal erythro- and leukonychia, distal V-shaped notching, longitudinal fissuring and ridging, and subungual hyperkeratotic fragments [157]. Interestingly, several neuropsychiatric conditions have been documented in a subset of patients with DD. Mild mental retardation, seizures, schizophrenia, bipolar disorder, major depression, and suicidal attempts have been reported [156, 158, 159].

Oral Signs and Symptoms

The incidence of oral lesions in DD varies between 15% (24/163) [156] and 50% (12/24) [160]. Lesions are painless, whitish, coalescing papules, primarily present on the palate (most common location), followed by the gingiva, oral mucosa, and tongue [160]. The severity of oral involvement seems to mirror that of cutaneous disease. Parotid gland swelling has also been described but only in patients with concomitant oral involvement [160]. Most recently, esophageal affliction, including carcinoma, has been noted [161, 162].

Differential Diagnosis

The differential diagnosis of oral lesions in DD are that in leukokeratosis/leukoplakia and includes morsicatio buccarum, candidiasis, leukoedema, leukokeratosis nicotina palate, dyskeratosis congenita, white sponge nevus, benign intraepithelial dyskeratosis and pachyonychia congenita.

Treatment Recommendations

Oral findings in DD are of no clinical significance, and treatment is not needed.

Ehlers-Danlos Syndrome

Epidemiology

The prevalence of Ehlers-Danlos syndrome (EDS) is approximately 1 in 5000–10,000. There is no racial predilection [163].

Etiopathogenesis

Mutations in collagen and collagen-processing enzymes are responsible for the various phenotypes of the disease. EDS types 1 and 2 are caused by mutations in either the collagen alpha-1(V) gene (COL5A1) on chromosome 9q34 or the collagen alpha-2(V) gene (COL5A2) on chromosome 2q31. EDS type 3 is caused by mutation in the tenascin-XB or COL3A1 genes. Mutations in COL3A1 genes are also responsible for EDS type 4. EDS type 6 is due to mutations in lysyl hydroxylase (PLOD1) on chromosome 1. Lastly, mutations in COL1A1, COL1A2, and procollagen protease ADAMTS2 cause EDS type 7A, 7B, and 7C, respectively [163]. EDS can be inherited in an autosomal or recessive fashion.

Clinical Manifestations

EDS is a group of connective tissue disorders with shared features including skin hyperextensibility, joint hypermobility, and tissue fragility. Each EDS type has one or more defining findings. A detailed description is beyond the scope of this chapter and can be found in the Online Mendelian Inheritance in Men website (www.omim.org). Briefly, patients have a variety of skeletal (osteoarthritis, joint hypermobility, joint dislocation, pes planus), cutaneous (fragile and velvety skin, easy bruisability, poor wound healing, molluscoid pseudotumors, spheroids, wide and cigarette-paper scars), cardiovascular (mitral valve prolapse, aortic root dilatation), ocular (blue sclerae, epicanthal folds, ectopia lentis, myopia, and eyelid extensibility), and oral manifestations.

Oral Signs and Symptoms

About 50% of EDS patients are able to touch their nasal tip with their tongue compared to 10% of the general population, the so-called Gorlin's sign. Absence of the inferior labial frenulum has a 100% sensitivity, whereas absence of the lingual frenulum has a 100% specificity for the EDS types I, II, and III [164].

The most comprehensive review on the oral manifestations of EDS is by Abel and Carrasco [163]. Patients may present with periodontal disease with early-onset periodontitis, gingival fibrinoid deposits, and bleeding as well as increased tooth mobility, congenital absence of teeth, and supernumerary teeth. Teeth can be small, irregularly placed with short, malformed, or dilacerated roots. Enamel hypoplasia and dentin structural irregularities are also observed and may render teeth prone to dental caries [165]. Hemorrhagic bulla of the oral mucosa as an early manifestation of EDS type 4 (vascular type) has been reported [166]. KCOTs can be found in association with supernumerary teeth [167]. Patients with EDS type 4 may also experience tooth loss following orthodontic treatment due to severe destruction of the periodontal support [168].

Hypermobility of the temporomandibular joint (TMJ) is a frequent sign [169] as is pain in the masticatory muscles upon mouth opening.

Increased mobility of the joints can also cause permanent locking of the TMJ [170].

Differential Diagnosis

Due to the heterogeneous presentation with several oral and mucosal findings, the differential diagnosis matches that of each individual condition or symptom. For example, KCOTs are major diagnostic criteria for basal cell nevus syndrome but can also be found in EDS. Periodontal disease is a feature of Papillon-Lefevre, supernumerary teeth are seen in Job syndrome, and Gorlin's sign may be a physiologic variant. Therefore, when considered in isolation, these individual findings may lead to an erroneous diagnosis. Nonetheless, their occurrence in association with skin and other organ system abnormalities along with a compatible pedigree or family history should help distinguish EDS cases.

Treatment Recommendations

Oral care in EDS is complex and requires a multidisciplinary approach with input from dental hygienists, general dentists, endodontists, orthodontists, orthopedic surgeons, and physical therapists [163]. These patients may develop complications during standard orthopedic treatment such as rapid migration and increased tooth mobility. Similarly, the gingiva is more prone to inflammation and the TMJ to subluxation [171].

Down Syndrome

Epidemiology

Down syndrome (DS) is estimated to occur in approximately 1 in 732 infants in the United States, but there is racial and ethnic variability [172].

Etiopathogenesis

DS is the most common numeric chromosome abnormality due to trisomy 21. Dosage imbalance of many genes is responsible for the phenotype.

Clinical Manifestations

Almost every organ system is affected in DS. Characteristically, patients have brachycephaly, short stature, flat facies, small ears, folded helices, conductive hearing loss, epicanthal folds, iris Brushfield spots, and upslanting palpebral fissures. Congenital heart disease, duodenal atresia, imperforate anus, and Hirschsprung disease are additional features. Patients are prone to Alzheimer, leukemia, and hypothyroidism (www.omim.org).

Oral Signs and Symptoms

DS patients present with a variety of dental anomalies. In one series the most common abnormality was taurodontism (vertical enlargement of the tooth and pulp, usually most striking in the molars), followed by rotation, hypodontia, tooth impaction, ectopic eruption, microdontia, and hyperdontia, in that order [173]. In another series, although the crown-to-root ratio was maintained, microdontia and progressive reduction in tooth size with senesce were documented [174]. Microdontia affects both primary and permanent dentitions [175]. In addition, there is a higher prevalence of malocclusion (anterior cross bite, anterior open bite) probably due to skeletal and soft tissue abnormalities [176]. Interestingly, DS patients are more resistant to dental caries but have a higher prevalence of gingival and periodontal disease.

Tonsillar hyperplasia has been implicated in the pathogenesis of sleep-disordered breathing in children with DS [177]. Due to small craniofacial parameters, patients with DS have relative rather than true macroglossia [178]. Cleft lip and/or palate and broad, dry, and fissured lips are observed [179].

Differential Diagnosis

Healthcare professionals are very well aware of the classic clinical findings associated with DS. Moreover, prenatal diagnosis is available. Therefore, in developed countries, the diagnosis has already been established by the time oral manifestations arise (i.e., primary dentition). In areas where neonatal screening is not universal, congenital hypothyroidism may be considered in the differential diagnosis.

Treatment Recommendations

Due to poor oral hygiene and high levels of periodontal disease in patients with DS, adequate oral health education for patients, their families, and other caregivers is an important priority [180]. Retrognathia, hypotonia, and macroglossia can lead to obstructive sleep apnea; therefore, overnight polysomnograph should be obtained and early referral to otolaryngology made, if indicated [181]. As with EDS patients, an interdisciplinary approach is necessary to achieve functional, phonetic, and esthetic outcomes [182].

Xeroderma Pigmentosum (XP)

Epidemiology

Xeroderma pigmentosum (XP) has an estimated incidence of 1 in 20,000 in Japan to 1 in 250,000 in the United States [183].

Etiopathogenesis

XP is a rare autosomal recessive genetic condition characterized by hypersensitivity to ultraviolet radiation and carcinogenic agents due to defective DNA repair after ultraviolet radiation damage. Nine different gene mutations are accountable for the XP phenotype. Eight of them belong to the nucleotide excision repair pathway (NER), a group of enzymes involved in DNA repair and one is involved in error-free replication of UV damaged DNA. Characterization of each individual XP group and variant is beyond the scope of this chapter.

Clinical Manifestations

The vast majority of XP clinical manifestations occur in sun-exposed areas of the skin including increased photosensitivity, development of ephelides, poikiloderma, skin atrophy, telangiectasias, angiomas, actinic keratoses, and, importantly, cutaneous malignancies (keratoacanthoma, squamous cell carcinoma, basal cell carcinoma, and melanoma). Up to 70% of patients with XP are diagnosed with a malignant skin neoplasm at a median age of 8 years [184, 185]. Additionally, patients present with photophobia, conjunctivitis, keratitis, ectropion, entropion, early cataracts, decreased visual acuity, corneal neovascularization, and tumors of the eyelid and cornea. Microcephaly, sensorineural hearing loss, and central nervous system abnormalities are also a features in some types of the disease [186].

Oral Signs and Symptoms

The oral manifestations are mainly due to sun-induced damage of the lips, exposed oral mucosa, and tip of the tongue and include actinic cheilitis and basal cell and squamous cell carcinomas. Perioral scarring from repeated episodes of actinic cheilitis and reconstruction of skin defects around the mouth (after excision of cutaneous malignancy) may result in microstomia. In such cases, limitation of the oral aperture may lead to poor oral hygiene and sequelae of periodontal disease and tooth decay. Enamel hypoplasia has also been reported [187].

Differential Diagnosis

Suspicious lesions may be white or red and should be biopsied for definitive diagnosis. The differential diagnosis is usually restricted to malignant neoplasms given that the diagnosis of XP has typically already been established by the time oral and dental complications arise.

Treatment Recommendations

Periodic dental exams are mandatory for early detection and treatment of precancerous and malignant lesions. Caution should be taken when treating dental caries in XP patients. It is recommended that glass-ionomer or auto-cure filling material be substituted for light-cure fillings as there is potential for light-induced malignant transformation of the epithelium and connective tissue [188]. Mouthwashes with a high alcohol concentration should also be avoided.

Papillon-Lefevre Syndrome

Epidemiology

The prevalence of Papillon-Lefevre syndrome (PLS) is approximately 1–4 cases per 1,000,000 [189, 190].

Etiopathogenesis

PLS is a rare autosomal recessive disorder with an increased rate of consanguinity in parents of affected patients [191]. Most cases are due to mutations of the cathepsin C gene on chromosome 11q14 [191].

Clinical Manifestations

Papillon-Lefevre syndrome (PLS) is a very rare genetic condition characterized by well-demarcated palmoplantar hyperkeratosis. Periodontitis separates PLS from other inherited palmoplantar keratodermas [191]. The features of the condition usually first become apparent between the age of 2 and 4 [192]. The palmoplantar hyperkeratosis has been reported to improve with time [192].

Oral Signs and Symptoms

Severe, inflammatory periodontitis results in complete loss of deciduous teeth by age 4. The same process results in complete loss of the permanent teeth. Late-onset periodontitis (age 12) has been documented as a rare phenotypic variation [193]. The wisdom teeth, however, are spared [192]. It has recently been proposed that deficits of antimicrobial and immunomodulatory functions of gingival LL-37 allow infection with *Aggregatibacter actinomycetemcomitans* leading to severe periodontal disease [194].

Differential Diagnosis

Mutations in cathepsin C also cause Haim-Munk syndrome with palmoplantar keratoderma, aggressive periodontitis, acroosteolysis, arachnodactyly, atrophic nail changes, and deformity of the fingers [195].

Treatment Recommendations

For years, prosthodontic rehabilitation has been the cornerstone of therapy in PLS [196]. Unfortunately, despite aggressive post-implant care, patients are at high risk of peri-implantitis and implant loss [197]. Recent advances in treatment suggest that low-dose acitretin improves periodontitis and results in increased alveolar bone height and periodontal attachment [198].

References

1. Orphanet Report Series, Prevalence of rare diseases: Bibliographic Data. 2014.
2. Landy SJ, Donnai D. Incontinentia pigmenti (Bloch-Sulzberger syndrome). J Med Genet. 1993;30(1):53–9.
3. Minic S, Trpinac D, Obradovic M. Incontinentia pigmenti diagnostic criteria update. Clin Genet. 2014;85(6):536–42.
4. Equi RA, Bains HS, Jampol L, Goldberg MF. Retinal tears occurring at the border of vascular and avascular retina in adult patients with incontinentia pigmenti. Retina. 2003;23(4):574–6.
5. Kim BJ, Shin HS, Won CH, Lee JH, Kim KH, Kim MN, et al. Incontinentia pigmenti: clinical observation of 40 Korean cases. J Korean Med Sci. 2006;21(3):474–7.
6. Minic S, Trpinac D, Obradovic M. Systematic review of central nervous system anomalies in incontinentia pigmenti. Orphanet J Rare Dis. 2013;8:25.
7. Wu HP, Wang YL, Chang HH, Huang GF, Guo MK. Dental anomalies in two patients with incontinentia pigmenti. J Formos Med Assoc. 2005;104(6):427–30.
8. Minic S, Trpinac D, Gabriel H, Gencik M, Obradović M. Dental and oral anomalies in incontinentia pigmenti: a systematic review. Clin Oral Investig. 2013;17(1):1–8.
9. Bergendal B. Orodental manifestations in ectodermal dysplasia-a review. Am J Med Genet A. 2014;164A(10):2465–71.
10. Holmstrom G, Bergendal B, Hallberg G, Marcus S, Hallén A, Dahl N. Incontinentia pigmenti. A rare disease with many symptoms. Lakartidningen. 2002;99(12):1345–50.

11. Doruk C, Bicakci AA, Babacan H. Orthodontic and orthopedic treatment of a patient with incontinentia pigmenti. Angle Orthod. 2003;73(6):763–8.
12. Yamashiro T, Nakagawa K, Takada K. Case report: orthodontic treatment of dental problems in incontinentia pigmenti. Angle Orthod. 1998;68(3):281–4.
13. McLean WH, Hansen CD, Eliason MJ, Smith FJ. The phenotypic and molecular genetic features of pachyonychia congenita. J Invest Dermatol. 2011;131(5):1015–7.
14. Dahl PR, Daoud MS, Su WP. Jadassohn-Lewandowski syndrome (pachyonychia congenita). Semin Dermatol. 1995;14(2):129–34.
15. Smith FJ, Coleman CM, Bayoumy NM, Tenconi R, Nelson J, David A, et al. Novel keratin 17 mutations in pachyonychia congenita type 2. J Invest Dermatol. 2001;116(5):806–8.
16. Shah S, Boen M, Kenner-Bell B, Schwartz M, Rademaker A, Paller AS. Pachyonychia congenita in pediatric patients: natural history, features, and impact. JAMA Dermatol. 2014;150(2):146–53.
17. Eliason MJ, Leachman SA, Feng BJ, Schwartz ME, Hansen CD. A review of the clinical phenotype of 254 patients with genetically confirmed pachyonychia congenita. J Am Acad Dermatol. 2012;67(4):680–6.
18. Leachman SA, Kaspar RL, Fleckman P, Florell SR, Smith FJ, McLean WH, et al. Clinical and pathological features of pachyonychia congenita. J Investig Dermatol Symp Proc. 2005;10(1):3–17.
19. Su WP, Chun SI, Hammond DE, Gordon H. Pachyonychia congenita: a clinical study of 12 cases and review of the literature. Pediatr Dermatol. 1990;7(1):33–8.
20. da Silva Santos PS, Mannarino F, Lellis RF, Osório LH. Oral manifestations of pachyonychia congenita. Dermatol Online J. 2010;16(10):3.
21. Karen JK, Schaffer JV. Pachyonychia congenita associated with median rhomboid glossitis. Dermatol Online J. 2007;13(1):21.
22. Hannaford RS, Stapleton K. Pachyonychia congenita tarda. Australas J Dermatol. 2000;41(3):175–7.
23. Rondon Lugo AJ. Congenital pachyonychia treated by oral retinoid. Med Cutanea Ibero-Lat-Am. 1982;10(6):395–8.
24. Gruber R, Edlinger M, Kaspar RL, Hansen CD, Leachman S, Milstone LM, et al. An appraisal of oral retinoids in the treatment of pachyonychia congenita. J Am Acad Dermatol. 2012;66(6):e193–9.
25. Kirwan M, Dokal I. Dyskeratosis congenita: a genetic disorder of many faces. Clin Genet. 2008;73(2):103–12.
26. Lamm N, Ordan E, Shponkin R, Richler C, Aker M, Tzfati Y. Diminished telomeric 3′ overhangs are associated with telomere dysfunction in Hoyeraal-Hreidarsson syndrome. PLoS One. 2009;4(5):e5666.
27. Vulliamy T, Beswick R, Kirwan M, Marrone A, Digweed M, Walne A, et al. Mutations in the telomerase component NHP2 cause the premature ageing syndrome dyskeratosis congenita. Proc Natl Acad Sci U S A. 2008;105(23):8073–8.
28. Dokal I. Dyskeratosis congenita: recent advances and future directions. J Pediatr Hematol Oncol. 1999;21(5):344–50.
29. Solder B, Weiss M, Jäger A, Belohradsky BH. Dyskeratosis congenita: multisystemic disorder with special consideration of immunologic aspects. A review of the literature. Clin Pediatr. 1998;37(9):521–30.
30. Atkinson JC, Harvey KE, Domingo DL, Trujillo MI, Guadagnini JP, Gollins S, et al. Oral and dental phenotype of dyskeratosis congenita. Oral Dis. 2008;14(5):419–27.
31. Fernandez Garcia MS, Teruya-Feldstein J. The diagnosis and treatment of dyskeratosis congenita: a review. J Blood Med. 2014;5:157–67.
32. Yavuzyilmaz E, Yamalik N, Yetgin S, Kansu O. Oral-dental findings in dyskeratosis congenita. J Oral Pathol Med. 1992;21(6):280–4.
33. Vohra F, Al-Kheraif AA, Qadri T, Hassan MI, Ahmed A, Warnakulasuriya S, et al. Efficacy of photodynamic therapy in the management of oral premalignant lesions. A systematic review. Photodiagn Photodyn Ther. 2015;12(1):150–9.
34. Tambuwala A, Sangle A, Khan A, Sayed A. Excision of oral leukoplakia by CO2 lasers versus traditional scalpel: a comparative study. J Maxillofac Oral Surg. 2014;13(3):320–7.
35. Kitao S, Shimamoto A, Goto M, Miller RW, Smithson WA, Lindor NM, et al. Mutations in RECQL4 cause a subset of cases of Rothmund-Thomson syndrome. Nat Genet. 1999;22(1):82–4.
36. Mann MB, Hodges CA, Barnes E, Vogel H, Hassold TJ, Luo G. Defective sister-chromatid cohesion, aneuploidy and cancer predisposition in a mouse model of type II Rothmund-Thomson syndrome. Hum Mol Genet. 2005;14(6):813–25.
37. Simon T, Kohlhase J, Wilhelm C, Kochanek M, De Carolis B, Berthold F. Multiple malignant diseases in a patient with Rothmund-Thomson syndrome with RECQL4 mutations: case report and literature review. Am J Med Genet A. 2010;152A(6):1575–9.
38. Pujol LA, Erickson RP, Heidenreich RA, Cunniff C. Variable presentation of Rothmund-Thomson syndrome. Am J Med Genet. 2000;95(3):204–7.
39. Wang LL, Levy ML, Lewis RA, Chintagumpala MM, Lev D, Rogers M, et al. Clinical manifestations in a cohort of 41 Rothmund-Thomson syndrome patients. Am J Med Genet. 2001;102(1):11–7.
40. Thomson MS. Poikiloderma congenitale: two cases for diagnosis. Proc R Soc Med. 1936;29(5):453–5.
41. Kraus BS, Gottlieb MA, Meliton HR. The dentition in Rothmund's syndrome. J Am Dent Assoc. 1970;81(4):895–915.
42. Starr DG, McClure JP, Connor JM. Non-dermatological complications and genetic aspects of the Rothmund-Thomson syndrome. Clin Genet. 1985;27(1):102–4.

43. Haytac MC, Oztunç H, Mete UO, Kaya M. Rothmund-Thomson syndrome: a case report. Oral Surg Oral Med Oral Pathol Oral Radiol Endod. 2002;94(4):479–84.
44. Roinioti TD, Stefanopoulos PK. Short root anomaly associated with Rothmund-Thomson syndrome. Oral Surg Oral Med Oral Pathol Oral Radiol Endod. 2007;103(1):e19–22.
45. Kant SG, Baraitser M, Milla PJ, Winter RM. Rapadilino syndrome – a non-Finnish case. Clin Dysmorphol. 1998;7(2):135–8.
46. Vargas FR, de Almeida JC, Llerena Júnior JC, Reis DF. Rapadilino syndrome. Am J Med Genet. 1992;44(6):716–9.
47. Faughnan ME, Palda VA, Garcia-Tsao G, Geisthoff UW, McDonald J, Proctor DD, et al. International guidelines for the diagnosis and management of hereditary haemorrhagic telangiectasia. J Med Genet. 2011;48(2):73–87.
48. McDonald JE, Miller FJ, Hallam SE, Nelson L, Marchuk DA, Ward KJ. Clinical manifestations in a large hereditary hemorrhagic telangiectasia (HHT) type 2 kindred. Am J Med Genet. 2000;93(4):320–7.
49. Wooderchak-Donahue WL, McDonald J, O'Fallon B, Upton PD, Li W, Roman BL, et al. BMP9 mutations cause a vascular-anomaly syndrome with phenotypic overlap with hereditary hemorrhagic telangiectasia. Am J Hum Genet. 2013;93(3):530–7.
50. Schwenter F, Faughnan ME, Gradinger AB, Berk T, Gryfe R, Pollett A, et al. Juvenile polyposis, hereditary hemorrhagic telangiectasia, and early onset colorectal cancer in patients with SMAD4 mutation. J Gastroenterol. 2012;47(7):795–804.
51. Austin GB, Quart AM, Novak B. Hereditary hemorrhagic telangiectasia with oral manifestations. Report of periodontal treatment in two cases. Oral Surg Oral Med Oral Pathol. 1981;51(3):245–51.
52. Hopp RN, de Siqueira DC, Sena-Filho M, Jorge J. Oral vascular malformation in a patient with hereditary hemorrhagic telangiectasia: a case report. Spec Care Dent. 2013;33(3):150–3.
53. Haitjema TJ, van Snippenburg R, Disch FJ, Overtoom TT, Westermann CJ. Recurrent epistaxis: sometimes Rendu-Osler-Weber disease. Ned Tijdschr Geneeskd. 1996;140(44):2157–60.
54. Mylona E, Vadala C, Papastamopoulos V, Skoutelis A. Brain abscess caused by Enterococcus faecalis following a dental procedure in a patient with hereditary hemorrhagic telangiectasia. J Clin Microbiol. 2012;50(5):1807–9.
55. Corre P, Perret C, Isidor B, Khonsari RH. A brain abscess following dental extractions in a patient with hereditary hemorrhagic telangiectasia. Br J Oral Maxillofac Surg. 2011;49(5):e9–11.
56. Brancati F, Valente EM, Tadini G, Caputo V, Di Benedetto A, Gelmetti C, et al. Autosomal dominant hereditary benign telangiectasia maps to the CMC1 locus for capillary malformation on chromosome 5q14. J Med Genet. 2003;40(11):849–53.
57. Galletta A, Amato G. Hereditary hemorrhagic telangiectasia (Osler-Rendu-Weber disease) management of epistaxis and oral hemorrhage by Nd-Yag laser. Minerva Stomatol. 1998;47(6):283–6.
58. Schallreuter KU, Frenk E, Wolfe LS, Witkop CJ, Wood JM. Hermansky-Pudlak syndrome in a Swiss population. Dermatology. 1993;187(4):248–56.
59. Wildenberg SC, Oetting WS, Almodóvar C, Krumwiede M, White JG, King RA. A gene causing Hermansky-Pudlak syndrome in a Puerto Rican population maps to chromosome 10q2. Am J Hum Genet. 1995;57(4):755–65.
60. Oh J, Bailin T, Fukai K, Feng GH, Ho L, Mao JI, et al. Positional cloning of a gene for Hermansky-Pudlak syndrome, a disorder of cytoplasmic organelles. Nat Genet. 1996;14(3):300–6.
61. Oh J, Ho L, Ala-Mello S, Amato D, Armstrong L, Bellucci S, et al. Mutation analysis of patients with Hermansky-Pudlak syndrome: a frameshift hot spot in the HPS gene and apparent locus heterogeneity. Am J Hum Genet. 1998;62(3):593–8.
62. Kinnear PE, Tuddenham EG. Albinism with haemorrhagic diathesis: Hermansky-Pudlak syndrome. Br J Ophthalmol. 1985;69(12):904–8.
63. Theuring F, Fiedler J. Fatal bleeding following tooth extraction. Hermansky-Pudlak-syndrome. Dtsch Stomatol. 1973;23(1):52–5.
64. Feliciano NZ, Rivera E, Agrait E, Rodriguez K. Hermansky-Pudlak syndrome: dental management considerations. J Dent Child. 2006;73(1):51–6.
65. Valera MC, Kemoun P, Cousty S, Sie P, Payrastre B. Inherited platelet disorders and oral health. J Oral Pathol Med. 2013;42(2):115–24.
66. Keebaugh AC, Sullivan RT, Thomas JW. Gene duplication and inactivation in the HPRT gene family. Genomics. 2007;89(1):134–42.
67. Torres RJ, Puig JG. Hypoxanthine-guanine phosphoribosyltransferase (HPRT) deficiency: Lesch-Nyhan syndrome. Orphanet J Rare Dis. 2007;2:48.
68. Limeres J, Feijoo JF, Baluja F, Seoane JM, Diniz M, Diz P. Oral self-injury: an update. Dent Traumatol. 2013;29(1):8–14.
69. Bodner L, Woldenberg Y, Pinsk V, Levy J. Orofacial manifestations of congenital insensitivity to pain with anhidrosis: a report of 24 cases. ASDC J Dent Child. 2002;69(3):293–6.. 235
70. Rojahn J. Self-injurious and stereotypic behavior of noninstitutionalized mentally retarded people: prevalence and classification. Am J Ment Defic. 1986;91(3):268–76.
71. Brunner J, Lotschutz D. Kelley-Seegmiller syndrome. Klin Padiatr. 2008;220(1):21–3.
72. Cusumano FJ, Penna KJ, Panossian G. Prevention of self-mutilation in patients with Lesch-Nyhan syndrome: review of literature. ASDC J Dent Child. 2001;68(3):175–8.
73. Amos CI, Bali D, Thiel TJ, Anderson JP, Gourley I, Frazier ML, et al. Fine mapping of a genetic locus for Peutz-Jeghers syndrome on chromosome 19p. Cancer Res. 1997;57(17):3653–6.
74. Kitagawa S, Townsend BL, Hebert AA. Peutz-Jeghers syndrome. Dermatol Clin. 1995;13(1):127–33.
75. Boardman LA, Thibodeau SN, Schaid DJ, Lindor NM, McDonnell SK, Burgart LJ, et al. Increased risk

for cancer in patients with the Peutz-Jeghers syndrome. Ann Intern Med. 1998;128(11):896–9.
76. Li Y, Tong X, Yang J, Yang L, Tao J, Tu Y. Q-switched alexandrite laser treatment of facial and labial lentigines associated with Peutz-Jeghers syndrome. Photodermatol Photoimmunol Photomed. 2012;28(4):196–9.
77. Xi Z, Hui Q, Zhong L. Q-switched alexandrite laser treatment of oral labial lentigines in Chinese subjects with Peutz-Jeghers syndrome. Dermatol Surg. 2009;35(7):1084–8.
78. Chang CJ, Nelson JS. Q-switched ruby laser treatment of mucocutaneous melanosis associated with Peutz-Jeghers syndrome. Ann Plast Surg. 1996;36(4):394–7.
79. Finger RP, Charbel Issa P, Ladewig MS, Götting C, Szliska C, Scholl HP, et al. Pseudoxanthoma elasticum: genetics, clinical manifestations and therapeutic approaches. Surv Ophthalmol. 2009;54(2):272–85.
80. Bergen AA, Plomp AS, Schuurman EJ, Terry S, Breuning M, Dauwerse H, et al. Mutations in ABCC6 cause pseudoxanthoma elasticum. Nat Genet. 2000;25(2):228–31.
81. Spinzi G, Strocchi E, Imperiali G, Sangiovanni A, Terruzzi V, Minoli G. Pseudoxanthoma elasticum: a rare cause of gastrointestinal bleeding. Am J Gastroenterol. 1996;91(8):1631–4.
82. Goette DK, Carpenter WM. The mucocutaneous marker of pseudoxanthoma elasticum. Oral Surg Oral Med Oral Pathol. 1981;51(1):68–72.
83. Sayin MO, Atilla AO, Esenlik E, Ozen T, Karahan N. Oligodontia in pseudoxanthoma elasticum. Oral Surg Oral Med Oral Pathol Oral Radiol Endod. 2007;103(5):e60–4.
84. Utani A, Tanioka M, Yamamoto Y, Taki R, Araki E, Tamura H, et al. Relationship between the distribution of pseudoxanthoma elasticum skin and mucous membrane lesions and cardiovascular involvement. J Dermatol. 2010;37(2):130–6.
85. Sherer DW, Sapadin AN, Lebwohl MG. Pseudoxanthoma elasticum: an update. Dermatology. 1999;199(1):3–7.
86. Shibuya Y, Zhang J, Yokoo S, Umeda M, Komori T. Constitutional mutation of keratin 13 gene in familial white sponge nevus. Oral Surg Oral Med Oral Pathol Oral Radiol Endod. 2003;96(5):561–5.
87. Rugg EL, McLean WH, Allison WE, Lunny DP, Macleod RI, Felix DH, et al. A mutation in the mucosal keratin K4 is associated with oral white sponge nevus. Nat Genet. 1995;11(4):450–2.
88. Richard G, De Laurenzi V, Didona B, Bale SJ, Compton JG. Keratin 13 point mutation underlies the hereditary mucosal epithelial disorder white sponge nevus. Nat Genet. 1995;11(4):453–5.
89. Lamey PJ, Bolas A, Napier SS, Darwazeh AM, Macdonald DG. Oral white sponge naevus: response to antibiotic therapy. Clin Exp Dermatol. 1998;23(2):59–63.
90. Otobe IF, de Sousa SO, Matthews RW, Migliari DA. White sponge naevus: improvement with tetracycline mouth rinse: report of four cases. Clin Exp Dermatol. 2007;32(6):749–51.
91. Otobe IF, de Sousa SO, Migliari DA, Matthews RW. Successful treatment with topical tetracycline of oral white sponge nevus occurring in a patient with systemic lupus erythematosus. Int J Dermatol. 2006;45(9):1130–1.
92. Satriano RA, Errichetti E, Baroni A. White sponge nevus treated with chlorhexidine. J Dermatol. 2012;39(8):742–3.
93. Dufrasne L, Magremanne M, Parent D, Evrard L. Current therapeutic approach of the white sponge naevus of the oral cavity. Bull Group Int Rech Sci Stomatol Odontol. 2011;50(1):1–5.
94. Kinzler KW, Nilbert MC, Su LK, Vogelstein B, Bryan TM, Levy DB, et al. Identification of FAP locus genes from chromosome 5q21. Science. 1991;253(5020):661–5.
95. Petersen GM, Slack J, Nakamura Y. Screening guidelines and premorbid diagnosis of familial adenomatous polyposis using linkage. Gastroenterology. 1991;100(6):1658–64.
96. Traboulsi EI, Maumenee IH, Krush AJ, Giardiello FM, Levin LS, Hamilton SR. Pigmented ocular fundus lesions in the inherited gastrointestinal polyposis syndromes and in hereditary nonpolyposis colorectal cancer. Ophthalmology. 1988;95(7):964–9.
97. Jagelman DG. Extracolonic manifestations of familial polyposis coli. Semin Surg Oncol. 1987;3(2):88–91.
98. Fader M, Kline SN, Spatz SS, Zubrow HJ. Gardner's syndrome (intestinal polyposis, osteomas, sebaceous cysts) and a new dental discovery. Oral Surg Oral Med Pathol. 1962;15:153–72.
99. Ida M, Nakamura T, Utsunomiya J. Osteomatous changes and tooth abnormalities found in the jaw of patients with adenomatosis coli. Oral Surg Oral Med Pathol. 1962;15:153–72.. 1981. 52(1):2–11
100. Kubo K, Miyatani H, Takenoshita Y, Abe K, Oka M, Iida M, et al. Widespread radiopacity of jaw bones in familial adenomatosis coli. J Craniomaxillofac Surg. 1989;17(8):350–3.
101. Wijn MA, Keller JJ, Giardiello FM, Brand HS. Oral and maxillofacial manifestations of familial adenomatous polyposis. Oral Dis. 2007;13(4):360–5.
102. Lew D, DeWitt A, Hicks RJ, Cavalcanti MG. Osteomas of the condyle associated with Gardner's syndrome causing limited mandibular movement. J Oral Maxillofac Surg. 1999;57(8):1004–9.
103. Jones EL, Cornell WP. Gardner's syndrome; review of the literature and report on a family. Arch Surg. 1966;92(2):287–300.
104. Payne M, Anderson JA, Cook J. Gardner's syndrome – a case report. Br Dent J. 2002;193(7):383–4.
105. Wijn MA, Keller JJ, Brand HS. Oral and maxillofacial manifestations of familial adenomatosis polyposis. Gardner's syndrome. Ned Tijdschr Tandheelkd. 2005;112(9):340–4.
106. Boffano P, Bosco GF, Gerbino G. The surgical management of oral and maxillofacial manifestations of Gardner syndrome. J Oral Maxillofac Surg. 2010;68(10):2549–54.

107. Stevenson DA, Carey JC, Byrne JL, Srisukhumbowornchai S, Feldkamp ML. Analysis of skeletal dysplasias in the Utah population. Am J Med Genet A. 2012;158A(5):1046–54.
108. Stoll C, Dott B, Roth MP, Alembik Y. Birth prevalence rates of skeletal dysplasias. Clin Genet. 1989;35(2):88–92.
109. Harrington J, Sochett E, Howard A. Update on the evaluation and treatment of osteogenesis imperfecta. Pediatr Clin N Am. 2014;61(6):1243–57.
110. Bodian DL, Chan TF, Poon A, Schwarze U, Yang K, Byers PH, et al. Mutation and polymorphism spectrum in osteogenesis imperfecta type II: implications for genotype-phenotype relationships. Hum Mol Genet. 2009;18(3):463–71.
111. Paterson CR, Monk EA, McAllion SJ. How common is hearing impairment in osteogenesis imperfecta? J Laryngol Otol. 2001;115(4):280–2.
112. Bonita RE, Cohen IS, Berko BA. Valvular heart disease in osteogenesis imperfecta: presentation of a case and review of the literature. Echocardiography. 2010;27(1):69–73.
113. Charnas LR, Marini JC. Communicating hydrocephalus, basilar invagination, and other neurologic features in osteogenesis imperfecta. Neurology. 1993;43(12):2603–8.
114. O'Connell AC, Marini JC. Evaluation of oral problems in an osteogenesis imperfecta population. Oral Surg Oral Med Oral Pathol Oral Radiol Endod. 1999;87(2):189–96.
115. Majorana A, Bardellini E, Brunelli PC, Lacaita M, Cazzolla AP, Favia G. Dentinogenesis imperfecta in children with osteogenesis imperfecta: a clinical and ultrastructural study. Int J Paediatr Dent. 2010;20(2):112–8.
116. Barron MJ, McDonnell ST, Mackie I, Dixon MJ. Hereditary dentine disorders: dentinogenesis imperfecta and dentine dysplasia. Orphanet J Rare Dis. 2008;3:31.
117. Abukabbos H, Al-Sineedi F. Clinical manifestations and dental management of dentinogenesis imperfecta associated with osteogenesis imperfecta: case report. Saudi Dent J. 2013;25(4):159–65.
118. Sapir S, Shapira J. Dentinogenesis imperfecta: an early treatment strategy. Pediatr Dent. 2001;23(3):232–7.
119. Mars M, Smith BG. Dentinogenesis imperfecta. An integrated conservative approach to treatment. Br Dent J. 1982;152(1):15–8.
120. Bencharit S, Border MB, Mack CR, Byrd WC, Wright JT. Full-mouth rehabilitation for a patient with dentinogenesis imperfecta: a clinical report. J Oral Implantol. 2014;40(5):593–600.
121. Evans DG, Howard E, Giblin C, Clancy T, Spencer H, Huson SM, et al. Birth incidence and prevalence of tumor-prone syndromes: estimates from a UK family genetic register service. Am J Med Genet A. 2010;152A(2):327–32.
122. Shanley S, Ratcliffe J, Hockey A, Haan E, Oley C, Ravine D, et al. Nevoid basal cell carcinoma syndrome: review of 118 affected individuals. Am J Med Genet. 1994;50(3):282–90.
123. Smith MJ, Beetz C, Williams SG, Bhaskar SS, O'Sullivan J, Anderson B, et al. Germline mutations in SUFU cause Gorlin syndrome-associated childhood medulloblastoma and redefine the risk associated with PTCH1 mutations. J Clin Oncol. 2014;32(36):4155–61.
124. Fujii K, Miyashita T. Gorlin syndrome (nevoid basal cell carcinoma syndrome): update and literature review. Pediatr Int. 2014;56(5):667–74.
125. Kimonis VE, Goldstein AM, Pastakia B, Yang ML, Kase R, DiGiovanna JJ, et al. Clinical manifestations in 105 persons with nevoid basal cell carcinoma syndrome. Am J Med Genet. 1997;69(3): 299–308.
126. Levine DJ, Robertson DB, Varma VA. Familial subconjunctival epithelial cysts associated with the nevoid basal cell carcinoma syndrome. Arch Dermatol. 1987;123(1):23–4.
127. Gorlin RJ, Goltz RW. Multiple nevoid basal-cell epithelioma, jaw cysts and bifid rib. A syndrome. N Engl J Med. 1960;262:908–12.
128. Evans DG, Sims DG, Donnai D. Family implications of neonatal Gorlin's syndrome. Arch Dis Child. 1991;66(10. Spec No):1162–3.
129. Lile HA, Rogers JF, Gerald B. The basal cell nevus syndrome. Am J Roentgenol Radium Ther Nucl Med. 1968;103(1):214–7.
130. Wright JM, Odell EW, Speight PM, Takata T. Odontogenic tumors, WHO 2005: where do we go from here? Head Neck Pathol. 2014;8(4):373–82.
131. Lo Muzio L, Nocini P, Bucci P, Pannone G, Consolo U, Procaccini M. Early diagnosis of nevoid basal cell carcinoma syndrome. J Am Dent Assoc. 1999;130(5):669–74.
132. Brannon RB. The odontogenic keratocyst. A clinicopathologic study of 312 cases. Part I. Clinical features. Oral Surg Oral Med Oral Pathol. 1976;42(1):54–72.
133. Habibi A, Saghravanian N, Habibi M, Mellati E, Habibi M. Keratocystic odontogenic tumor: a 10-year retrospective study of 83 cases in an Iranian population. J Oral Sci. 2007;49(3):229–35.
134. Evans DG, Ladusans EJ, Rimmer S, Burnell LD, Thakker N, Farndon PA. Complications of the naevoid basal cell carcinoma syndrome: results of a population based study. J Med Genet. 1993;30(6):460–4.
135. Kimonis VE, Singh KE, Zhong R, Pastakia B, Digiovanna JJ, Bale SJ. Clinical and radiological features in young individuals with nevoid basal cell carcinoma syndrome. Genet Med. 2013;15(1):79–83.
136. Leonardi R, Sorge G, Caltabino M. Bilateral hyperplasia of the mandibular coronoid processes associated with the nevoid basal cell carcinoma syndrome in an Italian boy. Br Dent J. 2001;190(7):349–50.
137. Roopak B, Singh M, Shah A, Patel G. Keratocystic odontogenic tumor: treatment modalities: study of 3 cases. Niger J Clin Pract. 2014;17(3):378–83.
138. Sembronio S, Albiero AM, Zerman N, Costa F, Politi M. Endoscopically assisted enucleation and curettage of large mandibular odontogenic keratocyst.

Oral Surg Oral Med Oral Pathol Oral Radiol Endod. 2009;107(2):193–6.
139. Terranova F, Trevisiol L, Nocini PF, Bissolotti G, Bondì V, De Santis D, Bertossi D, D'agostino A. Keratocyst, conservative treatment: case report. Minerva Stomatol. 2013;62(8 Suppl 1):71–8. Epub 2013 Aug 1.
140. Nakayama T, Otori N, Asaka D, Okushi T, Haruna S. Endoscopic modified medial maxillectomy for odontogenic cysts and tumours. Rhinology. 2014;52(4):376–80.
141. Gene Reviews. Nevoid basal cell carcinoma syndrome. 2013. 12/08/2014. Available from: http://www.ncbi.nlm.nih.gov/books/NBK1151/.
142. Hallett L, Foster T, Liu Z, Blieden M, Valentim J. Burden of disease and unmet needs in tuberous sclerosis complex with neurological manifestations: systematic review. Curr Med Res Opin. 2011;27(8):1571–83.
143. Osborne JP, Fryer A, Webb D. Epidemiology of tuberous sclerosis. Ann N Y Acad Sci. 1991;615:125–7.
144. Curatolo P, Bombardieri R, Jozwiak S. Tuberous sclerosis. Lancet. 2008;372(9639):657–68.
145. Cutando A, Gil JA, Lopez J. Oral health management implications in patients with tuberous sclerosis. Oral Surg Oral Med Oral Pathol Oral Radiol Endod. 2000;90(4):430–5.
146. Gomez MR. History of the tuberous sclerosis complex. Brain Dev. 1995;17(Suppl):55–7.
147. Teng JM, Cowen EW, Wataya-Kaneda M, Gosnell ES, Witman PM, Hebert AA, et al. Dermatologic and dental aspects of the 2012 International Tuberous Sclerosis Complex Consensus Statements. JAMA Dermatol. 2014;150(10):1095–101.
148. Tillman HH, De Caro F. Tuberous sclerosis. Oral Surg Oral Med Oral Pathol. 1991;71(3):301–2.
149. Flanagan N, O'Connor WJ, McCartan B, Miller S, McMenamin J, Watson R. Developmental enamel defects in tuberous sclerosis: a clinical genetic marker? J Med Genet. 1997;34(8):637–9.
150. Valerio RA, de Queiroz AM, Romualdo PC, Brentegani LG, de Paula-Silva FW. Mucocele and fibroma: treatment and clinical features for differential diagnosis. Braz Dent J. 2013;24(5):537–41.
151. Ammari MM, Ribeiro de Souza IP, Maia LC, Primo LG. Oral findings in a family with tuberous sclerosis complex. Spec Care Dent. 2014. [Epub ahead of print].
152. Sakuntabhai A, Ruiz-Perez V, Carter S, Jacobsen N, Burge S, Monk S, et al. Mutations in ATP2A2, encoding a Ca2+ pump, cause Darier disease. Nat Genet. 1999;21(3):271–7.
153. MacLennan DH, Brandl CJ, Korczak B, Green NM. Amino-acid sequence of a Ca2+ + Mg2+-dependent ATPase from rabbit muscle sarcoplasmic reticulum, deduced from its complementary DNA sequence. Nature. 1985;316(6030):696–700.
154. Ruiz-Perez VL, Carter SA, Healy E, Todd C, Rees JL, Steijlen PM, et al. ATP2A2 mutations in Darier's disease: variant cutaneous phenotypes are associated with missense mutations, but neuropsychiatric features are independent of mutation class. Hum Mol Genet. 1999;8(9):1621–30.
155. Munro CS. The phenotype of Darier's disease: penetrance and expressivity in adults and children. Br J Dermatol. 1992;127(2):126–30.
156. Burge SM, Wilkinson JD. Darier-White disease: a review of the clinical features in 163 patients. J Am Acad Dermatol. 1992;27(1):40–50.
157. Burge S. Darier's disease – the clinical features and pathogenesis. Clin Exp Dermatol. 1994;19(3):193–205.
158. Craddock N, Dawson E, Burge S, Parfitt L, Mant B, Roberts Q, et al. The gene for Darier's disease maps to chromosome 12q23-q24.1. Hum Mol Genet. 1993;2(11):1941–3.
159. Gordon-Smith K, Jones LA, Burge SM, Munro CS, Tavadia S, Craddock N. The neuropsychiatric phenotype in Darier disease. Br J Dermatol. 2010;163(3):515–22.
160. Macleod RI, Munro CS. The incidence and distribution of oral lesions in patients with Darier's disease. Br Dent J. 1991;171(5):133–6.
161. Thiagarajan MK, Narasimhan M, Sankarasubramanian A. Darier disease with oral and esophageal involvement: a case report. Indian J Dent Res. 2011;22(6):843–6.
162. Shimizu H, Tan Kinoshita MT, Suzuki H. Darier's disease with esophageal carcinoma. Eur J Dermatol. 2000;10(6):470–2.
163. Abel MD, Carrasco LR. Ehlers-Danlos syndrome: classifications, oral manifestations, and dental considerations. Oral Surg Oral Med Oral Pathol Oral Radiol Endod. 2006;102(5):582–90.
164. De Felice C, Toti P, Di Maggio G, Parrini S, Bagnoli F. Absence of the inferior labial and lingual frenula in Ehlers-Danlos syndrome. Lancet. 2001;357(9267):1500–2.
165. Majorana A, Facchetti F. The orodental findings in the Ehlers-Danlos syndrome. A report of 2 clinical cases. Minerva Stomatol. 1992;41(3):127–33.
166. Colebatch AN, Shaw EC, Foulds NC, Davidson BK. Hemorrhagic bullae of the oral mucosa as an early manifestation of vascular-type ehlers-danlos syndrome. J Clin Rheumatol. 2011;17(7):383–4.
167. Ferreira O Jr, Cardoso CL, Capelozza AL, Yaedú RY, da Costa AR. Odontogenic keratocyst and multiple supernumerary teeth in a patient with Ehlers-Danlos syndrome – a case report and review of the literature. Quintessence Int. 2008;39(3):251–6.
168. Badauy CM, Gomes SS, Sant'Ana Filho M, Chies JA. Ehlers-Danlos syndrome (EDS) type IV: review of the literature. Clin Oral Investig. 2007;11(3):183–7.
169. Letourneau Y, Perusse R, Buithieu H. Oral manifestations of Ehlers-Danlos syndrome. J Can Dent Assoc. 2001;67(6):330–4.
170. Hagberg C, Korpe L, Berglund B. Temporomandibular joint problems and self-registration of mandibular opening capacity among adults with Ehlers-Danlos syndrome. A questionnaire study. Orthod Craniofac Res. 2004;7(1):40–6.
171. Norton LA, Assael LA. Orthodontic and temporomandibular joint considerations in treatment of

patients with Ehlers-Danlos syndrome. Am J Orthod Dentofac Orthop. 1997;111(1):75–84.
172. Sherman SL, Allen EG, Bean LH, Freeman SB. Epidemiology of Down syndrome. Ment Retard Dev Disabil Res Rev. 2007;13(3):221–7.
173. Sekerci AE, Cantekin K, Aydinbelge M, Ucar Fİ. Prevalence of dental anomalies in the permanent dentition of children with Down syndrome. J Dent Child. 2014;81(2):78–83.
174. Abeleira MT, Outumuro M, Ramos I, Limeres J, Diniz M, Diz P. Dimensions of central incisors, canines, and first molars in subjects with Down syndrome measured on cone-beam computed tomographs. Am J Orthod Dentofac Orthop. 2014;146(6):765–75.
175. Oredugba FA, Eigbobo JO, Temisanren OT. Tooth crown dimensions in a selected population of Nigerians with Down syndrome. West Afr J Med. 2014;33(2):146–50.
176. Rao D, Hegde S, Naik S, Shetty P. Malocclusion in individuals with mental subnormality – a review. Oral Health Dent Manag. 2014;13(3):786–91.
177. de Miguel-Diez J, Villa-Asensi JR, Alvarez-Sala JL. Prevalence of sleep-disordered breathing in children with Down syndrome: polygraphic findings in 108 children. Sleep. 2003;26(8):1006–9.
178. Guimaraes CV, Donnelly LF, Shott SR, Amin RS, Kalra M. Relative rather than absolute macroglossia in patients with Down syndrome: implications for treatment of obstructive sleep apnea. Pediatr Radiol. 2008;38(10):1062–7.
179. Anuthama K, Prasad H, Ramani P, Premkumar P, Natesan A, Sherlin HJ. Genetic alterations in syndromes with oral manifestations. Dent Res J. 2013;10(6):713–22.
180. Al-Sufyani GA, Al-Maweri SA, Al-Ghashm AA, Al-Soneidar WA. Oral hygiene and gingival health status of children with Down syndrome in Yemen: a cross-sectional study. J Int Soc Prevent Commun Dent. 2014;4(2):82–6.
181. Chin CJ, Khami MM, Husein M. A general review of the otolaryngologic manifestations of Down syndrome. Int J Pediatr Otorhinolaryngol. 2014;78(6):899–904.
182. Ribeiro CG, Siqueira AF, Bez L, Cardoso AC, Ferreira CF. Dental implant rehabilitation of a patient with Down syndrome: a case report. J Oral Implantol. 2011;37(4):481–7.
183. Lehmann AR, McGibbon D, Stefanini M. Xeroderma pigmentosum. Orphanet J Rare Dis. 2011;6:70.
184. Kraemer KH, Lee MM, Andrews AD, Lambert WC. The role of sunlight and DNA repair in melanoma and nonmelanoma skin cancer. The xeroderma pigmentosum paradigm. Arch Dermatol. 1994;130(8):1018–21.
185. Li C, Hu Z, Liu Z, Wang LE, Strom SS, Gershenwald JE, et al. Polymorphisms in the DNA repair genes XPC, XPD, and XPG and risk of cutaneous melanoma: a case-control analysis. Cancer Epidemiol Biomark Prev. 2006;15(12):2526–32.
186. Anttinen A, Koulu L, Nikoskelainen E, Portin R, Kurki T, Erkinjuntti M, et al. Neurological symptoms and natural course of xeroderma pigmentosum. Brain. 2008;131(Pt 8):1979–89.
187. Wayli HA. Xeroderma pigmentosum and its dental implications. Eur J Dent. 2015;9(1):145–8.
188. Lopes-Cardoso C, Paes da Silva Ramos Fernandes LM, Ferreira-Rocha J, Teixeira-Soares C, Antônio-Barreto J, Humberto-Damante J. Xeroderma Pigmentosum – a case report with oral implications. J Clin Exp Dent. 2012;4(4):e248–51.
189. Gorlin RJ, Sedano H, Anderson VE. The syndrome of palmar-plantar hyperkeratosis and premature periodontal destruction of the teeth. A clinical and genetic analysis of the Papillon-Lefevre syndrome. J Pediatr. 1964;65:895–908.
190. Cury VF, Costa JE, Gomez RS, Boson WL, Loures CG, De ML. A novel mutation of the cathepsin C gene in Papillon-Lefevre syndrome. J Periodontol. 2002;73(3):307–12.
191. Zhang Y, Lundgren T, Renvert S, Tatakis DN, Firatli E, Uygur C, et al. Evidence of a founder effect for four cathepsin C gene mutations in Papillon-Lefevre syndrome patients. J Med Genet. 2001;38(2): 96–101.
192. Wiebe CB, Häkkinen L, Putnins EE, Walsh P, Larjava HS. Successful periodontal maintenance of a case with Papillon-Lefevre syndrome: 12-year follow-up and review of the literature. J Periodontol. 2001;72(6):824–30.
193. Ragunatha S, Ramesh M, Anupama P, Kapoor M, Bhat M. Papillon-Lefevre syndrome with homozygous nonsense mutation of cathepsin C gene presenting with late-onset periodontitis. Pediatr Dermatol. 2015;32(2):292–4.
194. Eick S, Puklo M, Adamowicz K, Kantyka T, Hiemstra P, Stennicke H, et al. Lack of cathelicidin processing in Papillon-Lefevre syndrome patients reveals essential role of LL-37 in periodontal homeostasis. Orphanet J Rare Dis. 2014;9:148.
195. Hart TC, Hart PS, Michalec MD, Zhang Y, Firatli E, Van Dyke TE, et al. Haim-Munk syndrome and Papillon-Lefevre syndrome are allelic mutations in cathepsin C. J Med Genet. 2000;37(2):88–94.
196. Ahmed B. Prosthodontic rehabilitation of Papillon-Lefevre syndrome. J Coll Phys Surg Pak JCPSP. 2014;24(Suppl 2):S132–4.
197. Nickles K, Schacher B, Ratka-Krüger P, Krebs M, Eickholz P. Long-term results after treatment of periodontitis in patients with Papillon-Lefevre syndrome: success and failure. J Clin Periodontol. 2013;40(8):789–98.
198. Sarma N, Ghosh C, Kar S, Bazmi BA. Low-dose acitretin in Papillon-Lefevre syndrome: treatment and 1-year follow-up. Dermatol Ther. 2015;28(1): 28–31.

Index

N. Fazel (ed.), *Oral Signs of Systemic Disease*, https://doi.org/10.1007/978-3-030-10863-2

D

I

R

S

W

X

Y

Z

GPSR Compliance

The European Union's (EU) General Product Safety Regulation (GPSR) is a set of rules that requires consumer products to be safe and our obligations to ensure this.

If you have any concerns about our products, you can contact us on ProductSafety@springernature.com

In case Publisher is established outside the EU, the EU authorized representative is:

Springer Nature Customer Service Center GmbH
Europaplatz 3
69115 Heidelberg, Germany

Batch number: 10731344

Printed by Printforce, the Netherlands